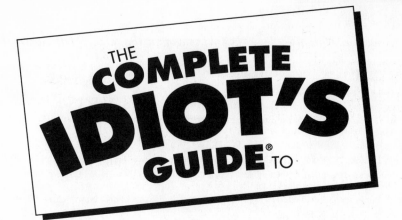

THE
COMPLETE
IDIOT'S
GUIDE® TO

Natural Remedies

by Chrystle Fiedler

ALPHA

A member of Penguin Group (USA) Inc.

To my mother, Marion Fiedler, who first taught me the value of natural remedies

ALPHA BOOKS

Published by the Penguin Group

Penguin Group (USA) Inc., 375 Hudson Street, New York, New York 10014, USA

Penguin Group (Canada), 90 Eglinton Avenue East, Suite 700, Toronto, Ontario M4P 2Y3, Canada (a division of Pearson Penguin Canada Inc.)

Penguin Books Ltd., 80 Strand, London WC2R 0RL, England

Penguin Ireland, 25 St. Stephen's Green, Dublin 2, Ireland (a division of Penguin Books Ltd.)

Penguin Group (Australia), 250 Camberwell Road, Camberwell, Victoria 3124, Australia (a division of Pearson Australia Group Pty. Ltd.)

Penguin Books India Pvt. Ltd., 11 Community Centre, Panchsheel Park, New Delhi—110 017, India

Penguin Group (NZ), 67 Apollo Drive, Rosedale, North Shore, Auckland 1311, New Zealand (a division of Pearson New Zealand Ltd.)

Penguin Books (South Africa) (Pty.) Ltd., 24 Sturdee Avenue, Rosebank, Johannesburg 2196, South Africa

Penguin Books Ltd., Registered Offices: 80 Strand, London WC2R 0RL, England

Copyright © 2009 by Chrystle Fiedler

International Standard Book Number: 978-1-59257-748-4
Library of Congress Catalog Card Number: 2007941482

11 10 09   8 7 6 5 4 3 2 1

Interpretation of the printing code: The rightmost number of the first series of numbers is the year of the book's printing; the rightmost number of the second series of numbers is the number of the book's printing. For example, a printing code of 09-1 shows that the first printing occurred in 2009.

Printed in the United States of America

Note: This publication contains the opinions and ideas of its author. It is intended to provide helpful and informative material on the subject matter covered. It is sold with the understanding that the author and publisher are not engaged in rendering professional services in the book. If the reader requires personal assistance or advice, a competent professional should be consulted.

The author and publisher specifically disclaim any responsibility for any liability, loss, or risk, personal or otherwise, which is incurred as a consequence, directly or indirectly, of the use and application of any of the contents of this book.

Most Alpha books are available at special quantity discounts for bulk purchases for sales promotions, premiums, fund-raising, or educational use. Special books, or book excerpts, can also be created to fit specific needs.

For details, write: Special Markets, Alpha Books, 375 Hudson Street, New York, NY 10014.

Publisher: *Marie Butler-Knight*
Editorial Director/Acquiring Editor: *Mike Sanders*
Senior Managing Editor: *Billy Fields*
Senior Development Editor: *Phil Kitchel*
Senior Production Editor: *Janette Lynn*
Copy Editor: *Krista Hansing Editorial Services, Inc.*

Cartoonist: *Steve Barr*
Cover Designer: *Kurt Owens*
Book Designer: *Trina Wurst/Kurt Owens*
Indexer: *Angie Bess*
Layout: *Ayanna Lacey*
Proofreader: *John Etchison*

Contents at a Glance

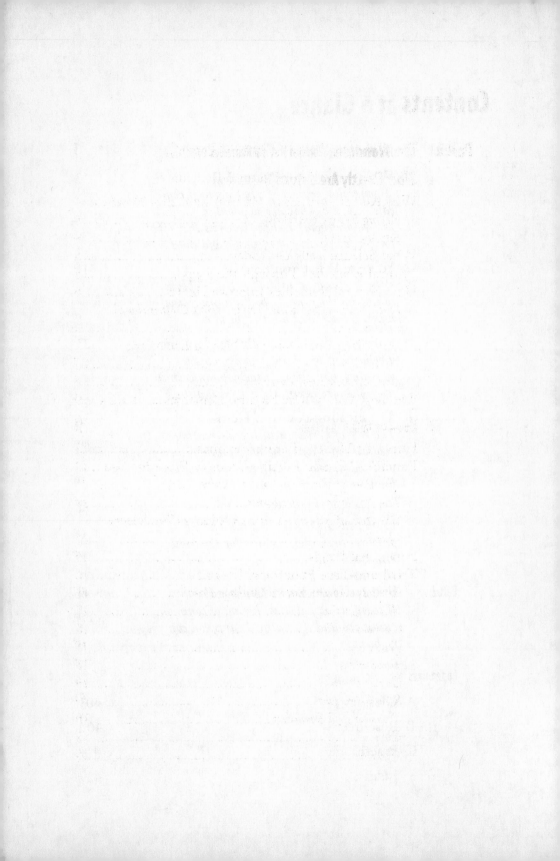

Contents

Introduction

Chances are, you've already tried a natural remedy, maybe without knowing it. Put aloe on a burn? Check. Popped a piece of ginger gum to ease nausea? Check. Iced a sore ankle? Check. Natural remedies are all around us. Once we tap into their power, it's amazing what can happen. But how do we use them to achieve results? That's what this book is all about.

Because you are reading this book, you obviously have questions about natural remedies and how they may work for you, whether you have a specific condition or complaint, want to be prepared, or want to improve your overall health. What are the benefits of natural remedies? What should you take for your condition? And finally, when should you see your doctor? We'll cover all of that here and more.

How This Book Is Organized

This book is divided into two major parts.

Part 1, "The Wonderful World of Natural Remedies," is five chapters that give you an overview of everything to do with natural remedies. To help you understand natural remedies better, I've provided introductory chapters that give you a general foundation. These chapters introduce you to the ins and outs of natural remedies, including how food can be used as medicine, when supplements can be useful, important herbs to be aware of, and alternative therapies that are most effective.

We start with an introduction to natural remedies, to give you a feel for the topic. We discuss the differences between natural and conventional medicine and what you can expect when you use natural remedies. We consider the important role food plays as a foundational component and how supplements can help provide a safety net for missing nutrients. We also list the herbs used most often, with a little history so you learn more about what they can do to improve health. We cover the benefits of alternative therapies that are discussed throughout the book, including acupuncture, aromatherapy, homeopathy, flower essences, qigong, and yoga.

Part 2, "Directory of Conditions and Natural Remedies," is a listing of more than 50 conditions, everything from acne to insomnia to varicose veins. For each condition, we provide a reader-friendly solution made of natural remedies. We talk about the condition and its symptoms; the role of food, supplements, and herbs; and which alternative therapies can be helpful. At the end of each chapter, you'll find remedies listed alphabetically, to make them easier to find and put into practice. I also tell you when you should see your doctor: natural remedies aren't a substitute for medical care—they're a helpful adjunct. At the end of each condition, you'll find "Natural Rx," a listing of supplements and dosages for each condition and, in some cases, where to find specific supplements. All of this makes it easier to put what you've learned into practice.

Helpful Sidebars

Throughout this book, you'll find four different sidebars, providing you more help and information.

dial your doc

When you need to check with your doctor before using a natural remedy.

def•i•ni•tion

Terms and jargon related to conditions, the body, and natural health.

risky remedy!

Warnings or precautions associated with the use of a remedy, including drug interactions.

natural news

Tidbits of information, as well as anecdotes, helpful hints, and insights from natural doctors about particular issues.

Acknowledgments

My thanks go to all the naturopathic doctors and other alternative health experts who made this book possible. Special thanks go to Deborah Wiancek, N.D.; Holly Lucille, N.D.; Beverly Yates, N.D.; Brigitte Mars, A.H.G.; Alan Logan, N.D.; Jacob Teitelbaum, M.D.;

Stephen Hartman; Jade Shutes; Nancy Buono, BFRP; Amanda McQuade Crawford, A.H.G.; Richard Shames, M.D.; Marc Grossman, O.D., L.Ac.; Pamela Hannaman, N.D.; Gary Rebstock; and Brenda Watson, N.D., C.N.C., for their generosity in sharing their expertise. Thanks also to Susan Zingraf, Phil Kitchel, Krista Hansing, and Janette Lynn, my astute editors, and to Mike Sanders for the opportunity to share this information with readers. My appreciation also goes to Gina Mehalakes for her help with manuscript preparation.

Special Thanks to the Technical Reviewer

The Complete Idiot's Guide to Natural Remedies was reviewed by experts who double-checked the accuracy of what you'll learn here, to help us ensure that this book gives you everything you need to know about natural remedies. Special thanks are extended to Deborah Wiancek, N.D., and Holly Lucille, N.D.

Trademarks

Part 1

The Wonderful World of Natural Remedies

So you want to learn more about natural ways to reduce pain, heal, live longer, and feel better? You've come to the right place! Part 1 introduces you to the basics of natural remedies. We'll talk about why there is so much interest in natural remedies today, what benefits they provide, how natural medicine differs from conventional medicine, and the best way to use them for positive results. One of the most important things to keep in mind is that although natural remedies can be a very useful alternative, they are not a substitute for proper medical care. See your doctor if you have any questions.

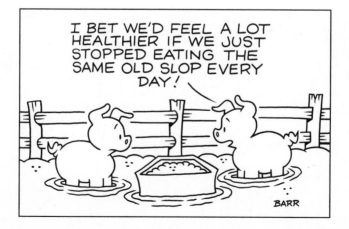

What Exactly Are Natural Remedies?

In This Chapter

- ◆ Why natural remedies are important
- ◆ What science tells us today
- ◆ How natural remedies can make you healthier
- ◆ Understanding the best way to use natural remedies

If you haven't used natural remedies, you're in for a treat! When you go "back to nature," you'll discover an amazing array of healers in nutrients, practices, and therapies: from vitamins, minerals, herbal supplements, and flower essences, to yoga and tai chi, to alternative therapies like aromatherapy, homeopathy, hydrotherapy, acupuncture, and massage therapy.

What do all these things have in common? When used correctly, natural remedies help address different health conditions and enhance your overall well-being. Some natural remedies are do-it-yourself; with others, you'll need to find a practitioner for best results. In this book, we'll help you learn about what natural remedies you can use for different conditions, and when and how to find the right person when you need a professional to help you.

Why All the Interest in Natural Remedies Now?

More people are joining the natural-remedy revolution. According to the National Center for Complementary and Alternative Medicine, more than 42 percent of Americans are turning to integrative medicine (a combination of alternative and conventional medicine). Some do it because they haven't found the results they want with conventional medicine alone. Courtney Gilardi, N.D., a naturopathic doctor who practices at the Kripalu Center for Yoga & Health in Stockbridge, Massachusetts, echoes the sentiments of many alternative practitioners when she says, "It's because the conventional health system doesn't provide people with the answers they need to make lasting changes." Conventional doctors can also be overwhelmed and overworked in an already overburdened health-care system, so it can be difficult to keep up with the latest alternative therapies.

Paying Your Own Way

For some people, it's worth it to pay out of pocket to see a naturopathic physician, even when their insurance won't cover it. "People feel like it's worth it if they get 50 minutes of uninterrupted time rather than leave with a prescription and a lot of unanswered questions," says Dr. Gilardi. "It makes you feel like you can make a difference. You feel empowered because you learn where the rubber meets the road in terms of diet and lifestyle changes in view of your genetic susceptibilities." Often getting five minutes with a traditional doctor can leave you feeling helpless, without a clear strategy of what to do next.

Saving Money

Other people might want to try natural remedies because they're looking for a way to address their needs in a less expensive way than with prescription medicines. Often folks don't like the side effects of the prescription medications they take. This may prevent them from consistently treating a condition that needs attention. Still others want to take control of their own health and feel empowered by using natural remedies to help treat their health conditions.

What Science Tells Us Today

Many studies have shown that certain natural remedies work to improve health. Of course, companies can't patent and sell a natural product, so pharmaceutical companies conduct far more studies on their own products. Fortunately, in 2004 the U.S. National Center for Complementary and Alternative Medicine of the National Institutes of Health began to fund research studies on herbal medicine. This adds to the already burgeoning wealth of knowledge we have about natural medicines. Many studies have come out of Europe—specifically, Germany: in 1978, West Germany appointed a panel of experts, called Commission E, to study herbs for different health conditions, to help guide medical doctors.

Natural Remedies Through the Ages

Since prehistoric times, herbs (all plants that serve a useful purpose are herbs) have been used to treat conditions from mosquito bites to menstrual cramps. The healing properties of herbs can be traced back 5,000 years ago to the Sumarians, a nomadic tribe that lived by the Tigris and Euphrates Rivers, who used thyme, laurel, and caraway. A little over 2,000 years later, the Chinese began to use herbs medicinally. We can thank the Egyptians for the discovery of antibacterial and antiviral herbs like garlic. The Greeks and Romans were also movers and shakers when it came to evolving herbal use; Hippocrates, in particular, played a key role by encouraging a whole-body approach, with rest, fresh air, and good food (he famously said, "Let your food be your medicine and your medicine be your food") to bring about good health. Later, colonists schooled in European folk medicine traditions crossed the Atlantic Ocean to North America. There they encountered Native Americans, who had their own medicinal cures that they shared with the new settlers.

These traditions and many others have been handed down over the centuries, evolving into folk and natural remedies. Today, while many of us in the United States are still discovering the value of natural remedies, in China, herbal medicines account for up to half of total medicines used, according to the World Health Organization. In Africa, 80 percent of the population uses natural remedies for primary health care.

How Natural Remedies Improve Health

Natural remedies work in different ways. But the main goal is to use the body's own processes to speed healing and boost overall health. The choices are endless, whether you focus on practices to keep you young (see "Healthy Aging"), use probiotics to improve digestion (see "Heartburn" and "Irritable Bowel Syndrome"), or tap ginger to ease motion and morning sickness (see "Nausea").

natural news

Natural products are everywhere today. According to Dr. Deborah Wiancek, N.D., a naturopathic physician of The Riverwalk Natural Health Clinic in Colorado's Vail Valley, it has become a kind of hype. "They put 'natural' on everything, and not everything is natural. Herbs come from nature because they grow from plants. So, too, do food sources like fruits and vegetables. Anything that grows in the earth is from nature and is, therefore, a natural substance. So be sure that what you are buying is from natural sources, not chemical substitutes."

How Natural Remedies Differ from Conventional Medicine

"Conventional medicine" is the mainstream or Western medicine practiced by medical doctors, nurses, and pharmacists. They diagnose and treat conditions based on symptoms using drugs, surgery, or radiation. If you have a cold or flu, you go to the doctor, who prescribes a nasal spray, antibiotic, and so on. *Naturopathic* doctors, *homeopaths*, those who practice *ayurvedic* medicine, and even traditional medical doctors who integrate alternative methods into their practice take a more preventive approach.

Naturopathy, or naturopathic medicine, focuses on the power of nature to prevent illness and create whole-body wellness. It supports the body's ability to heal itself through the use of natural healing approaches, which can include diet and lifestyle changes, herbal medicine, acupuncture, Chinese medicine, detoxification, and homeopathy. A doctor of naturopathic medicine receives a four-year degree at one of four accredited schools in the United States. Want to find an N.D. in your area? Call the American Association of Naturopathic Physicians at 206-298-0125, or visit www.naturopathic.org.

Homeopathic medicine is based on the principle that "like cures like," that the substances that produce symptoms of sickness in healthy people will have a healing effect when given in very diluted quantities to sick people who exhibit those same symptoms. Specific homeopathic remedies are used to stimulate the body's own healing processes.

Ayurvedic medicine (*ayurveda* means "science of life") has its origins in India. Using a whole-body approach and specific practices such as herbal medicines and massage, a practitioner works to cleanse the body and balance body, mind, and spirit.

def•i•ni•tion

Naturopathic medicine supports the body's ability to heal itself through the use of natural healing approaches. **Homeopathic** medicine uses specific homeopathic remedies to stimulate the body's own healing processes. **Ayurvedic medicine** takes a whole-body approach and specific practices to cleanse and balance body, mind, and spirit.

The best of these practitioners (many of whom you'll meet through the course of this book) view their patients in a holistic way, taking into account the physical, emotional, and spiritual aspects of their beings. When they use natural remedies, they try to design their treatments so that they work with the body's own processes to make patients feel better.

Don't Prescription and OTC Drugs Come from Nature, Too?

True, more than half of all prescription drugs have their origins in plants. But there isn't much that's natural about them. You could think of a prescription or OTC (over-the-counter) drug as a sort of bionic herb. For example, when a pharmaceutical company wants to make aspirin, it uses salicylic acid (a compound that comes from white willow bark) because of its anti-inflammatory properties. Unlike the herb, though, aspirin is far more potent. This also makes it much more likely to cause side effects, like stomach ulcers and bleeding of the stomach. All drugs affect the liver, to some degree, because the liver has to metabolize them.

On the other hand, natural remedies, like white willow bark, are not as strong as a drug like aspirin, but they are less likely to cause side effects. They may take longer to work because they're weaker, but they don't have the side effects and they're easier for the body to assimilate. They're also less likely to cause liver problems.

natural news

Serious and fatal adverse drug reactions in hospital patients are the fourth and sixth causes of death, according to the *Journal of the American Medical Association*. By the age of 50, on average, people are on 10 drugs. "Often the pharmaceutical companies and doctors don't know fully how the drugs will interact, especially if the drugs are new," says Dr. Wiancek. "Also, many doctors don't know the other drugs people are taking, so they may give them a drug that may be treating the side effects from another drug."

Are Natural Remedies Safe?

"Natural remedies generally have fewer side effects because they're not as concentrated as prescription drugs, which are synthesized with a chemical to make them really strong," says Dr. Wiancek. "Most natural remedies are safe when used as directed because they are designed to work with the body." Of course, if you overdo anything, it can be harmful. It's all about balance. We'll be noting as we go along when you should be extra careful about a remedy and any interactions with medications you're taking now.

dial your doc

If you have any concerns about adding new nutrients, supplements, or treatments, it's a good idea to talk with your doctor about what's right for you.

The Best Way to Use Natural Remedies

If you've never used natural remedies, you may want to keep it simple and start by using them for colds and minor problems. Yet natural remedies can also be helpful if you've already been diagnosed by your medical doctor with certain conditions, such as type 2 diabetes or osteoarthritis, and you want to improve your treatment.

Natural remedies can be a helpful adjunct but should never be used in place of proper medical treatment. If you have a health problem that is getting worse, with significant pain, redness, swelling (which could be an infection), high fever, unexplained headaches, or abdominal pain, it's important that you see your doctor immediately. Always be careful about treating yourself. When in doubt about anything to do with your health, ask your doctor for guidance.

The Least You Need to Know

- ◆ Natural remedies offer a valuable alternative to conventional medicine.

- ◆ Many studies show that specific natural remedies are effective.

- ◆ Natural remedies use the body's own processes to speed healing and improve overall health.

- ◆ If you've never used natural remedies, use them for colds and minor problems first.

Chapter 2

You Are What You Eat

In This Chapter

- ◆ Why food is good medicine
- ◆ How to start eating healthier
- ◆ Making food functional
- ◆ The importance of vitamins and minerals
- ◆ The purpose of antioxidants

You are what you eat. We've all heard this saying, but do you know why it's true? Well, one of the most important reasons to eat well is to keep your immune system strong. The immune system is our defender against infection. To do its job, you have to give it the right nutrients to keep it (and everything else in your body) in tip-top shape. If you're always getting sick, it could be a signal that you aren't giving your immune system what it needs to keep you safe.

"Our cells, tissues, and organs only function as well as they are nourished," says Judy Stone, C.N., M.S.W., and author of *Take Two Apples and Call Me in the Morning: A Practical Guide to Using the Power of Food to Change Your Life* (www.taketwoapples.com). "Our health is dependent on what we eat, drink, and breathe."

Things like a poor diet (going to the drive-through a little more than you should?), stress (which depletes certain vitamins, like B's and C's), a lack of exercise, and bad habits (like smoking and alcohol) all put your immune system in debit status. When you eat healthfully, though, you take back your power to prevent numerous diseases, including heart disease, cancer, stroke, hypertension, diabetes, and more. Making smart choices can make a difference in how you feel today and may make a difference in how long you live—and live well.

Harvard's Healthy Eating Pyramid

One way to change your eating habits is to follow an eating plan. The USDA developed its first food pyramid in 1992 and recently revised it. The new pyramid, called My Pyramid, allows you to customize food choices based on how old you are and how active you are in an average day. It offers 12 different eating plans, but it doesn't differentiate among different types of carbohydrates and proteins.

The nutrition experts at Harvard had a problem with that. In fact, they challenged the new USDA pyramid because placing all fats in the top implied that all fats are bad. We know this just isn't true. Most unsaturated fats from plants and fish are good, whereas fats from animals (saturated fats) and fats in processed foods (trans fats) are not.

Harvard scientists decided to develop their own pyramid and compare the two head to head. After examining the diets of more than 100,000 adults, they found that men who followed Harvard's Healthy Eating Pyramid lowered their overall risk of certain diseases by 20 percent, compared to 11 percent for men who followed the original USDA food pyramid. Women lowered their risk by 11 percent with the Healthy Eating Pyramid, compared to just 3 percent for those who followed the USDA food pyramid.

The base of Harvard's Healthy Eating Pyramid is daily exercise and weight control. From there, the pyramid builds up in order as follows:

◆ Whole-grain foods at most meals and plant oils (olive, canola, soy, sunflower, and other vegetable oils).

◆ Vegetables in abundance and fruits two to three times per day. At least 5–12 different veggies a day.

- Nuts and legumes one to three times per day. (Eighteen nuts is one serving. Remember, though, nuts can be fattening.)

- Fish, poultry, and eggs zero to two times per day.

- Dairy one to two servings per day, or calcium supplement: 1,200 mg daily.

- Red meat, butter, white rice, white bread, white pasta, potatoes, soda, and sweets all used sparingly.

- Alcohol in moderation (if appropriate), and daily multivitamin (for most people).

You can find more information about Harvard's Healthy Eating Pyramid online at www.hsph.harvard.edu/nutritionsource/pyramids.

Functional Foods: Putting Foods to Work for You

When you have the basics of a healthy diet down, you can take food and your diet one step further. Functional foods like fruits and vegetables, whole grains, and beverages are used for specific conditions or to enhance overall health and wellness. According to the Food Marketing Institute, 69 percent of Americans have already jumped on the bandwagon and are incorporating foods into a preventive lifestyle, while 27 percent are utilizing food as a treatment to manage a preexisting health condition, like high cholesterol, high blood pressure, osteoporosis, or diabetes. The key to functional foods are the nutrients or compounds they contain that either nurture health, speed healing, or prevent illness. Today you'll find a wide variety of functional foods in your grocery store, which makes it easier than ever to reap their benefits. You'll find ways to eat for wellness throughout this book.

The Role of Vitamins and Minerals

When we choose functional foods, we are giving the body what it needs for optimal wellness. An important part of wellness is the 30 vitamins, minerals, and dietary components the body needs that it can't make on its own. These micronutrients found in foods include water-soluble vitamins, fat-soluble vitamins, major minerals, and trace minerals.

Each micronutrient has a job to do. The calcium and vitamin D in dairy products can help to reduce the risk of osteoporosis. The potassium you find in whole grains or bananas can help lower blood pressure. The magnesium you eat in spinach and pumpkin seeds and Brazil nuts can help maintain normal muscle and nerve functions. These nutrients play various roles throughout the body and serve important functions—helping to do everything from building bones to converting food into energy, to helping repair cellular damage from free radicals.

The Power of Antioxidants

Out of the vitamins and minerals we need, antioxidants are some of the most important and functional nutrients because they work as free-radical scavengers, neutralizing those unstable molecules before they can damage your DNA, thus keeping your tissues young and vital longer. You can find antioxidants in citrus fruits (vitamin C), almonds (vitamin E), carrots (beta carotene that can be converted into vitamin A), and garlic (selenium).

Bioflavonoids are big on antioxidant activity. You'll find them in fruits and vegetables like citrus fruits, berries, onions, parsley, legumes, green tea, red wine, sea buckthorn, and dark chocolate (with a cocoa content of 70 percent or greater). You'll also find them in plants, fulfilling many functions, including producing yellow or red/blue pigmentation in flowers and protecting against attack by microbes and insects. Catechins are bioflavonoids, a type of antioxidants found in plant compounds that may help stop the growth of cancer cells. You'll find high amounts of catechins in tea, chocolate, and red wine.

Many studies have shown that the antioxidants found in fruits and vegetables can help prevent age-related conditions such as heart disease and cancer. Antioxidants help neutralize free radicals, which are a byproduct of normal metabolism and can damage DNA and lead to cancer. Phytochemicals in soy act as "lite" estrogens and help ease the symptoms of menopause. Plant chemicals, like garlic, also have antibacterial qualities. Making phytochemicals a part of your diet (aim for five to nine servings of fruits and veggies, for best effect) can help prevent many other conditions and diseases, too, including heart disease and high blood pressure. You'll find out more about the wonderful properties of phytochemicals throughout this book.

Antioxidants also stop the free radicals associated with age-related memory loss and can help keep the brain young. Studies at Tufts University have found that deep purple prunes have more than twice the antioxidant properties of many other fruits and vegetables. Close seconds are blueberries (freeze them for a tasty snack), blackberries, and strawberries. Other good choices are raisins, oranges, plums, kale, broccoli, and spinach. Herbs such as ginger and turmeric have potent antioxidant properties, too. You'll find that antioxidants play a key role in many of the foods we mention here.

The Role of Inflammation and Anti-Inflammatory Foods

If you keep up with health news, you've probably seen numerous articles about inflammation and the inflammatory response. Why is this topic such a hot-button? Well, researchers at universities like the Massachusetts Institute of Technology have discovered that chronic inflammation plays a role in diseases such as cancer and atherosclerosis. When an infection occurs, immune cells flock to the area and secrete large amounts of highly reactive chemicals to combat the invader. But these inflammatory chemicals also attack normal tissue surrounding the infection and damage critical components of cells, including DNA. When the body is in a state of chronic inflammation, this damage to DNA can occur in the form of mutations or cell death and may lead to bigger problems like cancer and other diseases.

Inflammation can be promoted in the body because of what you eat. The biggest saboteur of health in the body is inflammation, says Judy Stone. Foods that are proinflammatory tend to be flour products, refined products, and sugar. Foods that are less inflammatory are lean proteins, vegetables, and healthy fats. "Eating in a way that calms inflammation in the body is good for everyone, but it's especially critical for people who are dealing with chronic conditions like IBS (irritable bowel syndrome), arthritis, and fibromyalgia," says Stone.

Functional Foods

The more functional foods you eat, the healthier you'll be. But supplements can help, too. (More about these in the next chapter!) For now, let's take a closer look at some functional foods that can improve your health. Why not jot down a few of these foods (some are new and some are tried and true) on your shopping list and put them to work for you?

natural news

It's important to consider how much nutrition is actually in the food you eat. Studies show that there are actually fewer nutrients in some foods today than in years past. Consider not just what to eat, but actually what kind of soil the produce you buy is grown in. You also need to think about how long it was in transport, how long it was on the shelf, and the best way to cook it to retain the most nutritional value. Debate has arisen over whether there are more nutrients in organic foods, but one thing is for sure: with organic foods, you won't be exposed to pesticides and herbicides. "Focus more on eating locally," says Judy Stone. "You'll get more nutrition in the food because it loses less value in transit."

Tried-and-True Functional Foods

You probably know that berries—particularly blueberries—are some of the best sources of antioxidants you can eat. They also may help to improve brain function. But you may not know that frozen foods are as good as fresh. That's important because you can keep them on hand more easily. Dried fruits can be part of the mix as well. Berries help the immune system, lowering blood cholesterol, getting rid of carcinogens (substances involved in the promotion of cancer in the body), and protecting the cells. If you can, buy organic berries; otherwise, they can be heavily treated with pesticides, and this just adds to the toxins your liver has to deal with.

Broccoli and the Entire Cabbage Family

You can add cruciferous vegetables in the cabbage family (plants with flowers of four petals and long, narrow seed pods) like cauliflower, kale, turnips, Brussels sprouts, spinach, leafy greens like collards, bok choy, and broccoli to your stir-fry. Broccoli and the cabbage family provide fiber and protect against damage from free radicals to DNA, too. Some studies show that people who eat cruciferous vegetables have lower-than-average risks for bladder and colon cancers. Broccoli, cauliflower, cabbage and kale, Brussels sprouts, and horseradish also contain the compound sulforaphane, which may also help to detox the body.

Whole Grains

By now, you've surely heard of the benefits of whole grains. But you may not know that whole grains, like whole-wheat bread and brown rice, contain *phytochemicals* that can reduce the cancer-causing effects of free radicals. "Whole grains are also packed with fiber and slow the release of carbohydrates, so that's why they tend to be lower on the glycemic index," says Bradley J. Willcox, M.D., a clinical scientist and geriatrician at the Pacific Health Research Institute at the University of Hawaii in Honolulu and co-author of *The Okinawa Program: How the World's Longest-Lived People Achieve Everlasting Health and How You Can, Too.* "This is important because when foods are lower on the glycemic index, there is evidence that this may lower the risk of cancer. Mostly it has to do with insulin, thought to be one of the growth factors for these hormone-dependent cancers such as breast, prostate, ovarian, and colon. If you're eating a lot of high-glycemic foods you are always triggering that insulin response."

Foods high on the glycemic index tend to be fluffy—think cotton candy or white bread. Harder foods are lower on the glycemic index. Whole-grain pasta, for example, is lower on the glycemic index because the carbohydrates are really packed in and your stomach has to work to break it down. So avoid the white pastas; eat spinach or whole-grain pastas instead.

Whole grains also help lower blood cholesterol and can prevent colon cancer. Fiber binds to the bad fat and plays an important role in the body, helping to eliminate toxins more quickly. This can have a protective effect against breast cancer, studies show. Whole grains and fiber like the beta glucan found in oatmeal and oat bran, and soluble fiber found in psyllium seed husks and beans can also help protect against heart disease.

Whole grains also contain an abundance of B vitamins, including vitamin B_1 (thiamin) and B_6 (pyridoxine), both of which help to regulate metabolism.

Coldwater Fish

The sea contains bountiful nutrients to promote a healthy heart, to improve mental functioning and clarity, and to alleviate depression. So be sure to include salmon, tuna, and mackerel in your diet. All these coldwater fish contain essential omega-3 fatty acids, DHA and EPA. "Omega-3 fatty acids have been associated with a lower risk for a number of hormone-associated cancers, like breast, for example," says Dr. Willcox. "Unless you are eating fish or flax several times a week, you're probably not getting enough." He also advises aiming for a high intake of healthy monounsaturated fats, like canola oil, olive oil, and tree nuts, as these can help reduce the risk of cardiovascular disease.

Tea

It's a good idea, too, to get in the habit of brewing a nice pot of tea. Green and black teas (also called sanpin, jasmine, or oolong tea) are filled with *bioflavonoids* known as *catechins*, which, because they are antioxidants, can act as powerful free-radical fighters. Overall, research shows that drinking three cups of tea a day has a moderate effect of helping to improve heart health by reducing the risk of heart attack. In other words, you shouldn't count on it as a sole form of therapy, but it may be helpful.

If you want to find the highest levels of catechins, go for tender white tea leaves, which come from the plant Camellia Sinensis. You can even find this in mainstream tea products now. Look in your grocery and health food store.

Tomatoes

Like pasta? (Whole wheat, of course!) Then you can reap the benefits of lycopene, a phytonutrient found in tomatoes that acts as an antioxidant and is absorbed optimally in sauce form. Research shows that the protective effect of tomato consumption is strongest for cancers of the prostate, lung, and stomach, and, to a lesser degree, the pancreas, colon, rectum, esophagus (throat), mouth, breast, and cervix.

Citrus Fruits

Blood oranges may be the new kid on the block when it comes to citrus fruits, but there are plenty of others to choose from when you need vitamin C—and we all do. Oranges, tangerines, and grapefruit all contain phytochemicals, which act as antioxidants to scavenge free radicals. You can also find vitamin C in strawberries!

Sweet Potatoes

Sweet potatoes and other yellow-orange fruits and vegetables contain carotenoids, pigments that give them their distinctive color. They also provide important anticancer compounds, vitamin A, and beta carotene. Besides sweet potatoes, you can find all of these nutrients in carrots, cantaloupe, apricots, squash, and yams.

Flaxseed and Soybeans

We know that bioflavonoids are powerful antioxidants. But two plants, soybeans and flaxseed, have pharmacological levels of these compounds, says Dr. Willcox, co-author of *The Okinawa Program: How the World's Longest-Lived People Achieve Everlasting Health and How You Can, Too.* "The levels exceed those in other plants as much as 1,000 times and work to inhibit the actions of powerful estrogens at the breast and other areas that might be responsible in part for breast cancer."

Kiwi

The refreshing kiwi is originally native to southern China and tastes like a mixture of strawberry, banana, and pineapple. Kiwi is a rich source of vitamin C that has been shown to reduce the inflammatory response. It can be helpful in reducing the severity of conditions like osteoarthritis, rheumatoid arthritis, and asthma, and can help prevent conditions such as colon cancer, atherosclerosis, and diabetic heart disease.

You'll also find vitamin E in kiwi, along with potassium and vitamin A, in the form of beta carotene. Studies show that kiwi can help respiratory problems like wheezing associated with asthma, shortness of breath, and night coughing. Need to add fiber to your diet? Although the kiwi is small, it's a good source of roughage that can help keep you regular.

Walnuts

One reason the Mediterranean diet may work so well could be the nut factor—walnuts, that is, say researchers at Barcelona's Hospital Clinic. A study in the *Journal of the American College of Cardiology* showed that eating walnuts with a fatty meal helped protect arteries from the damaging effects (inflammation and oxidation) of saturated fats. Researchers think this is due to the fact that walnuts contain alpha linolenic acid, a plant-based fatty acid like the "good fats," omega-3 fatty acids found in coldwater fish.

New Functional Foods

We all know that an apple a day is, well, a good idea, but other fruits and vegetables may not be so obvious when it comes to eating for good health. The Food Marketing Institute has identified these foods as up-and-comers. Think about adding them to your grocery list.

Blood Oranges

You may not have eaten one (yet!) but they are so full of nutrients that you really need to, especially if you feel a cold coming on. Juicy and sweet, this mildly acidic snack with a slight raspberry taste, from Italy and Spain (although they are being grown in the United States now, too), is packed with vitamin C. This means both the red flesh of the orange and the deep red juice are packed with healthful antioxidants. Blood oranges contain the pigment anthocyanin, which gives them their vibrant color. You can drink blood oranges as a juice or slice one up and put it in a salad.

Goji Berries

Tangy Goji berries look like red raisins but are packed with powerful antioxidants. Used in herbal medicine for thousands of years, they are rich in carotenoids, such as beta carotene and zeaxanthin, which can help keep your vision healthy. Eating foods that are high in zeaxanthin is especially important if you have an AARP card, as they can help your eyesight by preventing age-related macular degeneration. Goji berries also contain vitamins B_1 (thiamin), B_2 (riboflavin), B_6 (Pyridoxine), and E.

Seabuckthorn

If you need to ease a digestive-tract ailment, like an ulcer, or soothe your skin, try seabuckthorn. Not only do the phytochemicals in this plant ease pain, but they are also anti-inflammatory and help tissues heal. Seabuckthorn is also chock-full of beneficial antioxidant nutrients like vitamin C, vitamin E, beta carotene, and bioflavonoids, along with omega-9 fatty acid (oleic acid).

Mangosteens

It doesn't look or taste like a mango. It looks like a purple tennis ball. It's a mangosteen. And the taste? Awesome! Besides its delicate flavor, it's packed with antioxidants. The powerful phytonutrients responsible for the health benefits in mangosteens are known as xanthones, which can boost immune health. Mangosteens were just recently imported into the United States, so the price can be high for this delectable fruit—but one bite and you may think it's worth it!

Garbanzo Beans

Want to lower your cholesterol? Get into the habit of eating garbanzos, or chickpeas. The soluble fiber in garbanzos forms a kind of gel that helps to move cholesterol out of your body. In fact, a 2001 study in the *Archives of Internal Medicine* showed that high-fiber foods like garbanzo beans can help prevent heart disease. The insoluble fiber in garbanzos doesn't affect cholesterol, but it can help prevent constipation and, in turn, digestive problems like irritable bowel syndrome. The fiber in garbanzos (also a good protein source) can also help to keep your blood sugar stable if you have diabetes or hypoglycemia. Garbanzo beans are high in potassium and low in sodium, which means they can lower blood pressure. Want an easy way to add these to your diet? Toss them onto a salad.

Specialty Mushrooms

Shiitake, maitake, and reishi are the three best-known specialty mushrooms, known for their polysaccharide and beta-glucan compounds and cancer-preventative properties. But did you know that portabellas, criminis, and even the lowly button mushroom also have potent antioxidant powers, thanks to the phytochemical L-ergothioneine? Criminis also contain selenium; B complex vitamins like riboflavin (B_2) and niacin (B_3); iron; and zinc, an important mineral for immune function. If you want to incorporate these into your diet, try a nice stir-fry. These mushrooms are just as potent cooked as they are raw.

The Least You Need to Know

◆ Think of food as good medicine. Eating well keeps your immune system strong and prevents many diseases.

◆ Using the Harvard Healthy Eating Pyramid is a good way to learn healthy eating habits.

◆ Functional foods can help you boost health, treat conditions, and prevent illnesses.

◆ Chronic inflammation can contribute to many diseases. Eating certain foods like lean proteins, vegetables, and healthy fats can promote less inflammation in the body.

◆ The body needs 30 vitamins, minerals, and dietary components that it can't make on its own.

◆ Studies have shown that the antioxidants found in fruits and vegetables help prevent heart disease and cancer. Adding a variety of foods ensures the intake of these and other important nutrients.

Chapter 3

Filling in the Gaps with Supplements

In This Chapter

- What exactly is a supplement?

- Which nutrients are most important

- How probiotics, plant sterols, and green foods can help

- The difference between whole-food vitamins and vitamin supplements

In a perfect world, you would get all the nutrients you need from your diet. But this isn't the reality for most of us. When the job, the commute, and a busy schedule lead to processed foods, nutrient-poor foods, and the drive-through, we may constantly come up short. The result? We're left with the nagging feeling that we're doing something wrong—and, worse, that we're putting our health at risk. This can happen when the immune system (which we talked about in the previous chapter) doesn't have the nutrients it needs to protect us from illness both now and in the future. That's why if, in spite of your best efforts to eat a healthy diet, you still need help (and most of us do), you may want to add supplements to fill in the nutritional gap. First, let's learn more about exactly what supplements are and do.

What Is a Supplement, Anyway?

Here's how Congress defines a dietary supplement in the Dietary Supplement Health and Education Act, which became law in 1994. It's a product that ...

◆ Is intended to supplement the diet

◆ Contains one or more dietary ingredients (including vitamins, minerals, herbs or other botanicals, amino acids, and other substances) or their constituents

◆ Is intended to be taken by mouth as a pill, capsule, tablet, or liquid

◆ Is labeled on the front panel as being a dietary supplement

Okay, that's fine, but dietary supplements are regulated more like foods, not like drugs, right? Unlike new drugs, dietary supplements don't have to go through review by the FDA for safety and effectiveness, or be "approved" before they can be marketed. Recently, though, the FDA established Current Good Manufacturing Practice requirements (CGMPs—say that three times fast!) for dietary supplements. Now supplement manufacturers must report all serious adverse side effects of dietary supplements to the FDA. This is good news for consumers.

The FDA will also now be able to check out dietary supplements to evaluate their identity, purity (to make sure they're free of contaminants like lead and bacteria), quality, strength, and composition. Robert E. Brackett, Ph.D., director of the FDA's Center for Food Safety and Applied Nutrition, stated, "The dietary supplement CGMPs should increase consumers' confidence in the quality of the dietary supplement products that they purchase. These regulations provide more accountability in the manufacturing process so that consumers can be confident that the products they purchase contain what is on the label." Supplements will also be evaluated for health benefits and safety risks through studies and reviews of studies that have already been done.

natural news _____

When it comes to buying supplements, use your noggin. Read the latest health magazines and cruise health websites. You may also find it very helpful to talk to a nutritionally oriented doctor, like a naturopath, who knows about the latest studies on supplements and knows what works for specific conditions and what doesn't. Most important, an expert will work with you to tailor treatment for your needs, keeping in mind how certain supplements work together and making sure they don't interact in a negative way. Once you have a regimen, update your regular M.D. on your next visit. He or she needs to know all the medicines and supplements you're taking, especially if you are scheduled for surgery, so there are no complications.

Nutrients You Need Now

Okay, now that we've covered the background of supplements, let's take a closer look at the nutrients most of us need right now on a daily basis (known as the *RDA*, which stands for Recommended Dietary Allowance). You can get quite a few of these nutrients through common foods (we discussed some of these in the previous chapter and go into more detail here), but this assumes that you eat a varied diet, and many of us don't. This is no reason to get down on yourself. Like we said, it can be a challenge to eat right! That's why you may want to pick up a multivitamin that contains these nutrients or individual supplements. The RDA or Retinal equivalent (RAE) will tell you how much you need to take each day.

def•i•ni•tion _____

RDA stands for Recommended Dietary Allowance and was first used as a dietary guideline in 1941. The RDAs are revised every 5 to 10 years. Many alternative health practitioners think dosage amounts for supplements are often far too conservative. The RDA only provides the amount of a nutrient needed to not get sick—for example, the amount of vitamin C needed to avoid scurvy. It is conservative when considering optimal nutritional status.

Vitamin A: About half of us get the vitamin A we need every day. We need to do better. Why? Beta carotene, an antioxidant that is converted into vitamin A, can help lower the risk for cancer and heart disease. "Vitamin A is important for vision, cell development and differentiation, and immune function," says Karen Collins, M.S., R.D., a registered dietitian and advisor to the American Institute for Cancer Research. Major sources of vitamin A include dark, leafy greens and dark orange veggies—think spinach, collard greens, kale, carrots, winter squash, sweet potatoes, red peppers, and cantaloupe. Retinal equivalent (RAE): 700–900 mcg. daily.

Vitamin C: Approximately half of adults and up to 20 percent of children don't get enough vitamin C through the diet. This potent antioxidant can neutralize harmful free radicals and help make collagen (a tissue needed for healthy bones, teeth, gums, and blood vessels). To make up the shortfall, think citrus, but also think outside the orange. Vitamin C is in kiwi, strawberries, papaya, cantaloupe, and even veg-etables like broccoli and green and red peppers. RDA: Women, 75 mg; men, 90 mg.

Vitamin E: Eighty percent of the population doesn't meet the RDA for this antioxidant. Foods high in vitamin E include sunflower, cot-tonseed, canola, and safflower oil. Sunflower and pumpkin seeds are rich in vitamin E, as are hazelnuts and almonds. Cereals fortified with vitamin E can provide up to 17 mg. Still, it can be tough to get enough vitamin E from foods alone. You may want to supplement the gap. RDA: 15 mg, or 22–33 IU (international units).

Calcium: Fewer than half of women consume enough milk for bone health. To turn over a new leaf, aim for three servings a day of dairy products. This will also supply vitamin D, which helps keep bones and cells healthy. Choose nonfat and low-fat dairy products like skim milk and reduced-fat cheese. A supplement can also help, in 500 mg doses for optimal absorption. RDA: 1,000 mg; women over 50 should have 1,200 mg.

Magnesium: Studies show that when people meet the RDA for mag-nesium, the risk of diabetes drops because the magnesium interacts with how insulin functions. It also works with calcium to prevent osteoporosis and is linked to better blood pressure control. It can also help to prevent migraine headaches. RDA: Women, 310–320 mg; men, 400–420 mg.

Potassium: Although the RDA for potassium is 4,700 mg, most of us consume only 2,100 mg to 3,200 mg. When in balance with sodium, potassium helps control blood pressure. Bananas are a no-brainer for potassium, but higher sources include white and sweet potatoes, legumes such as kidney beans (a major source of magnesium and fiber), dark-green leafy vegetables, and dairy products such as yogurt, along with all types of fish. RDA: 4,700 mg.

natural news

Probiotics, which means "for life," are supplements that contain billions of health-promoting bacteria that help to support healthy microbial balance in the gastrointestinal (GI) tract. The majority of the immune system is located in the GI tract, and "friendly" intestinal bacteria are vital to our bodily defenses. They also aid digestion and nutrient absorption. When beneficial flora occupy the intestinal lining, potentially harmful micro-organisms are deprived of both space and nutrients. A lack of beneficial bacteria in your diet can result in a lack of support for your immune system.

Friendly bacteria also help manufacture certain B vitamins (including niacin [B3], pyridoxine [B6], folic acid, and biotin), reduce cholesterol, and aid in synthesizing short-chain fatty acids. They can be useful in the treatment of acne, psoriasis, eczema, allergies, migraines, gout (by reducing uric acid levels), rheumatic and arthritic conditions, cystitis, candidiasis, and some forms of cancer. You can take probiotics as a supplement, found at your local health food store. It is important to look for a product that has a delivery system that makes certain the bacteria reach the intestines without being killed off by the stomach acid.

Fiber: Average fiber consumption is half of what it should be. "Fiber is important in terms of heart disease, intestinal function, digestive problems like diverticulosis, and potentially colon cancer," says Collins. "It also helps to control cholesterol and blood sugar in people who have diabetes." Use a fiber supplement or eat foods like legumes, nuts, and whole grains. Suggested intake: Women, 25 g per day; over 50, 21 g per day. Men, 38 g per day; over 50, 30 g per day.

Folate: This water-soluble B vitamin occurs naturally in food. Folic acid is the synthetic form of folate that is found in supplements and added to fortified foods. It's especially important during periods of rapid cell division and growth, such as infancy and pregnancy, because folate is necessary to make DNA and RNA, the building blocks of cells. For this reason, it can also help protect cells from changes that can lead to cancer. We also need folate to help make red blood cells and prevent anemia. You'll find folate in leafy greens, citrus fruits, and fortified breads and cereals, or in supplement form. RDA: Ages 19 and over, 400 mg; women during pregnancy, 600 mg (in lactation, reduce to 500 mg). See your doctor with any questions.

Vitamin B12: Needed to help make DNA, vitamin B12 helps maintain healthy nerve and red blood cells. It is found in foods that come from animals, including fish, meat, poultry, eggs, milk, and milk products, along with fortified breakfast cereals. RDA: Ages 14 and over, 2.4 mg.

Vitamin B6: The nervous and immune systems need vitamin B6 to function efficiently, and it's also needed for the conversion of tryptophan (an amino acid) to niacin (a vitamin). Hemoglobin in red blood cells carries oxygen to tissues. Vitamin B6 also boosts the amount of oxygen hemoglobin (in red blood cells) carries to cells. Vitamin B6 also boosts immunity, regulates metabolism, and helps keep blood glucose (sugar) stable. You can find vitamin B6 in beans, nuts, legumes, whole grains, and vegetables like spinach and garbanzo beans. RDA: Ages 19–50, 1.3 mg; men over 50, 1.7 mg; women over 50, 1.5 mg.

Vitamin D: This vitamin is a rising star in the vitamin world. It can do everything from promoting calcium absorption to help form strong bones, to protecting against lung cancer. Also, a recent report in the *Archives of General Psychiatry* showed that older individuals with low blood levels of vitamin D may have a higher risk of depression. Sunshine is a significant source of vitamin D because UV rays from sunlight trigger vitamin D synthesis in the skin. A few minutes of exposure on a summer day can generate huge quantities of vitamin D.

Fortified foods like milk are common sources of vitamin D. According to the National Institutes of Health Office of Dietary Supplements, 1 cup of vitamin D–fortified milk supplies half of the recommended daily intake for adults between the ages of 19 and 50, one quarter of the recommended daily intake for adults between the ages of 51 and 70, and approximately 15 percent of the recommended daily intake for adults age 71 and over. Recommended intake: 800 I.U.

Iron: We need iron so our blood can deliver oxygen from our lungs to all the cells in our body. When we don't have enough, it can result in anemia (see the chapter on anemia) and we can feel tired and sluggish. Most of the iron in the body is found in hemoglobin, the protein in red blood cells that carries oxygen to tissues. You'll find iron in foods like red meat, fish, and poultry, and in plant foods such as lentils and beans. RDA: Women, 18 mg; men 19–50, 8 mg; men and women over 50, 8 mg.

natural news

You can also find supplements in your food, so to speak. Plant sterols are a class of natural, fatlike plant compounds with chemical structures similar to cholesterol, so they block its absorption. The FDA has approved the addition of plant sterols to a wide variety of foods, such as orange juice, dairy substitutes, cheese, granola bars, bread, and cereal, as one way to lower your cholesterol. Research shows that plant sterols lower "bad" (LDL) cholesterol by 8 to 15 percent, while lowering total cholesterol by 10 percent. "It's a wonderful addition to restrictive diets because it's a whole variety of foods to eat to add to the benefit of cholesterol reduction," says Dr. Joseph Keenan, a professor of family medicine at the University of Minnesota (he also holds a joint professorship in the University of Minnesota School of Food Science and Nutrition). "For folks with mild cholesterol problems, adding foods with plant sterols to the diet can keep them from going on a drug."

Aim for 1–2 g of plant sterols a day with your main meal for a cholesterol-lowering effect (not recommended for pregnant women). For more information on plant sterols and a listing of products, visit www.corowise.com.

Selenium: This important antioxidant helps protect our cells from free-radical damage and boosts overall immune function. Major sources of selenium include walnuts and Brazil nuts, but you can also find this nutrient in fish, liver, garlic, and eggs. You can also easily add this nutrient through supplementation. RDA: Over age 19, at least 55 mcg.

Vitamin K: This vitamin, which refers to a group of fat-soluble compounds called naphthoquinones, is necessary for the liver to make what it needs for the blood to clot properly. The type we get through the diet is vitamin K1 (phytonadione), found in green leafy vegetables like spinach, broccoli, asparagus, watercress, cabbage, and cauliflower, as well as green peas, beans, olives, canola, soybeans, meat, cereals, and dairy products. Vitamin K deficiencies should be managed under medical supervision.

natural news

According to the U.S. Department of Agriculture, less than 9 percent of American adults consume the recommended five to six servings of fruits and vegetables a day. To fill the gap, it's a good idea to go for the greens—a green supplement, that is. When we eat green foods, we make the body's pH more neutral or alkaline, which enables it to operate at its best. Green foods include young cereal grasses like wheat, kamut, barley, oats, alfalfa, dandelion grasses; sea vegetables like sea kelp and sea dulse; sprouted sesame and sunflower seeds; grains; and legumes. You'll find that these foods are rich in nutrients like beta carotene, which is converted into vitamin A and vitamin C.

The chlorophyll found in green foods like spirulina, chorella, kelp, and other blue-green algae is also very important. Research indicates that chlorophyll assists in protection from carcinogens, toxic chemicals, and radiation, and helps stimulate the repair of damaged tissues and the synthesis of red blood cells—accelerates wound healing and inhibits the growth of bacteria. One brand of chlorophyll supplement to check out is Garden of Life's Perfect Food (www.gardenoflifeusa.com). You'll find others in your health food store.

Zinc: This antioxidant trace mineral found in almost every cell is essential for life. More than 300 enzymes in our bodies need this nutrient to function effectively. We need zinc for immune health, which is why you'll find it in lozenges designed to short-circuit colds and flu. It's also important for proper thyroid function and wound healing, and it improves our sense of smell and taste. The oyster tops the list when it comes to zinc content. But you'll also find this nutrient in dairy products, wheat germ, beans, lentils, nuts, and whole-grain cereals. RDA: Women over 19, 8 mg; men over 19, 11 mg.

dial your doc

Taking a combination of supplements or using these products together with medications (whether prescription or OTC drugs) could produce adverse effects, some of which could be life-threatening. For example, Coumadin (a prescription medicine), ginkgo biloba (an herbal supplement), aspirin (an OTC drug), and vitamin E (a vitamin supplement) can each thin the blood, and taking any of these products together can increase the potential for internal bleeding.

So if you are taking any prescription or over-the-counter medicines, make sure they are compatible with any supplements you may be interested in trying. In some cases, such as with mild depression, a supplement like St. John's wort may be able to replace an antidepressant, but you shouldn't make this switch on your own. See a qualified health practitioner to ensure that the supplements you want to take are compatible with the drugs you are already taking.

The Least You Need to Know

◆ Supplements can be a valuable adjunct to help us meet our nutritional needs.

◆ The FDA has established Current Good Manufacturing Practice requirements, which will help guarantee the safety of dietary supplements.

◆ The Recommended Daily Allowance helps us know how much of each nutrient we need on a daily basis. But many alternative health practitioners think dosage amounts for supplements are too conservative.

◆ Less than 9 percent of American adults consume the recommended five to six servings of fruits and vegetables a day. To fill the gap, it's a good idea to add a green supplement.

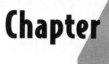

The Healing Power of Herbs

In This Chapter

- ◆ How herbal medicine can be helpful for many common health conditions
- ◆ The therapeutic qualities of herbs to treat symptoms
- ◆ The anti-inflammatory, antioxidant, antifungal, and anticancer properties of herbs
- ◆ The many different ways you can use herbs to get results

Herbal medicine has been used around the world for thousands of years to heal the body and calm the mind. In academic circles, especially in Europe, Australia, New Zealand, Asia, South Africa, South America, and increasingly North America, the term used is *phytotherapy*, from the Greek *phyton*, for "plant." This specifies the use of herbs for their therapeutic value.

Herbal medicine means you have another choice in how you care for your body and your health. There are herbal equivalents for many prescription drugs on the market right now. A fruit, flower, leaf, stem, root, seaweed, or bark may be just as effective—and safer.

Plants and their roots, leaves, flowers, or berries can help with mild problems, aid in preventing and treating chronic problems, and strengthen and detoxify certain organs or the entire body. As you'll see in the pages ahead, the herbs mentioned here can be used to treat everything from common health issues like acne to bug bites, from colds and flu to more chronic problems like heartburn, constipation, type 2 diabetes, and arthritis. One thing is certain: herbs can effectively prevent and treat illness. We'll show you how.

Popular Herbs and Their Characteristics

Information on herbs you'll be reading about in this chapter comes from the National Center for Complementary and Alternative Medicine (nccam.nih.gov/health/herbsataglance.htm). For additional information, visit these sources:

◆ The American Botanical Council: www.herbalgram.org

◆ The American Herbal Products Association: www.ahpa.org

Aloe vera (Aloe barbadensis): Ah, aloe. You may have this plant on your windowsill. If you do, you know that aloe leaves contain a clear gel that you can use to soothe and help heal minor burns and sunburns. In recent trials, the gel and its derivatives have been shown to have antifungal, antioxidant, and wound-healing properties.

Astragalus (Astragalus membranaceus, Astragalus mongholicus): Often used in Chinese medicine to bolster the immune system, astragalus is also commonly used to treat the common cold and other upper respiratory infections. Only the water-extracted form in liquid, capsule, or tablet is considered medicine. This is because the polysaccharides thought to be responsible for immune benefits are at full potency in this form, as opposed to traditional preparations that include soup, tea, or cooked foods, such as rice, that do not provide the same medicinal benefit.

Bilberry (Vaccinium myrtillus): Used for nearly 1,000 years in traditional European medicine, today the fruit is used to prevent cataracts, varicose veins, and other circulatory problems. Bilberry leaf is used for treating diabetes. Read more about the benefits of bilberry in the "Cataracts" section later in Part 2.

Black cohosh (Cimicifuga Racemosa): This herb is often used to treat the symptoms of menopause, like vaginal dryness, night sweats, and, of course, hot flashes. "Its value for reducing hot flashes safely is not due to hormone activity like that of prescription hormone-replacement therapy, and evidence supports the view of traditional practitioners that black cohosh root is protective rather than problematic for women at risk of breast cancer," says Amanda McQuade Crawford, *Dip. Phyto., MNIMH, RH (AHG), MNZAMH*, a consultant medical herbalist in Los Angeles. It's also used to help menstrual irregularities and premenstrual syndrome. Black cohosh also relaxes tension and is a vasodilator, opening peripheral vessels. This effect can lower high blood pressure or, in sensitive women, cause a frontal headache and even dizziness upon standing up too quickly.

Recent concerns over possible liver toxicity have largely been laid to rest by reviews of numerous human and animal studies. However, herbalists have always cautioned against large doses or using this potent root as a general women's tonic.

natural news

Ever wonder what all those initials are after experts' names? For example, with Amanda McQuade Crawford, here's what they mean:

Dip. Phyto: Diploma of Phytotherapy

MNIMH: Member of the National Institute of Medical Herbalists

RH: Registered Herbalist

AHG: Professional member and founding member of the American Herbalists Guild

MNZAMH: Member of the New Zealand Association of Medical Herbalists

Cranberry (Vaccinium macrocarpon): This berry is used to prevent urinary tract infections, or what is known as *Helicobacter pylori* infections. Cranberry has also been reported to have antioxidant and anticancer activity. Read more about the benefits of cranberry in the "Bladder Infection" section in Part 2.

Dandelion (Taraxacum officinale): Native American and traditional Arabic medicine often use dandelion. Dandelion greens are edible and a rich source of vitamin A. Some people use dandelion as a liver or kidney "tonic." The root, which is very difficult to dig up, is called "earth-nail," according to Amanda Crawford, because it helps flighty people to be grounded. In addition, it's good for the skin because dandelion helps the liver detoxify and the kidneys eliminate waste products. Dandelion root is also used as a diuretic and for minor digestive problems. You can find the leaves and roots of the dandelion plant in teas, capsules, or extracts.

Echinacea (Echinacea purpurea): This herb, commonly called purple coneflower or coneflower, has traditionally been used to treat or prevent colds, flu, and upper-respiratory infections by stimulating the immune system. A review of more than 700 research studies published in the medical journal *The Lancet* in 2007 concluded that echinacea is effective at preventing colds and limiting their length.

natural news

During the westward expansion of the United States in the nineteenth century, echinacea was called "Prairie Doctor" because it helped with so many infectious diseases that plagued families in covered wagons. The nation's first people to cross the plains boiled roots for external washes and internal healing, including snake bites, from which echinacea got the name "Kansas Snake Root."

Evening primrose oil (Oenothera biennis): Extracted from the seeds of evening primrose, a wildflower common from coast to coast, this oil contains gamma-linolenic acid (GLA), an essential fatty acid you need for growth and development. Good for conditions that involve inflammation, such as rheumatoid arthritis, evening primrose oil can also be helpful for women with PMS and with the breast pain associated with the menstrual cycle. Traditionally, Native Americans added the seeds to their meals to increase their nutritional value.

Feverfew (Tanacetum parthenium, Chrysanthemum parthenium): Feverfew can be helpful most commonly for migraine headaches and rheumatoid arthritis. Supplements of feverfew made of dried leaves, flowers, and stems have also been used in allergies and asthma, sporiasis, tinnitus (ringing of the ears), dizziness, nausea, and vomiting. When eaten fresh, though it tastes bitter, one leaf a day of feverfew, even hidden in a sandwich with leafy greens, may be enough to reduce migraines, says Crawford. This pretty member of the daisy family grows easily in many climates, even as a potted plant on your kitchen countertop. So you may want to become a tabletop gardener!

Flaxseed and flaxseed oil (Linum usitatissimum): A plant with origins in ancient Egypt, flaxseed oil is often used for hot flashes, breast pain, and arthritis. Ground-up flaxseed contains lignans (phytoestrogens, or plant estrogens) made up of soluble fiber, like that found in oat bran, which, when sprinkled on cereal, acts as an effective laxative.

Garlic (Allium sativum): This edible bulb from the lily family is a common ingredient in chicken noodle soup for the cold or flu, with good reason (more about these conditions in Part 2). This cousin of the onion and leek has antibacterial and antiviral properties. Allicin is the potent phyto or plant chemical you'll find in garlic, but it also contains many other healthful compounds. Garlic is heart friendly. Not only does it help reduce high cholesterol, but it also helps cut back on sticky plaque in arteries. This small but mighty herb also has been shown in studies to lower high blood pressure.

natural news

Worried about garlic breath? Eating garlic with parsley or crunching on a fragrant cardamom seed clears the breath of garlic odor.

Ginger (Zingiber officinale): The phytochemicals known as gingerols and shogaols are responsible for ginger's antinausea properties. This traditional Asian remedy also helps ease digestive upset, diarrhea, and the urge to vomit. You may also find relief with ginger if you have rheumatoid arthritis or osteoarthritis, or common joint and muscle pain.

Ginkgo (Ginkgo biloba): The ginkgo tree is one of the oldest types of trees in the world. Fossil records show that the tree with this fan-shaped leaf has not changed for ages. In China, and the United

risky remedy!

As a potential blood thinner, herbalists recommend to stop taking ginkgo biloba three days or more before major surgery.

States now, too, ginkgo is used as a memory booster to keep the brain young. Since the natural compounds in ginkgo promote circulation and better blood flow to all parts of the body, especially the brain, it is recommended for everything from Alzheimer's disease and senility to tinnitus and macular degeneration.

Asian ginseng (Panax ginseng): One of several types of true ginseng (another is American ginseng, *Panax quinquefolius*), Asian ginseng supports overall health and boosts the immune system. It is also used to treat erectile dysfunction, hepatitis C, and menopause symptoms, and it can help control blood pressure and lower blood glucose.

Ginseng increases the production and upward flow of vital energy. In fact, it can make one's energy rise so well that, in sensitive people, it can lead to headaches or insomnia. On the plus side, it nourishes and rebuilds energy in those whose reserves are low.

Goldenseal (Hydrastis canadensis): This antibiotic and antiviral herb is often used with echinacea to fend off colds and flu. This is thanks to the phytochemical berberine, which motivates white blood cells to attack bacteria and viruses that are up to no good. According to Amanda Crawford, the botanical name hydrastis refers to *hydro* (water); this herb dries up watery secretions, whether from sinuses, lungs, or the digestive tract, or on the skin. Goldenseal is also used for infectious diarrhea, eye infections, and vaginitis (inflammation or infection of the vagina). Women who are pregnant or breastfeeding should avoid using goldenseal, and it should not be given to infants or young children.

Grape seed extract (Vitis vinifera): Grape seed extract is good for your heart and blood vessels. It's filled with procirculatory and anti-inflammatory phytochemicals that help protect the heart and prevent atherosclerosis, the hardening of the arteries. Grape seeds also contain resveratrol, which can help lower cholesterol. It's available in capsule and tablet forms.

Green tea (Camellia sinensis): Thanks to minimal processing (green tea is just steamed and dried, as opposed to black tea, which is dried, rolled, fermented, and roasted), green tea has more phytochemical punch. Today green tea and its extracts are some of the most widely used and most powerful herbs available.

Many studies have shown the benefits of green tea. Regularly drinking green tea may reduce heart attack risk or atherosclerosis. It can also be beneficial in reducing inflammation related to arthritis and slowing cartilage breakdown. In addition, a recent study found that older adults in Japan who drank green tea daily had better memories than those who didn't. Plus, green tea is one of the most affordable antioxidants: a regular habit of five cups of green tea (not tall mugs, like a latte!) provides just a little caffeine and a lot of anti-inflammatory protection.

Horse chestnut (Aesculus hippocastanum): The seed extract from horse chestnuts (also called buckeyes) contains the phytochemical aescin, which, among other compounds, helps to strengthen veins and reduces inflammation. It also gets blood moving and eases chronic venous insufficiency, when veins in the legs don't return blood as well as they should to the heart. When blood doesn't make the round-trip in a normal amount of time, it can result in varicose veins and spider veins, which can be very uncomfortable, even painful. You can also use horse chestnut for hemorrhoids.

Lavender (Lavandula angustifolia): Ah, lavender! The soothing phytochemicals from lavender essential oil can help reduce stress by calming nerves, making it a good fix for anxiety and insomnia. You can also use this versatile herb as an antiseptic to disinfect wounds (more about this in the First Aid chapter in Part 2).

Licorice root (Glycyrrhiza glabra, Glycyrrhiza uralensis–Chinese licorice): Licorice root can be used for heartburn, stomach ulcers, bronchitis, and sore throat. The natural compounds in real licorice (which has nothing to do with the red or black candy you eat at the movies!) are 50 times sweeter than sugar. An herbal one-stop shop all on its own, licorice root combines antiviral properties with wound-healing and anti-inflammatory properties, plus cleansing effects to remove congestion from lungs and the digestive tract.

Peppermint oil (Mentha x piperita): Did you know that peppermint is a cross between water mint and spearmint? Menthol is the most important compound in this cool essential oil. Because it helps to calm muscle spasms and ease pain, studies show it is very helpful for irritable bowel syndrome, or IBS (see IBS in Part 2). Peppermint is also good for nausea and indigestion.

St. John's wort (Hypericum perforatum): This small-leaved plant with yellow flowers has long been used to ease mental troubles. Over the years, it was given internally and also used as an oil rubbed on externally to help damaged nerves. Today studies show that St. John's wort is helpful for mild to moderate depression. However, it can cause you to be sensitive to sunlight and may interact with certain drugs, including antidepressants and others:

dial your doc

If you have any concerns about interactions between the prescription or OTC drugs you are taking now and any herbs you're considering adding to your regimen, consult your physician.

♦ Indinavir and other drugs used to treat HIV

♦ Irinotecan and other cancer drugs

♦ Cyclosporine, a transplant rejection drug

♦ Digoxin, a heart drug that strengthens the heart muscle

♦ Warfarin and anticoagulants

♦ Birth-control pills

Turmeric (Curcuma longa): One of the nutrients that may help prevent Alzheimer's, turmeric is a spice you'd do well to add to your diet. This distinctive yellow herb is often used in Indian foods like curry and in mustards and cheeses. Grown throughout India and parts of Asia and Africa, this shrub is also helpful when it comes to indigestion and gallstones. Early research shows that one of the phytochemicals found in turmeric, curcumin, also has anti-inflammatory and anticancer properties. You'll find turmeric in capsules, liquid extracts, and teas. You can also make turmeric into a paste and use it on the skin to ease the pain of osteoarthritis.

The Different Ways to Use Herbs

Herbs are used in different ways, depending on the condition. Some may be more effective in extract form, while others may be more soothing to the system if they are obtained through a nice cup of tea.

We note these as we go along, but as always, if you have any questions about what is best for you, ask your natural health care practitioner.

- **Extracts**—Made by mixing an herb with alcohol. When the herb is removed or extracted, the "essential oil" remains. It is used this way or evaporated for use in capsules or tablets.

- **Powders**—A common form of herbal preparation for East Indian and Southeast Asian ayurveda populations. (*Ayurveda* means "the science of life." It is a 5,000-year-old ancient system of health care native to India that identifies and works with the unique energies present in each person to enhance overall health.)

- **Teas**—In this method, you add boiling water to fresh or dried herbs and steep them for 5 minutes before drinking. This is also known as infusion.

- **Decoction**—Boiling the denser or harder elements of an herb, such as the roots, bark, or stems, to release the important compounds and then straining it; the liquid that results is the decoction.

- **Tinctures**—An alcohol-based derivative of an herb. Tinctures are made in different strengths, which means botanical (weight of the dried herbs) to extract ratio (what is in the bottle). For example, a 1:2 ratio, often used by practitioners, is stronger than 1:5, the strength of most retail brands available.

The Least You Need to Know

- Herbal medicine gives you another choice in how you care for your body and your health.

- For many prescription drugs on the market right now, an herbal equivalent exists.

- Herbs can help with mild problems, aid in preventing and treating chronic problems, and strengthen and detoxify certain organs or the entire body.

- If you have any questions about interactions between the prescription or OTC drugs you're taking now and any herbs you're considering adding to your regimen, consult your physician.

Chapter 5

Alternative Therapies

In This Chapter

- ◆ Many alternative therapies that offer benefits for body, mind, and spirit
- ◆ Understanding different natural approaches to dealing with pain
- ◆ A closer look at acupuncture, aromatherapy, ayurvedic medicine, chiropractic treatments, craniosacral therapy, flower essences, homeopathy, massage therapy, and reflexology
- ◆ Using alternative therapies to soothe emotions
- ◆ Tapping into energy with qigong
- ◆ The power of yoga and mediation

Chances are, you've tried either yoga or meditation, since 16.5 million Americans now practice yoga and 10 million practice meditation. But why stop there? How about using flower power (flower essences) to lift your mood? Craniosacral therapy to adjust your back? Massage therapy to ease your aching head? These are all examples of alternative therapies we cover in the pages ahead.

Many people like alternative healing because of its mind-body connection and its individual approach, according to a study in the *Journal of the American Medical Association*. You may also find that alternative therapies are a more personal way to wellness. This chapter gives you an overview of different types of alternative therapies, and we reference these therapies to help treat different conditions in Part Two. So let's get started—and let the healing begin!

Acupuncture

An estimated 8.2 million U.S. adults have used acupuncture. Acupuncture originated over 2,000 years ago and is a practice from traditional Chinese medicine (TCM). To understand the healing nature of acupuncture, it's helpful to have some insight into TCM. TCM is based on the belief that disease results when "chi," or the vital life force in the body, is disrupted and an imbalance arises of two opposing yet complimentary forces, known as *yin* and *yang*, along pathways in the body known as meridians. TCM uses herbs, meditation, massage, and acupuncture to restore this balance.

def•i•ni•tion

Yin represents the cold, slow, or passive principle. **Yang** represents the hot, excited, or active principle.

According to TCM, there are 12 main meridians (6 yin and 6 yang) and 8 secondary meridians in which chi circulates in your body. Each meridian is associated with an organ or a function, such as the lungs (yin) or large intestine (yang). Acupuncture is the stimulation of these meridians, which are punctuated by 400 acupuncture points on the body by a variety of techniques, most commonly by inserting ultrathin metal needles into the skin. According to TCM, this relieves blockages to chi and improves health. Acupuncture is used on everything from migraine headaches to carpal tunnel syndrome, to back and neck pain. From the Western point of view, acupuncture may be beneficial because it releases endorphins, pain-relieving hormones, into the body. Acupressure stimulates these points, or acupoints, with the tips of the fingers.

Aromatherapy

More people are following their noses to discover the benefits of aromatherapy, the therapeutic application of essential oils to support health and well-being. Aromatherapy is also being used for a wide range of healing benefits in many therapeutic settings, including hospices, maternity wards, spas, and hospitals.

Plants produce essential oils for a variety of reasons—to attract pollinators, to protect against bacterial and/or fungal invasion, to deter pests, and to inhibit other plants from growing near them. A process known as distillation extracts the essential oil from the plant for therapeutic concentration.

natural news

Essential oils from citrus oils are most often extracted through expression—the use of pressure to squeeze the essential oil from the peel of the fruit.

Essential oils can be extracted from the leaves (eucalyptus), grass (lemongrass), seeds (fennel), fruit/zest (mandarin), flowers (rose), wood/trunk of tree (cedarwood), roots (ginger), resins (frankincense), and herbs (rosemary). Genuine aromatherapy utilizes only essential oils derived directly from plants. Synthetics are a no-no. The effectiveness of aromatherapy depends on the quality and wholeness of the essential oils you use, so it's important to use the very best essential oils possible. Keep in mind that all essential oils should be kept away from infants, toddlers, and children. They can be highly toxic and even fatal if taken internally.

Using Aromatherapy

It's easy to begin experiencing the benefits of aromatherapy. Holistic aromatherapist Jade Shutes, B.A., Diploma AT, owner of the East West School for Herbal and Aromatic Studies (www.TheIDA.com) in Willow Spring, North Carolina, suggests hopping into a tub and adding 7 to 10 drops of an essential oil and inhaling the aroma. (Adding the oil when you are already in the tub allows you to fully experience its potency.) Take caution with citrus oils, and use in moderation because they may irritate the skin. Add three to five drops total. Avoid essential oils from peppermint and lemongrass completely because they may be too irritating to the skin.

Diffusion is a very effective way of using aromatherapy. You can use an electronic diffuser, for example, to disperse essential oils throughout your home or workspace. It works by sending small aromatic particles into the air. A diffuser can help with respiratory problems, enhance immune response and emotional well-being, and act as an air antiseptic. A candle diffuser is used by placing 5 to 10 drops of essential oil in water in the diffuser and lighting the candle. This method is wonderful for enhancing room ambiance and emotional well-being.

Unscented shampoos and soaps can be used for aromatherapy as well by adding 5 to 10 drops of essential oil per ounce. Adjust as necessary to either strengthen or reduce the aroma. The same is true for face creams: add three to five drops of essential oil per ounce of cream.

To make an aromatic spritzer, add 10 to 25 drops per 4 ounces of water in a squirt bottle. Be sure to shake it each time before use. Use it as a room spray, to reduce microbes in the air and enhance emotional well-being.

You can also make your own aromatic massage oil by combining vegetable oil with essential oils. Use organic, cold-pressed oils such as sunflower, apricot kernel, sweet almond, or hazelnut for the vegetable oil, and add 15 drops of essential oil (total) per ounce of vegetable oil. Here's Jade Shutes's recipe to soothe muscular aches and pains:

- 4 drops peppermint oil
- 6 drops rosemary oil
- 5 drops lavender oil
- 1 oz. sweet almond oil

Essential Oils Medicine Cabinet

Keep these essential oils on hand for when you need a little relief from a variety of different aches, pains, or stresses.

Roman chamomile (Anthemis nobilis syn, Chamaemelum nobile): Soothing, relaxing; good for inflammations, insomnia, PMS, stress, tension, hyperactivity in children, and general anxiety. This is *not* the chamomile from which chamomile tea is made. Chamomile tea is made from German Chamomile, *Matricaria recutita.*

German chamomile (Matricaria recutita): Anti-inflammatory; sedative; good for eczema, insomnia, wound healing, and acne.

Clary sage (Salvia sclarea): Euphoric; antispasmodic, relaxor; good for PMS, cramps, irritability, anxiety, stress, and muscle cramps or spasms. Known as a feminine oil.

Eucalyptus (Eucalyptus globules): Enhances the immune system; good for cold and flu (preventative), respiratory congestion, and sinusitis. Only adults should use this eucalyptus species. For children and adolescents, use Eucalyptus radiata.

Frankincense (Boswellia carterii): All-around healer; balancing, immune enhancing, calming, soothing; good for the skin and wound healing.

Geranium (Pelargonium graveolens): Feminine oil for balancing (with hormones, jet lag, or anything that throws the body, mind, and spirit out of balance); calming; good for PMS. Use geranium only in small amounts because it can be overwhelming in high dilutions.

Ginger (Zingiber officinale): Aphrodisiac; good for nausea, muscular aches and pains, morning sickness, and motion sickness.

Helichrysum (Helichrysum italicum): Bruises, wound healing.

Lavender (Lavandula angustifolia): A must-have essential oil, lavender is of benefit to almost any condition. It's calming and soothing, and good for burns, insomnia, diaper rash, cuts, tension headache, PMS, and cramps (use with Clary sage and Roman chamomile).

Neroli (Citrus aurantium): All-around stress and anxiety buster; nurturing, antidepressant, cell regenerative; good for mature skin.

Peppermint (Mentha x piperita): Stimulating; good for muscular aches and pains, headaches/migraines, colds, flu, upset stomach, and nausea. *Do not use on infants or toddlers under 3 years of age.*

Rosemary (Rosmarinus officinalis): Stimulant, expectorant; cleansing; good for muscular aches and pains, short-term memory, bronchitis, and poor circulation.

Mandarin/tangerine (Citrus reticulata): Calming, soothing; has a gentle aroma; great for young toddlers and children; can be uplifting without being stimulating; safe for all ages.

Tea tree (Melaleuca alternifolia): Antiseptic, antibacterial; cleansing; good for nail fungus, athlete's foot; medicinal aroma; use as a mouthwash as a preventative (mix with myrrh in one-half water, one-half apple cider vinegar blend).

Ylang ylang (Cananga odorata): Floral, feminine; nurturing; aphrodisiac; great for stress relief.

Ayurvedic Medicine

Ayurveda means "the science of life" (*veda*: "knowledge," *ayus*: "life"). It is a 5,000-year-old system that identifies and works with the unique energies present in each person to enhance overall health. "Ayurveda, with its individualized focus, its ancient roots, and its systematic approach to health, helps you take more control of all aspects of your physical, mental, and spiritual well-being in an increasingly stressful world," says Hilary Garavaltis, an ayurvedic practitioner and dean of curriculum for the Kripalu School of Ayurveda. "Ayurveda teaches that we all have the ability to heal ourselves, but it's our job to find harmony, it's our responsibility to pay attention to our lives."

Ayurvedic medicine works from the premise that each person has a predominant "dosha," roughly translated as "body type." Body-type analysis is simply a study of each person's traits and characteristics, including body shape and coloring. It has been found through time that certain body types function more efficiently under certain parameters, such as temperature, climate, activity level, and diet. Ayurveda uses this quantitative analysis to help design individual strategies for health.

The three doshas—vata, pitta, and kapha—are bodily humors or energies that are present in one's body and psychoemotional being. They reflect the principal forces of nature—space, air, fire, water, and earth—and how they are combined uniquely within each of us.

- **Vata:** Space and air. This governs movement in the body.

- **Pitta:** Fire and water. This influences the transformational processes in the body.

- **Kapha:** Water and earth. This is responsible for structure and growth in the body.

Once you know your predominant dosha, it helps in evaluating your other traits, such as appetite, stamina, temperament, and even tolerance for climate.

An ayurvedic practitioner may recommend herbal formulas to bring the body back into balance. Herbs are also used in ayurveda to help awaken the body's own healing response. The body's bioreceptors are designed to recognize the vibration of other biological organisms, such as plants. These receptors lock and recognize one another, and stimulation occurs, reminding the body to work toward maintaining harmony. Ayurvedic herbs and herbal formulas are a gentle and highly powerful therapeutic tool used with great reverence in the ayurvedic tradition.

Chiropractic Treatments

Chiropractic treatments can be an important way to help the back heal itself and the body as a whole. The chiropractor uses gentle force to realign misaligned vertebrae, freeing pinched nerves and sending proper nerve flow from the spine throughout the body. "Chiropractic is not just for neck and back pain, but it's to balance out the whole system," says Lisa Cowley, D.C. Her practice, Alternative Healthcare, is in Southold, New York. "It's another way of turning on the light switch of energy." Holistic chiropractors like Dr. Cowley incorporate exercise, strength training, stress reduction, nutrition, and stretching into their treatment programs.

Some of the many benefits of chiropractic include ...

- Relief from acute and chronic neck and lower-back pain.

- Enhanced immune system function.

- Improved respiratory function.

- Greater nerve supply to heart and coronary arteries.

- Improved circulation.

Craniosacral Therapy

Craniosacral therapy is used for a wide range of problems, including chronic back pain. Developed in the 1970s by osteopathic physician and surgeon John E. Upledger, craniosacral therapy is designed to release restrictions in the membranes that surround and protect the brain and spinal cord so the central nervous system can perform at optimum efficiency. The craniosacral system consists of the membranes and cerebrospinal fluid that surround and protect the brain and spinal cord. It extends from the bones of the skull, face, and mouth (cranium) down to the tailbone area (sacrum).

Craniosacral therapy is performed while you recline fully clothed (although shoes are usually removed for comfort) on a massage or treatment table, and lasts between 15 minutes and one hour. Using a light touch (starting with the weight of a nickel), the practitioner tests for restrictions in the craniosacral system by monitoring the rhythm of the cerebrospinal fluid as it flows through the system. The practitioner then uses delicate manual techniques to release restrictions and help strengthen the body's ability to heal itself. Physical, mental, and emotional stresses can be reflected in the body and show up in the tissue for practitioners to evaluate. Because of this, craniosacral therapy can also help restore emotional balance.

Flower Essences

Discovered by noted homeopath and bacteriologist Edward Bach, M.D., in England over 75 years ago, Bach Flower Remedies are now used in 66 countries worldwide. Bach Flower Remedies are made from "sun tea" of specific wildflowers or trees known for their healing properties, and are then diluted (similar to homeopathic remedies in that regard). "They work to balance negative emotions, freeing the body's energy to heal itself," says Nancy Buono, a Bach Foundation Registered Practitioner (BFRP) and director of Bach Flower Education. Bach

Flower Remedies are dispensed over the counter and have no contraindications or side effects. They're nontoxic, nonaddictive, and safe even for infants, the elderly, plants, and animals.

Here we've included a listing of the Bach Flower Remedies. You can find out more by visiting www.bachremedies.com. To find a Bach Foundation Registered Practitioner, visit www.bachcentre.com.

- ◆ **Agrimony:** Helps you hide your feelings.

- ◆ **Aspen:** Eases anxiety.

- ◆ **Beech:** Makes you more accepting and less critical.

- ◆ **Centaury:** Helps you just say "no."

- ◆ **Cerato:** Helps you believe in yourself and your decisions.

- ◆ **Cherry Plum:** Helps you stay in control.

- ◆ **Chestnut Bud:** Breaks bad patterns.

- ◆ **Chicory:** Helps you let go of loved ones.

- ◆ **Clematis:** Grounds you in reality.

- ◆ **Crab Apple:** Improves feelings of self-worth.

- ◆ **Elm:** Helps you feel able to take action.

- ◆ **Gentian:** Helps you be more resilient.

- ◆ **Gorse:** Gives you fortitude to keep on keeping on.

- ◆ **Heather:** Tempers too much talkativeness, which can lead to isolation.

- ◆ **Holly:** Heals wounded feelings, eases jealousy.

- ◆ **Honeysuckle:** Keeps you in the present moment.

- ◆ **Hornbeam:** Helps stop procrastination.

- ◆ **Impatiens:** Gives you patience.

- ◆ **Larch:** Improves self-confidence.

- ◆ **Mimulus:** Helps you to overcome shyness, eases anxiety.

- ◆ **Mustard:** Lifts your spirits.

- ◆ **Oak:** Builds on your natural strength.

- ◆ **Olive:** Boosts energy

- ◆ **Pine:** Eases guilt and blame.

- ◆ **Red Chestnut:** Helps you feel less anxious about someone else's safety.

- ◆ **Rock Rose:** Soothes terrors.

- ◆ **Rock Water:** Helps you not be so hard on yourself.

- ◆ **Scleranthus:** Helps you make up your mind.

- ◆ **Star of Bethlehem:** Eases shock or grief.

- ◆ **Sweet Chestnut:** Gives hope.

- ◆ **Vervain:** For burn-out. Renews enthusiasm.

- ◆ **Vine:** Helps you be a fair leader.

- ◆ **Walnut:** Helps you deal with change and other people's ideas.

- ◆ **Water Violet:** Eases loneliness even if you like solitude.

- ◆ **White Chestnut:** Stops mental chatter.

- ◆ **Wild Oat:** Helps you find your direction in life.

- ◆ **Wild Rose:** Helps you be more engaged in life.

- ◆ **Willow:** Good for resentment and the "poor me's."

Homeopathy

Homeopathy (from the Greek *homeo*, meaning "similar," and *pathos*, meaning "suffering or disease") is a therapeutic approach that is based on the principle of "like cures like." This means that it prevents or treats conditions by giving very small amounts of substances that produce symptoms in people (similar to vaccines in this regard) when given in larger doses. When the body mounts a response to this small substance, it heals itself. Most homeopathic remedies are derived from natural substances that come from plants, minerals, or animals.

Homeopaths or naturopathic doctors who practice homeopathy take a whole-body approach when it comes to prescribing homeopathic medicines for patients, meaning they take into account their mental, emotional, and spiritual well-being.

Homeopathic medicines are considered very safe and do not interfere with over-the-counter or prescription drugs. It's a good idea to consult with your doctor, though, if you don't see an improvement within a few days or if you are pregnant or nursing a baby. Keep homeopathic remedies out of the reach of children.

natural news

Homeopathy was created by Samuel Hahnemann, a physician, chemist, and linguist in Germany in the late 1700s. Hahnemann read about a treatment (cinchona bark) used to cure malaria. He took some cinchona bark and observed that, as a healthy person, he developed symptoms that were very similar to malaria symptoms. This led Hahnemann to consider that a substance may create symptoms that it can also relieve. This concept is called the "similia principle" or "like cures like."

Massage Therapy

One of the first forms of medical treatment, the ancient healing practice of massage was first practiced in China during the second century B.C.E. Massage was also often "prescribed" by physicians in ancient Greece and Rome for pain. Today massage is widely used in India as part of ayurvedic medicine. When you have a massage, a masseuse manipulates the soft tissue and muscles of the body.

Massage can be beneficial when it comes to relieving stress, enhancing immunity, improving circulation, easing tension-type headaches and migraine pain, soothing low-back pain and sore muscles, improving osteoarthritis, and more. Massage also drains the lymphatic system, which is important because it does not have its own "pump" to get rid of toxins that can accumulate in the body. Some of the specific types of massage therapy include shiatsu and Swedish massage.

Since so much of illness is stress related, massage can be incredibly important in boosting health. "Most people still consider massage a luxury, but you need touch. It's an essential aspect of our being," says Steven Hartman, the director of professional training and association at the Kripalu Center for Yoga & Health in Stockbridge, Massachusetts. "Just the act of being touched is good for our nervous system, our circulation, and our muscles, and for detoxification, but it's good for our spirit as mammals to be touched and connected to." One of the best things to do is get together with a friend for tea and a foot rub, says Hartman. "Have tea and trade feet. Talk and massage each other's feet!" You can give yourself a massage, too. If you're in the tub, instead of scrubbing yourself from head to toe, be gentle and give yourself a soothing soak.

More people are realizing that massage promotes good health. A new survey by the American Massage Therapy Association of hospitals and clinics revealed that the number of hospitals that now offer massage therapy as a patient service has increased by more than one third over the past two years. Seventy-one percent of hospitals are now offering massage therapy for stress management, patient comfort, improved joint and muscle mobility, pregnancy, physical therapy, and infant care as part of their post- and pre-operative regimens and to comfort those in hospice facilities:

- Sixty-seven percent now offer massage to patients experiencing chronic pain, such as fibromyalgia.

- Fifty-two percent have incorporated massage into their cancer care programs.

- Fifty-two percent now offer massage to physically challenged or rehab patients to improve mobility.

- Sixty-seven percent offer healing hands to their staff, to cut down on work-related stress and illnesses.

Visit www.massagetherapy101.com and www.massagetherapy.com for more information on massage and to find a massage therapist near you.

Reflexology

Reflexology, the practice of stimulating nerves on the feet, hands, and ears to improve health, dates back to ancient Egypt, India, and China. Practitioners work on the premise that pressure points in these areas correspond to areas of the body and that reflexology assists the self-healing process by balancing life energy, or qi. For example, when you rub the point between your index finger and your thumb, L4 (large intestine 4), you treat the pain of migraine headaches. For more information, visit www.reflexology-usa.org/index.html and www.reflexology-research.com/whatis.htm.

Meditation

Tired of constant mental chatter? Why not try meditation? As the yogis say, you can't stop the waves, but you can learn how to surf! Meditation is a mind-body practice that uses certain techniques such as focusing attention (for example, on a word, an object, or the breath), a specific posture, and a neutral attitude toward distracting thoughts to calm the mind and emotions.

"The ability to be in charge of our mind and thoughts is at the core of our ability to have a satisfying and happy life, which is no small thing," says Hartman. "Most people think they are their minds, that they are their thoughts. But it's all about what's outside of them. When we meditate, we start to become in charge of our attention. We start to choose where we direct it and what thoughts we're going to entertain, as opposed to being a victim of whatever thoughts enter our heads. We also start to realize that there is a true self behind the mind and behind the thoughts. Meditation helps us quiet our thoughts enough to get in touch with the voice that is behind our thoughts—that's who is really in charge."

Studies conducted by the Benson-Henry Institute for Mind-Body Medicine at Massachusetts General Hospital in Boston show that meditation can also help to alleviate anxiety, tension headache, high blood pressure, and even chronic pain.

To meditate, follow these steps:

1. **Still the body.** Sit up tall and straight. If you are lying down, make sure your spine is straight. Find a place of comfortable stillness.

2. **Deliberately calm the breath.** All day long, we breathe unconsciously and involuntarily. But the moment we make our body

breathe deliberately and voluntarily, we begin to immediately tap into the ability to calm the body and are able to direct our attention. Meditation begins the moment we do conscious breathing. The doorway to our unconscious comes from making our breath voluntary. That's why one of the main tools for meditation, no matter what the tradition, starts with deliberate breathing.

3. **Choose a practice to still the mind.** Focus on the breath and determine that you are going to do five minutes of conscious, deliberate breathing. When your attention wanders from the breath, simply bring it back to the breath. You can also use a mantra or a candle flame; when your attention wanders, simply bring it back to the mantra or candle flame. (Choose an object in the room and set a timer for two minutes, direct your attention toward it, and see what happens!) Another meditation method focuses on mandalas, which are meditation drawings. One of the most famous is the Shri Yantra. To see what it looks like, visit www.tantra-kundalini.com/sri-yantra.htm.

With all of these techniques, you're training your attention. You're leaning how to be deliberate and to get your attention to flow like a constant dripping or pouring of oil. You want to be able to have your attention flow that easily, uninterrupted on the breath, or on a mantra, a prayer, or even a visualization.

Say that you are dealing with cancer and are undergoing chemotherapy. Instead of living in fear, says Hartman, your meditation could be visualizing the chemotherapy as a positive action as it goes to the cancer cells and destroys and removes them, while seeing healthy cells filled with light. Whenever your mind is filled with fearful thoughts, bring them back to your positive visualization again. "There is untapped potential when our thoughts are joined with the innate knowledge of our body," says Hartman.

You can learn more about meditation and the Relaxation Response (you'll read more about this later in the book, too), a specific type of meditation created by Herbert Benson, M.D., of the Benson-Henry Institute at www.mbmi.org.

natural news

The ability to keep your mind on one point for 12 seconds without a break is called one concentration. Twelve concentrations, or two and a half minutes, equals one meditation. If you can keep your attention and concentration in an even flowing state for a half-hour (12 meditations), you have achieved the state of Samati, a state of peacefulness. But this takes time. Be gentle with yourself, says Hartman. It's like training a puppy. If your mind wanders, bring it back and say sit, stay. The rewards are well worth it!

Qigong

Qi (chi) means "energy" and *gong* (kung) means "a skill or a practice." Qigong started more than 5,000 years ago, when Chinese scholars, studying the workings of the universe, concluded that everything is energy. (A few millennia later, Albert Einstein reached the same conclusion.) Qigong teaches that sickness results from too much or too little energy in different parts of the body. Qigong practice is designed to help you redirect the flow of energy in your body to regain energy balance and regain or maintain optimal health and wellness. Thousands of different styles of qigong are practiced, many of which are very difficult to learn.

Spring Forest Qigong, created by Qigong Master Chunyi Lin, is one of the most accessible. After years of study with some of the finest qigong masters in his native China, Lin created a style that is simple enough for anyone to practice. "Many people think of energy in a very limited way," says Master Chunyi Lin. "They think of energy as being electricity or the gasoline that powers their car. Electricity and gasoline are indeed forms of energy, but everything in the universe is also a form of energy, including every cell in your body." Lin teaches that you can transform your energy by utilizing a combination of breathing techniques, mental focus, simple movements, and sound.

Numerous studies have found that simply by slowing your breathing to 10 breaths per minute or less for just 15 minutes a day, you can dramatically reduce high blood pressure without the need for medication. "Most folks breathe between 15 and 20 breaths per minute," says Gary Rebstock, co-author with Lin of *Born a Healer*, about Lin's journey and the creation of Spring Forest Qigong. "Breathing that rapidly keeps you from utilizing your full lung capacity." In fact, most folks use only about 60 percent of their lung capacity, which means that, at any given moment, 40 percent of the air in your lungs is stale air. (Doctors call this functional residual capacity.) "Energy breathing expands your lung capacity and dramatically increases the exchange rate of oxygen, which, of course, is the body's primary fuel," says Rebstock.

Even just five minutes can make a big difference in the way you feel. Why don't you try it right now and see?

1. Sit or lie down in a comfortable position. Smile to relax your mind and body.

2. Place the tip of your tongue gently against the roof of your mouth and breathe through your nose in slow, gentle, deep breaths. Picture in your mind that you are connected to the limitless energy of the universe.

3. As you breathe in, gently pull in your lower stomach a little. Imagine that you are using your entire body to breathe. Feel the air flowing into every part of your body.

4. As you breathe out, let your stomach out and visualize any tiredness or stress, pain or sickness, doubt or worries changing into smoke. Visualize it shooting out of your body to the ends of the universe.

5. To end your energy-breathing session, take one final, slow, gentle, deep breath. Slowly open your eyes, rub your hands together palm to palm, and gently massage your face, running your fingertips gently up each side of the bridge of your nose to your forehead, then out and down to your chin in a circular motion several times.

For more information, visit www.SpringForestQigong.com.

Yoga

You may think of yoga as twisting yourself into a pretzel, but it's actually a 5,000-year-old spiritual practice. True, it is done with asanas (postures), but approached in the right way and frame of mind, these poses can help bring you to a state of higher consciousness. Yoga also increases overall health and vitality. When we practice poses, the oxygen content in the body is improved, which helps balance the hormonal systems. This means it's a boon to anyone with menopause or thyroid disorders. Because the practice releases endorphins, it can ease depression as well. Yoga also improves flexibility, improves strength and muscle tone, and reduces stress. In 2007, research published in the medical journals *Diabetes Research* and *Clinical Practice* revealed that practicing yoga can even help reduce waist size, blood pressure, blood sugar, and triglycerides (the chemical form of fat cells), and improve HDL or so-called "good" cholesterol!

Yoga is catching on. The number of people who are practicing yoga and the number of people who say they are planning to take their first yoga class within the next year are growing exponentially. It seems to have no end, says Hartman. "People are seeing it as a form of exercise that can be done no matter how old you are. There's something in it for everyone. No matter what state of health you are in, you can get some benefit." For further resources about yoga, see Appendix B and visit:

www.yogajournal.com/poses/finder/browse_categories

www.yogasite.com/postures.html

The Least You Need to Know

- ◆ Alternative therapies are valuable tools because of their focus on mind-body connection and their individual approach to wellness.

- ◆ Many alternative therapies can ease pain, including acupuncture, acupressure, reflexology, massage, craniosacral therapy, and chiropractic treatments.

- ◆ Aromatherapy has a wide variety of uses, from PMS to anxiety to insomnia.

- ◆ Flower essences help to balance negative emotions, freeing the body's energy to heal itself.

- ◆ You can take homeopathic remedies in liquid, pellet, and tablet forms. They are generally considered safe and do not interfere with conventional drugs.

- ◆ Studies show that practicing yoga, meditation, and qigong can make you healthier.

Part 2

Directory of Conditions and Natural Remedies

In Part 2, you'll find a variety of different natural and alternative therapies for more than 60 common health conditions. These conditions are arranged alphabetically, and each is independent and self-contained, so feel free to read them in any order you want.

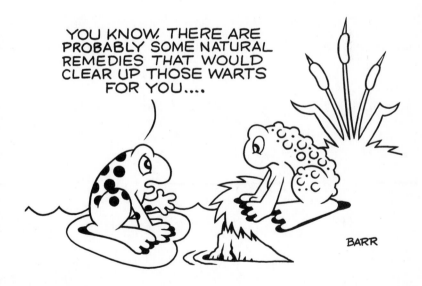

YOU KNOW, THERE ARE PROBABLY SOME NATURAL REMEDIES THAT WOULD CLEAR UP THOSE WARTS FOR YOU....

BARR

Acne

The dreaded zit. Zits happen when sebaceous, or oil, glands produce sebum that blocks your pores, usually on your face, neck, or back, and bacteria starts to grow. When it does, it results in pimples, blackheads, and whiteheads. Though we're not sure what causes acne, diet and food allergies may play a role—but so may stress and hormonal imbalances. Pimples usually appear when you have a big meeting or an important event. Or maybe it just seems that way! Fortunately, there's lots you can do about it.

The Importance of Diet

Teens love sugar and greasy foods like pizza and French fries, but they're some of the worst foods for acne. Why? Simple carbohydrates (carbs) are metabolized as sugar, and this can affect the hormone balance in the body. But cutting out these carbs (we know, it's not easy) and increasing protein, like lean meats and whole-wheat breads, can help prevent acne breakouts, as can eating regular meals and adding five servings of fruits and vegetables.

Green veggies especially help to clear the skin, and they're high in vitamins and minerals. Green food supplements are also very cleansing for the skin. Go for greens like chlorophyll, spirulina, and barley greens to help filter out toxins. Drinking lots of water also helps to remove toxins from the skin. Get in the habit of keeping your water bottle or glass full throughout the day.

Recognizing Food Allergies

Acne can also result from food allergies. When you have an allergic reaction to a particular food, like dairy or eggs, it's because the immune system perceives the food as a kind of "invader" and mounts a response resulting in inflammation and acne. To find out if this is what's happening to you (or your teen), have your doctor give you the *ELISA*

def•i•ni•tion _____

> ELISA stands for enzyme-linked immunosorbent assay. The test determines which antibodies your body is making. This helps identify which foods you are allergic to.

Blood Test (no, this has nothing to do with *My Fair Lady*), which tests for different food allergies, or try an elimination diet. To get a good response, you'll want to eliminate possible offending food products in your diet for two weeks to see if your skin clears.

Acidophilus to Prevent Outbreaks

When your digestive tract isn't functioning optimally, it shows on the skin. Taking acidophilus, a type of "friendly bacteria" or probiotic, can help your digestion by replenishing essential bacteria, similar to beneficial microorganisms found in the human gut that are lost to poor diet and overuse of antibiotics. You can find acidophilus in yogurt or sold as a capsule. The recommended dosage is 10 billion parts of acidophilus with bifidus, another type of helpful probiotic. Now you can buy multi-layer acidophilus with bifidus "pearls," which do not need to be refrigerated and deliver the bacteria intact and alive. Visit www.consumerlab.com or www.enzy.com for more information.

Topical Treatments for Blemishes

One of the best treatments for your zits has to be tea tree oil. That's because clinical studies prove its antiseptic effectiveness. It's readily absorbed by the skin, which means it can help dry up and heal pimples faster. Calendula (from marigold petals) with vitamin E is also excellent for healing skin with acne, and lavender essential oil is a good antibiotic and antiseptic. Antioxidants vitamins A (Retinol-A), C, and E in topical form, either separately or together, can be effective in battling acne, too. At health food stores, you'll find the available dosages for Retinol-A in cream form at 1 to 2 percent retinol. With a doctor's prescription, you can get up to 5 percent. Taking these vitamins as oral supplements can help, too.

Don't Fear Oil

If you have oily skin, the idea of adding more oil can seem, well, nuts. But the right kind can actually be helpful, says Barbara Close, an herbalist and founder of Naturopathic Holistic Health Spa in East Hampton, New York. "People are phobic of using oil on the skin, but creating a custom blend of lightweight astringent essential oils like juniper or rosemary oil can actually help to reduce sebum production." To make your own custom blend astringent, Close recommends filling a 1-ounce bottle with the following:

$\frac{1}{2}$ oz. hazelnut oil

4 drops juniper oil

3 drops tea tree oil

2 drops rosemary oil

Shake all ingredients together, then top off with another $\frac{1}{2}$ ounce of hazelnut oil. Apply two to three drops to a cotton pad and massage into clean skin twice daily.

Full Steam Ahead

For adults with acne, Close recommends putting a tea kettle on. Once the water is boiling, pour the contents into a plugged bathroom sink and create an herbal steam by adding a few drops of essential antiseptic oils like tea tree and juniper oil to soften pores. Pull up a chair and put a towel over your head to capture the steam around your face. Top off with more hot water as needed. Afterward, dab tea tree oil on any pimples you may have.

Cleansing Regime

When cleansing and toning the skin—an essential routine for those with acne—try the following natural regime from homeopathic aromatherapist Jade Shutes, B.A., Diploma AT, owner of the East West School for Herbal and Aromatic Studies (www.TheIDA.com) in Willow Spring, North Carolina.

Aromatic Cleanser:

> 2 oz. unscented cleansing base (you can use Dr. Bronner's liquid baby-mild soap—see www.drbronner.com)
>
> 7 drops tea tree oil (Melaleuca alternifolia)
>
> 5 drops lemon oil (Citrus limon)
>
> 5 drops lavender oil (Lavandula angustifolia)

Mix together all ingredients. Wash with cleanser two times a day, once in the morning and once in the evening.

Aromatic Toner:

> 4 oz. witch hazel hydrosol or extract
>
> 4 drops tea tree oil
>
> 2 drops lemon oil

Place all ingredients in a 4-ounce bottle with a spritzer top. Shake before each use. Apply by spritzing the face or mix 1 tablespoon into 2 ounces of unscented castile soap (find the soap at www.drbonner.com).

Most acne skin types are prone to dehydration due to the overuse of alcohol-based toners and cleansers. For this reason, individuals with acne can benefit from applying a soothing hydrating cream after cleansing and toning.

Aromatic Cream:

> 2 oz. unscented water-based cream
>
> 2 drops German chamomile oil
>
> 4 drops lavender oil
>
> 5 drops Frankincense oil

Mix together all ingredients. Apply to skin as a last step after cleansing and toning.

Helpful Herbal Teas

The liver is the primary organ of detoxification in the body, but if it's overwhelmed by the wrong food and drink or hormonal imbalances, it can cause an acne flare-up. Certain herbal teas help the liver detoxify, including burdock root, dandelion leaves, milk thistle, and red clover. Chaste tree berry tea is especially good for hormonal women.

Natural R$_x$

Acidophilus with bifidus multi-layer pearls: 10 billion parts

Burdock root tea

Calendula with vitamin E essential oil

Chaste tree berry tea

Dandelion leaves tea

Green food supplement: As directed

Juniper essential oil

Lavender essential oil

Milk thistle tea

Red clover tea

Tea tree oil essential oil

Tea tree oil with vitamins A and E topical salve

Vitamin A: 2,500 IU

Vitamin A: Retinol-A, C, and E cream

Vitamin C: 2,000 mg

Vitamin E: 400 IU

ADD/ADHD

Kids with attention-deficit disorder (ADD) or attention-deficit hyperactivity disorder (ADHD) can find it really difficult to sit still and pay attention, whether they are at home or in class at school. The fact that kids with ADD and ADHD fidget, lack focus, and tend to be hyperactive means they can also be disorganized and not as productive as they could be. It can also mean that they can be moody and out of sorts. None of this is their fault.

What We Know Today

Awareness has grown when it comes to ADD and ADHD, and we also have better diagnostic tools. But this doesn't tell the whole story when it comes to the explosion in the rate of these conditions. We know that in other brain-related disorders, such as depression, the increased number of people diagnosed since 1945 is due to many factors, not just because people know more about it. It's likely that this is the case with ADD and ADHD as well, says Alan Logan, author of *The Brain Diet* and an invited faculty member at Harvard University's Mind/Body Institute. He believes it's probably due to a combination of factors, including diet and environmental causes, including the overstimulated world we live in. Even video games can play a part.

The brain has two types of neurotransmission pathways: one that accelerates incoming stimuli and one that puts the brakes on, called inhibitory neurotransmitters. In today's world, in particular, with its lights, sounds, and colors everywhere, the inhibitory centers need to be working in top gear to dampen unwanted stimuli. Unfortunately, children with ADHD and other related conditions, like panic disorder, do not have properly working inhibition centers, so they can't filter out the unwanted material as readily.

natural news

Medications like Ritalin stimulate the inhibitory centers of the brain, the part that helps calms things. Now research shows that seeing green has the same effect. Outdoor green environments are grounding for kids with ADD and ADHD, says Dr. Logan. "As much as possible, you want to help support the areas of the brain that help to dampen things down." So consider spending more time with your child in nature or outdoors in a park, since unnatural stimuli is kept to a minimum in these settings.

The Role Food Plays

Foods take center stage when it comes to ADD and ADHD. Removing certain ones from your child's diet is a natural way to provide relief. Kids who have ADD and ADHD are particularly sensitive to fluctuations in blood sugar, more so than adults. "When kids have low blood sugar, adrenaline is released to bring blood sugar back to normal," says Mary Ann Block, D.O., the founder of The Block Center in the Dallas area of Texas. "Kids react to this fight-or-flight hormone by becoming hyperactive, unable to concentrate, fidgety, and aggressive. For this reason, it's critical to change the diet to remove as much sugar as you can." It's important not to substitute any artificial sweeteners because the brain still sees that as sugar and kids may still have a low blood sugar reaction to it.

To stabilize blood sugar, focus on foods like high-quality lean proteins (such as turkey, which contains tryptophans, a natural relaxant) and whole grains instead of foods that spike blood sugar, like the simple carbohydrates in white bread and sugary breakfast cereals. Be sure to give kids protein, like bacon and eggs, for breakfast and then provide a midmorning and midafternoon protein snack, like a handful of cashew or pistachio nuts or natural peanut butter on whole-wheat crackers.

Steer Clear of Dyes and Preservatives

Research shows that children with ADD and ADHD often have sensitivities, particularly to chemicals, food dyes, benzoates (food preservatives), aspartame (a sugar substitute), and sodium glutamate. So it's best to remove artificial food dyes, preservatives, artificial sweeteners, and artificial flavoring agents as much as possible. For a complete list of additives, visit Food and Behaviour Research at www.fabresearch.org.

Go Organic!

In addition, if your budget allows, eat organic food whenever possible. Doing so can reduce the toxic load on your child's developing body and brain. That's because when farmers grow organic foods, they can't use synthetic fertilizers or pesticides. To research produce containing the most pesticides, visit the Environmental Working Group at www.ewg.org. Mercury contamination is also an issue when it comes to ADD and ADHD. Avoid this as much as possible. The EWG provides up-to-date information on how much of a particular fish a child should eat, based on age and weight.

The Elimination Diet

Some kids are also sensitive to dairy and wheat. Using an elimination diet can help you find out which items in the diet may be causing symptoms. If you suspect that your child is reacting to dairy or wheat, try eliminating one of these items at a time from your child's diet for two weeks. When you reintroduce it, if you find it provokes symptoms again, you know that food group is a trigger for your child.

Research shows that when these foods are reintroduced in kids who have ADD or ADHD, food sensitivities can elevate immune cells called cytokines that can influence behavior. This inappropriate immune response can result in anxiety, depression, and brain fog.

It can be very helpful to have your child tested for food allergies one at a time so you can see which allergen is causing which symptom. Unfortunately, conventional allergists don't normally test for food allergies in relation to behavioral issues. But you can find support by contacting the Block Center (www.blockcenter.com) or by visiting the American Academy of Environmental Medicine (www.aaem.com) and the Pan American Allergy Society (www.paas.org).

natural news _____

If you do need to eliminate dairy from your child's diet, you'll need to supplement with calcium and vitamin D to make sure your child doesn't become deficient in these nutrients. You can find rice and soy beverages fortified with these nutrients at your health food store.

The Importance of Omega-3 Essential Fatty Acids

Children with ADD and ADHD have increased oxidative stress from free-radical damage in the brain, so they break down their essential fats more rapidly. For this reason, supplementing with omega-3 essential fatty acids from fish oil is especially important for learning and central nervous system development. Research shows that greater behavior problems, like temper tantrums and sleep problems, can be associated when kids don't get enough omega-3 fatty acids, too. The essential fatty acid DHA, especially is, well, "essential" for the brain to develop and function. DHA may also help modulate mood, helping kids with ADHD to seem more like their old selves.

natural news _____

A new study in the medical journal *Nutritional Neuroscience* reveals that the extract from the bark of a pine tree that grows along the French coastline can lower the stress hormones adrenaline and dopamine, easing ADHD. Pycnogenol also helps reduce hyperactivity and improves attention, concentration, and motor-visual coordination in children with ADHD. For more information, visit www.pycnogenol.com.

Flower Power

Bach Flower Remedies (see Chapter 5) are made from a "sun tea" of specific wildflowers or trees known for their healing properties, then diluted (similar to homeopathic remedies, in that regard). They work to balance negative emotions, freeing the body's energy to heal itself.

You can add two drops of the chosen remedy to a glass of water or juice and have your child sip it at intervals. You can also place two drops of a selected remedy into a 1-ounce dropper bottle filled three quarters with spring water. This personal formula can be taken by mouth a minimum of four times each day, four drops each time, especially in the morning and at bedtime. You can also apply the remedies externally by moistening the lips, wrists, and/or temples, or use them in an atomizer or tub of water.

Nancy Buono, a Bach Foundation Registered Practitioner (BFRP) and director of Bach Flower Education, recommends the following Bach Flower Remedies for these ADD/ADHD behaviors:

Behavior	Bach Flower Remedy
Spaced out, not paying attention	Clematis to help focus and concentration
Easily frustrated, irritable, fidgety	Impatiens for more patience and calmer demeanor
Easily discouraged, small problems make child give up and feel blue	Gentian for confidence to overcome obstacles

For more information, visit www.bachflowereducation.com and www. bachremedystore.com.

natural news

We assume that all kids learn the same way. Not so, says Mary Ann Block, D.O., the founder of The Block Center in the Dallas area of Texas. "Kids who have ADD and ADHD learn through touch. They don't learn as well through just listening or looking. They're tactile. A little trick that can help is for a child to have something in their hand while listening in class. I always recommend that they hold something like a rubber eraser, something that they can fiddle with in their hand that's not distracting to others that will help them focus and listen better."

Bust a Yoga Move

The Crane pose, a yoga asana, is particularly good for ADD/ADHD, says Stephen Hartman, the director of professional training and association at the Kripalu Center for Yoga & Health in Stockbridge, Massachusetts (www.Kripalu.org). It stimulates the nervous system;

balances right and left hemispheres of the brain; and develops concentration, coordination, balance, poise, strength, groundedness, and confidence. It also strengthens the ankles, thighs, knees, back, shoulders, and neck. You can see how the Crane pose is performed by visiting www.yogajournal.com/poses/468.

1. Shift your weight to the left leg and firm up the leg without locking the knee.

2. Inhale. Bend the right knee and lift the foot off the floor, bringing the thigh parallel to the floor. Flex the right ankle.

3. Inhale. Stretch the arms at each side, to shoulder height. Roll the shoulder blades down the back, and press up through the crown of the head.

4. Hold the posture and breathe.

5. To release, exhale and lower arms and leg. Relax.

Natural R$_x$

Where not noted, please check with your nutritionist or physician for specific dosages appropriate for your child:

American ginseng: 400 mg.

Calcium

Ginkgo biloba: 100 mg.

Magnesium: Also combined with vitamin B$_6$; dose set by body weight.

Omega-3 essential fatty acids from fish oil: Ages 5–12: 500 mg. Essential fatty acid EPA: 558 mg. Essential fatty acid DHA: 480 mg. Gamma Linoleic Acid: 96 mg. (Capsules can be punctured and rubbed on the skin; also comes in chewables.) One brand is Nordic Naturals Omega 3-6-9 Junior Lemon. Nordic Naturals also come in liquids, so you can add them to smoothies.

Vitamin A

Vitamin B$_1$ (thiamine)

Vitamin B$_3$ (niacin)

Vitamin B$_6$: Pyridoxine. Also combined with magnesium; dose set by body weight.

Vitamin D

Zinc sulfate: At least 15 mg, up to 45 mg of elemental (actual) zinc.

Allergies

Is it a cold? Or allergies? If your runny nose and sneezing linger for more than a week or two, there's a good chance it's allergies. If you have allergies, your immune system, your body's defense system against bacteria and viruses, is in overdrive. This means when it encounters a substance that normally wouldn't bother a nonallergic person, it reacts as if it's a foreign invader. Often your immune system will be bugged by more than one thing—pollen, dust mites, mold spores, pet dander, or even food.

To defend the body, the immune system produces *antibodies* called immunoglobulin E, or IgE. These antibodies attach to the body's mast or tissue cells and basophils, or blood cells. When an allergen like pollen encounters its unique IgE, it fits like a key into a lock and releases histamines that result in inflammation and all the uncomfortable symptoms of allergies: runny nose, sneezing, nasal congestion, itching, rash, swelling, and even asthma.

natural news

After noticing that some of his patients were hypersensitive to things like dust, pollen, and certain foods, Viennese pediatrician Clemens von Pirquet named this phenomenon *allergy* in 1906, from the Greek words *allos*, meaning "other," and *ergon*, meaning "work."

def•i•ni•tion

Antibodies are a kind of protein that the immune system produces to handle what it perceives as foreign substances like allergens, virus, and bacteria.

If your mom and pop are allergy prone, you may be, too. Or you can develop them when your resistance is low because of a virus or when you are pregnant. When a severe allergic reaction affects the entire body, it is known as anaphylaxis.

Food Allergies

Almost six million people have food allergies. One of the most common is dairy, but wheat, peanuts, corn, citrus (lemon, lime, orange), eggs, sugar, preservatives, additives, and food colorings can also be offenders. Common symptoms of food allergies include chronic nasal congestion, frequent ear infection, irritable bowel syndrome (IBS), constipation, chronic diarrhea, abdominal cramping, Crohn's disease, ulcerative colitis, acne, eczema, psoriasis, hives, arthritis, headaches, and even obesity.

"Basically, the foods that we crave are the ones that we're allergic to because those are the ones that stimulate us and make us feel good for a short period of time," says Dr. Deborah Wiancek, N.D., a naturopathic physician and author of *The Natural Healing Companion*.

 natural news _____

> Soy is becoming a common allergen because it's genetically modified and highly processed, so it's difficult to digest, says Dr. Wiancek. "We're also seeing this with farm-raised Atlantic salmon. If it's not wild, it's gray, so it's dyed pink. Besides dyes, there are also fertilizers and hormones in farm-raised salmon. All of these things can cause allergies."

If you suspect you may have food allergies, you can try an elimination diet. This means not eating the food that you think is triggering your symptoms for two weeks. If it is the cause, your symptoms should clear.

You can also get a blood test from a doctor who specializes in food allergies or a naturopathic doctor to tell you what foods you're allergic to. A health practitioner or nutritionist can then help you change the way you eat.

Often people who have food allergies are deficient in digestive enzymes, which can keep you from getting the nutrients you need. Taking digestive enzymes such as bromelin, which comes from the stems of pineapples, can help. Betaine hydrochloric (HCl) acid may be helpful if you have reduced levels of stomach acid production.

Environmental Allergies

When you suffer from food allergies and your immune system is depleted, usually you react to environmental allergens as well. You may be allergic to airborne allergens like pollen from trees, grasses, and weeds. In North America, ragweed is the number-one culprit. You also may be allergic to mold, which can be aggravated by the foods you eat, like cheeses processed with fungi and foods containing yeast, like soy sauce and vinegar. Two other common offenders are dust mites and animal dander.

Getting a skin test with an allergist can determine whether you have IgE antibodies in the skin that react to a specific allergen. Skin testing is the most sensitive and least expensive way to determine whether you have allergies.

When it comes to taming allergens, air conditioners and HEPA filters can be two of your best friends. Air conditioners help stop pollen and other allergens from entering your house. A good HEPA filter on your central heating and air-conditioning unit can help to filter out allergens, too. You can also put individual units in rooms you use most. To keep dust mites under control, use a vacuum with a special HEPA filter. Replace carpets with washable throw rugs, if you can.

Reducing the Inflammatory Response

Supplements and herbs can act as natural antihistamines without the drowsy side effects. One of the best is quercitin, a bioflavonoid. We know from research studies that quercitin is effective at stabilizing mast cells. No, this has nothing to do with a sailing ship. This means it inhibits the release of histamines, making you feel better. Bromelin, which comes from the enzymes in pineapple stems, is another powerful anti-inflammatory. Together these two nutrients can effectively reduce the allergy response.

Butterbur is another natural antihistamine. A recent study in the medical journal *The Archives of Otolaryngology—Head & Neck Surgery* showed that when patients took two tablets of a special butterbur leaf extract (Ze 339) for two weeks, their symptoms of seasonal allergic rhinitis, like sneezing, nasal congestion, itchy eyes and nose, red eyes, and skin irritation, improved by 90 percent. A study in the medical journal *Clinical & Experimental Allergy* showed butterbur works as well as fexofenadine (Allegra) at 180 mg per day. It may also be helpful for treating asthma and chronic bronchitis.

Regional Homeopathic Remedies

Since where you live determines what unique allergens you are exposed to, it's important to consider your specific environment when evaluating allergies and remedies. You can desensitize yourself with specific homeopathic mixes tailored to fit your environment. Dr. Wiancek often does this with her patients in her Rocky Mountain–area practice. "I use a Rocky Mountain mix of all the pollens and grasses in this area and desensitize patients by giving them homeopathy drops of specific allergens orally. When they go out, they don't react with allergies." Find a local homeopath (see Appendix C for help) to customize a mix for you, depending on where you live and what you are exposed to.

The Boiron Allergy Care Kit can also be helpful. One of the ingredients, Histaminum, will block most of the histamines that circulate. Another, Apis, prevents the swelling of the mucous membranes of the nose, and Gallphimia works well for hay fever. There are no side effects and it doesn't interfere with other medications. It's safe for kids, too.

Ways to Clear Your Head

When you have allergy-related sinus issues, they are often dairy related. Dairy products tend to cause mucus buildup in the sinuses, so it's smart to cut back on your dairy intake. Using a *Neti Lota Pot* with ½ teaspoon of noniodized salt dissolved into 1 cup of warm water with a pinch of baking soda daily can help clear your sinuses. Hilary Garavaltis, an ayurvedic practitioner and the dean of curriculum for the Kripalu School of Ayurveda in Stockbridge, Massachusetts, recommends following this remedy with nasal drops called nasya oil, which has specific herbs to balance and clear out excess mucus and open channels on a daily basis. Doing daily breathing exercises (see Chapter 5) can help, too.

def•i•ni•tion

The **Neti Lota Pot** comes from the practice of yoga and is often used to clear nasal passages to prepare for meditation. As a form of hydrotherapy, the water clears allergens from the sinuses, and the salt also draws fluid out of swollen mucous membranes, allowing sinuses to drain.

Filling your space with the wonderful smell of essential oils is another great way to clear your head. Using essential oils with a diffuser can help clear your space of airborne allergens, says Garavaltis. She recommends conifer oils, such as pine, cedar, or even eucalyptus, depending on what appeals to you. "Essential oils are good for enhancing the immune system because essential oils are actually the immune system of the plant," Garavaltis says. "A plant uses these scents and oil to send the bugs and pathogens away. Essential oils taken from the plant are a very concentrated form of this and can help build up your own immune system."

You can run a diffuser in your workspace, in your bedroom, or at specific times of the day or year when allergens are more prevalent, like on a windy day or when things are blooming all around you. Diffusers can even be set on timers. You'll find earth-friendly and worker-friendly organic essential oils and diffusers at www.floracopeia.com.

Ayurvedic Skin Allergy Relief

Natural remedies from ayurvedic medicine can also soothe skin allergies, which are thought to be related to what is called a *pitta* condition, or excess heat in the body—too much fire.

def•i•ni•tion

Pitta is one of three doshas, or body types, in ayurvedic medicine. They are bodily energies that reflect the principal forces of nature. Pitta is fire and water influencing the transformational processes in the body. (See Chapter 5.)

For hives or rashes, grind up fresh cilantro and squeeze out the juice; take 1 to 2 teaspoons three times a day. You can also apply the fresh paste directly to the rash. "There's almost immediate relief," says Garavaltis.

Drinking fresh coconut water is very cooling and soothing to pitta inflammation, specifically when there is excess heat. Sandalwood and/ or turmeric applied as a paste (one-half herb to one-half water) directly to the affected area can also soothe hot spots.

Relief Through Acupuncture

Acupuncture, an ancient Chinese healing practice, has been shown in studies to reduce the number of allergy-related immune system cells, which suggests that it moderates the immune system's response to whatever you're allergic to. It's the most popular form of alternative allergy treatment.

Some people find relief with Nambudripad's Allergy Elimination Technique (NAET), a form of acupuncture that desensitizes people to allergies. Using pressure points, the acupuncturist desensitizes you to the allergen. See Appendix C for help in finding a practitioner.

Natural R$_x$

Betaine hydrochloric acid (Hcl): Check with your health practitioner for dosage; may be helpful if you have reduced levels of stomach acid production.

Bromelin: 500 mg two times per day. For digestive purposes, take with a meal; for anti-inflammatory effects, take at least 20 minutes before or after eating.

Butterbur: 50 mg twice daily.

Lactase: 6,000–9,000 IU. Good if you are lactose intolerant and experience symptoms like abdominal cramping, bloating, diarrhea, and gas.

Pancreatin: 8,000–24,000 USP units before meals. Helps replace missing pancreatic enzymes to boost digestion.

Papaya: As directed, chewable tablets. Rich in an enzyme called papain, a protease that helps digest proteins.

Pepsin: 1,500 mg. A digestive protease released by cells in the stomach that helps break down food proteins into peptides.

Quercetin: 500 mg two to four times daily between meals.

risky remedy!

Bromelain may thin the blood if consumed in large amounts. So use caution if you take blood-thinning medications. Bromelain may increase the absorption of some antibiotics such as amoxicillin. Take it with meals to avoid digestive upset.

Betaine HCl taken in too-large amounts can cause ulceration of the stomach. Do not use it if you have a history of peptic ulcers, gastritis, or gastrointestinal symptoms, like heartburn, or if you are taking nonsteroidal anti-inflammatory drugs (NSAIDs) or cortisone-like drugs. Use only under medical supervision.

Pancreatin may interfere with some diabetes medications.

Alzheimer's Disease

When you have Alzheimer's disease, abnormal tissues and protein deposits in the cerebral cortex affect the brain's ability to function. This results in memory loss, depression, paranoia, and anxiety. Alzheimer's usually affects folks between the ages of 70 and 80. About five million people in the United States are living with Alzheimer's, and that number could grow to 13.2 million by 2050. If you have a close relative who has Alzheimer's, it could increase your risk for the disease.

Scientists are beginning to believe that diet is as important for brain health as it is for heart health. In this chapter, we look at the causes of damage to delicate brain cells and what you can do to take better care of them. For now, prevention remains our best tool.

natural news

Research in the *New England Journal of Medicine* in 2003 showed that engaging in leisure activities like doing crossword puzzles, reading books or newspapers, writing for pleasure, or playing board games or cards can help ward off dementia and keep your brain young. Studies also show that one hour of exercise five times a week will help prevent Alzheimer's disease, because it increases circulation, gets rid of stress, and keeps the fires of inflammation down.

Causes of Inflammation

Although inflammation is part of the healing process, it can go into overdrive, and when it does, it's considered to be one of the underlying mechanisms for Alzheimer's disease, Parkinson's disease, and depression. Why does this happen? One reason may be the food we eat, explains Dr. Alan C. Logan, N.D., FRSH, an invited faculty member of Harvard's Mind-Body Medicine courses and author of *The Brain Diet*.

Americans love to eat trans and saturated fats, and these foods are chock-full of omega-6 fatty acids that encourage the production of inflammatory chemicals called *prostaglandins*. These fats affect the production of immune chemicals called *cytokines*, which can really do a number on mood, cognition, and long-term brain health. This chronic inflammation takes a toll on our delicate brain cells and damages nerve cells. It is also involved in the initial stages of Alzheimer's disease.

def•i•ni•tion

> **Prostaglandins** are a type of hormone found in cells that serve different functions depending on how they are used. For example, omega-6 fatty acids, found in meats and most vegetable oils, stimulate the production of inflammatory prostaglandins, while the consumption of omega-3 fatty acids found in coldwater fish inhibits the production of these inflammatory prostaglandins.
>
> **Cytokines** are chemicals produced by the immune system that enable cells to communicate with each other so they can attack infections.

Where There's Smoke, There's Fire

When you have inflammation, you have oxidative damage because more free radicals are being generated than the brain cells can handle. Remember when Lucy and Ethel couldn't keep up with all those chocolates in that assembly line? Well, it's kind of like that.

Free radicals, unstable oxygen molecules that harm healthy cells, are generated by activities of the body—in this case, the brain—and all the thinking you're doing. If we eat enough of the good stuff, there's a good chance we'll have enough antioxidants to scavenge these bad boys and put them in their place. If not, and the production of free radicals overwhelms our antioxidant defenses, our delicate brain cells could be in for a bruising, resulting in plaque buildup and less-than-optimal brain function.

Unfortunately, research shows that Americans don't get the antioxidants we need to protect our brains. Research shows that most of us get half of our veggies by eating nutrient-poor potatoes and iceberg lettuce, canned tomatoes, and onions.

dial your doc

Short-term memory loss can be due to anemia, hormonal changes due to menopause, thyroid problems, or a vitamin B$_{12}$ deficiency. Ask your doctor for complete blood tests to get the whole picture if you are concerned.

How Diet Affects Brain Function

Until very recently, the dietary influence on the development and progression of neurological conditions like Alzheimer's disease has been underappreciated. But now that is beginning to change. "Choosing a diet rich in deeply colored fruits and vegetables, oily fish, high-fiber grains, green tea, spices such as turmeric, as well as select supplementation with synergistic antioxidant nutrients may help to decrease the inflammation and oxidative stress that characterize cognitive decline and Alzheimer's disease," says Dr. Logan. "DHA from fish oils is emerging as one of the stars in the long-term prevention of the structural brain changes that accompany Alzheimer's disease."

Fat Head

The brain, command central for everything we say and do, is made up of 60 percent fat. Because of this, omega-3 "fatty" acids are an important nutrient. That's because when we take omega-fatty acids we make it easier for nerve cells to talk to each other. In fact, studies show that the high amounts of DHA (docosahexaenoic acid) and EPA (eicosapentaenoic acid) in omega-3 fatty acids may prevent or slow Alzheimer's progression by protecting against damage to the area where brain cells communicate. Omega-3 fatty acids are also building blocks for important players like cell membranes, hormones, enzymes, and neurotransmitters. Neurons are also made up of fats and neurological tissue, or what we would call white or gray matter.

When we don't have enough essential fatty acids in our diet, it has a big impact on a wide range of mental functions, like learning and intelligence. It has also been associated with attention-deficit disorder (ADD), and it can affect your mood by bringing on the blues.

Can I Take Your Order?

Unfortunately, we're spending too much time at the drive-through. As a result, our diets are heavy in omega-6 fatty acids, not omega-3s. The current typical American diet contains up to 20 times more omega-6 than omega-3. We know that when omega-6s dominate in the body, it can create a situation that promotes chronic inflammation, cancer, heart disease, stroke, diabetes, arthritis, and auto-immunity. Sources of omega-6s include any foods that incorporate vegetable oils (corn, sunflower, soybean, safflower), such as baked goods, grains, and margarine.

natural news

Not a big fan of fish? Take fish oil by capsules or liquid instead. You can even get it lemon flavored! Concentrated fish oil contains about 600 mg per capsule. We currently take in only 130 mg of heart- and brain-healthy EPA and DHA from omega-3, while we need at least 650 mg, according to an expert panel at the National Institutes of Health that made the recommendation in 1999. For optimal results, aim for an EPA/DHA amount of 1,000 mg daily.

For maximum absorption and a reduced risk of a fishy aftertaste, take enteric-coated capsules with food. To find supplements that are molecularly distilled so they have no heavy metal or contamination, visit www.nutrasource.ca.

Parkinson's Disease

In a related category with Alzheimer's, Parkinson's disease (PD) is a degenerative disorder of the central nervous system. Almost one million folks in North America have PD. Symptoms include tremors at rest, slow movements, rigidity, and difficulty walking and maintaining posture. Parkinson's disease runs in families, and eating lots of animal fats increases risk for PD, as does increased iron intake and high cholesterol. Red meat is a source of animal fat, iron, and cholesterol—three good reasons to cut back on red meat.

On the plus side, says Dr. Logan, research is now showing that coenzyme Q10 (CoQ10) and creatine can be used as preventives against the progression of Parkinson's disease. "Both CoQ10 and creatine improve the efficiency of the energy packets of the cell's mitrochondria so the cell doesn't run out of gas," says Dr. Logan. "CoQ10 and creatine are specific fuel for that energy cell—the battery, if you will."

The greatest effect from CoQ10 affects activities of daily living, says Dr. Logan. In one study, those taking CoQ10 had 44 percent less decline in mental function, motor (movement) function, and the ability to carry out activities of daily living, such as feeding or dressing themselves.

Feed Your Brain

To effectively feed the brain, a good place to start is at your fish market, the seafood section at your supermarket, or your health food store. Cold saltwater fatty fish—such as cod, mackerel, salmon, tuna, haddock, lake trout, herring—and fish oil supplements are full of essential omega-3 fatty acids DHA and EPA—EPA is especially helpful for Parkinson's disease. (To learn about fish high in mercury that you should avoid, visit www.ewg.org.) We know that fatty acids EPA and DHA are converted into natural anti-inflammatory substances that help decrease inflammation and pain.

You can also get the benefit of plant-based alpha linolenic acid, an omega-3 fatty acid, from flaxseed, walnut, and hemp seed oil that is converted in the liver into DHA and EPA. The conversion rate is not spectacular—usually only 5 percent. With fish oil, it's ready for use, since the friendly fish has done the conversion for us. Most of the studies on prevention and intervention with omega-3 have focused on dietary fish or fish oil supplements. Here are other foods and supplements that you can incorporate into your diet to help dampen the fires of inflammation and reduce oxidative stress:

Green tea: This tea contains phytochemicals (from the Greek word meaning "plant") called catechins, which are potent antioxidants with powerful anti-inflammatory properties. "A growing body of evidence shows that green tea has properties which make it a strong candidate in the prevention of damage to nerve cells characteristic of such conditions as Alzheimer's and Parkinson's diseases," says Dr. Logan.

Nuts: New research by neuroscientists from the University of Illinois–Chicago shows that nuts, and almonds in particular, prevent age-induced mental decline. Almonds' fatty acid composition is most similar to that of olive oil, with a high proportion of monounsaturated fat and smaller proportions of polyunsaturated and saturated fats. An outstanding source of vitamin E (alpha-tocopherol), a valuable antioxidant with 10 IU per ounce, almonds are also good sources of nutrients such as magnesium, copper, calcium, and riboflavin.

A test tube study by the New York State Institute for Basic Research in Developmental Disabilities found that walnut extract was able to reduce the risk or delay the onset of Alzheimer's disease by inhibiting Abeta fibril formation. Abeta or fibrillar amyloid beta-protein is the principal component of amyloid plaques in the brains of patients with Alzheimer's disease.

Purple and red foods: When you eat blueberries, dark cherries, pomegranates, black grapes, and beets, you tap the power of anthocyanins, strong antioxidants that protect blood vessels, and enhance communication between nerve cells. A study in the *American Journal of Clinical Nutrition* (2005) showed that the phytochemicals such as anthocyanins in blueberries may enhance signaling between nerve cells. Blueberries may also make nerve cell receptors friendlier toward binding with the brain's chemical messengers.

Green foods: Dark green veggies contain magnesium that lowers levels of C-reactive protein (CRP), a blood marker of inflammation. Their antioxidant properties help protect the central nervous system from the damage caused by oxidation. They also improve memory.

natural news

One theory about Alzheimer's disease is that it can be caused when toxic and heavy metals accumulate and cause plaque to form on the brain, so it's a good idea to avoid aluminum in all its forms by not cooking in aluminum pots or using aluminum utensils or deodorants. Toxins such as mercury may play a role when we're exposed to it, too, whether on the job, in the atmosphere, in our fillings, in vaccines, and in our foods. So avoid them as much as possible, too.

Dark chocolate: You've probably heard that dark chocolate is high in antioxidants. And it's tasty, too! If you can, go for organic dark chocolate because it is free from pesticides. Go for low sugar, too, since sugar promotes an inflammatory response.

Sesame seeds: Tiny but mighty, sesame seeds work as an antioxidant to protect the fats that make up the walls of our cells. According to Dr. Logan, three studies show that black sesame seeds popular in Japan are even more effective than white sesame seeds in protecting cells against free-radical damage. Find more information at www.kenkonutrition. com.

Turmeric: A study in the *Journal of Biological Chemistry* shows that this natural anti-inflammatory yellow powder found in curry, a common and popular cooking additive, especially in Indian foods, could be an effective enhancer of an enzyme that protects the brain against oxidative conditions like Alzheimer's disease. You can also take it as a supplement.

natural news

An apple a day could help protect the brain from neurodegenerative diseases such as Alzheimer's and Parkinson's, according to a study in the *Journal of Food Science*. That's because the phytonutrients in apples, phenolic acids and flavonoids such as quercetin, are natural antioxidants that help stop the damage to cells from free radicals. In fact, Cornell University researchers found that quercetin works even better in protecting nerve cells than vitamin C, an antioxidant known to help prevent cell and tissue damage from oxidation. High amounts of quercetin are also found in berries, plums, and onions.

Vitamins E and C: Antioxidant vitamin E is one of the more powerful nutrients in delaying the onset of dementia. Researchers for the Okinawa Program in Japan studied vitamin E levels in Okinawan elders and found that their blood level of vitamin E was 30 percent higher than that of Americans. This is probably because the elders naturally reach for super foods like sweet potatoes and other foods that are high in vitamin E. They also cook in vitamin E–rich cooking oils. You can find vitamin E in foods like nuts, seeds, olives, olive oil, vegetable oils,

risky remedy!

If you take blood-thinning medication, check with your doctor before taking any vitamin E supplementation.

avocados, wheat germ, whole grains, and leafy green vegetables. If you don't get enough vitamin E from your diet, supplements can help.

Vitamin C can be found in fruits (especially citrus) and vegetables, including green and red peppers, tomatoes, potatoes, and green, leafy varieties like spinach and collard greens. Vitamins C and E work synergistically to protect against dementia.

Vitamin B12: Levels of vitamin B12 are usually lower than normal in Alzheimer's patients. B12 is an essential nutrient involved in the makeup of the myelin sheath. It also helps bring oxygen to the brain cells and reduces inflammation. When you're stressed, you go through your B12 in no time flat, so you need to replenish it on a daily basis. Highest sources of B12 are liver, blue-green algae like chorella, and brewer's yeast, but it can be difficult to get enough B12 nutrients from food alone. To make it easier, you may want to take B12 sublingually (under the tongue) or by injection.

Acetyl-L-Carnitine: Supplementing with this amino acid, a vitamin-like compound, improves memory by stabilizing membranes, boosting energy production, and making nerve transmission more effective.

Ginger: A study at RMG Biosciences of Baltimore, Maryland, showed that ginger (Zingiber officinale and Alpinia galanga) extract (GE) may help inhibit the manufacture of inflammatory brain chemicals, slowing the onset and progression of neurodegenerative disorders.

Natural Rx

For Alzheimer's Disease

Acetyl-L-Carnitine: 500 mg to 2 g, in two divided doses.

Alpha lipoic acid: 600–1,200 mg.

CoQ10: 100 mg three times daily; can help clear up brain fog and increase circulation and oxygenation in the brain. A good brand is www.vitalineformulas.com.

DHEA dehydroepiandrosterone: A steroid hormone made by the adrenal glands that decreases in the body as we age; see a holistic practitioner for the right dose for you.

Folic acid: 400 mcg daily. Low levels of folic acid are shown to be a factor in cognitive decline.

Ginger: 300 mg twice per day.

Ginkgo biloba: 240 mg daily. Improves blood flow to the brain, oxygenating brain cells.

Ginseng: As a stimulant, 100–600 mg divided doses standardized to 5 percent ginsenosides per dose. Helps with circulation, energy, and blood flow to the brain.

Huperzine A Hup A, Huperzia serrata: 400 mcg daily. Purified compound isolated from Chinese club moss. Boosts memory. U.S. studies in progress.

Phosphatidylserine: 300 mg. Building block for nerve cell membranes. Helps memory.

Selenium: 400 mg. Studies show this antioxidant inhibits aluminum absorption; taken with zinc and folic acid, it helps to metabolize omega-3 fatty acids so the body can use them more efficiently.

Turmeric: One 400–600 mg capsule—100 percent curcumin—three times a day.

Vitamin B$_{12}$: 2.4 mcg daily.

Vitamin C: 2–4 g daily in divided doses.

Vitamin E: 800–1,200 IU daily.

For Parkinson's Disease:

Acetyl-L-Carnitine and alpha lipoic acid: 2–4 capsules daily; Juvenon, www.juvenon.com.

Creatine: 10 g. Take *only* under the direction of a health practitioner.

EPA from omega-3 fatty acids: 1,000 mg daily; o3mega Joy by Genuine Health.

Nicotinamide adenine dinucleotide (NADH): 10–30 mg daily. Enada, www.enadh.com. Like CoQ10 and creatine, it improves mitochondrial function.

Taurine: 1,000 mg daily.

Anemia

Feeling too tired to finish your to-do list? You may have anemia. The word *anemia* means "without blood" in Greek. If you have anemia, your red blood cells, or hemoglobin, a protein that gives blood that red color, aren't able to carry enough oxygen from your lungs to the cells in your body. This can leave you feeling less than peppy. Because your heart has to work harder to pump more oxygen-rich blood to your body, you may also feel weak, dizzy, cold, or irritable.

Usually anemia is caused by a lack of iron, which you need to make hemoglobin. You may not have enough iron if you have heavy menstrual periods, uterine fibroids, or ulcers; regularly use aspirin; and have a deficiency of vitamin B_{12} and folic acid. Often if you're a vegetarian and give up meat but don't replace it with lentils, peas, beans, and iron-rich green leafy vegetables (collard greens, spinach, and broccoli), you may also be anemic.

The good news is, Courtney Gilardi, N.D., a naturopathic physician who practices at the Kripalu Center for Yoga & Health in Stockbridge, Massachusetts, has seen anemia improve overall in the past 15 years. "Women are paying more attention to their diet. Because of the new birth-control methods where women are having shorter and shorter periods or even not having a period for a whole year, anemia is on the decrease. It's not as big an issue as it was in the past."

But if you have unexplained fatigue, heavy bleeding from uterine fibroids, or endometriosis, or if your periods last longer than seven days, you may need to be tested for anemia. Anemia can also result from an underlying condition like colon cancer, which is why it's important to check with your doctor if you are feeling fatigued or weak, the two most common symptoms of anemia.

natural news

Naturopaths often look at the nail bed to see if someone may be anemic. Blue or very pale nail beds can be a sign of anemia, as can cold hands or feet.

Digestible Iron

If you are anemic, it's important to use the right kind of iron, one that your body can easily absorb. Dr. Gilardi recommends a plant-based, iron-rich liquid supplement called Floridix that is packed with nutrients like black strap molasses, green leafy vegetable extracts, and yellow dock. It contains iron, B vitamins, and vitamin C. "It's sweet, and it's also nonbinding, so it doesn't cause constipation, which can be especially good with our modern diets that tend to be heavy in sugars, white breads, and not enough fiber," says Dr. Gilardi. "It can be effective if you have heavy periods or fibroids, and after endometriosis or right after childbirth." You can also take it in tablets or capsules.

Iron-Rich Herbs

Pamela Hannaman-Pittman, N.D., a naturopathic physician from Richmond, Virginia, recommends an iron-rich, blood-building formula called Hematonic, which includes yellow dock, stinging nettle leaf, alfalfa, dandelion leaf, and lemongrass in a base of organic apple cider vinegar. You can find it at www.wisewomanherbals.com.

Metagenics (www.thenaturalonline.com) also makes an iron-rich compound called Hemagenics that treats anemia and builds blood; it contains iron glycenate, B_6, B_{12}, thiamine, and folate. You can also take important nutrients like vitamin B_6, vitamin B_{12}, and vitamin E separately.

It's very important that you take your iron separately from your zinc and calcium supplements because zinc interferes with absorption. Caffeine and cola drinks also decrease your iron absorption.

Natural R$_x$

Floridix: As directed

Hemogenic: As directed

Vitamin B_6: 2–200 mg daily

Vitamin B_{12}: 1,000 mcg daily

Vitamin E: 400 IU daily

Anxiety

If you're anxious, it can feel like you've had too many cups of coffee. Many people experience anxiety but may not experience it in the same way. That's because anxiety can include panic disorder, obsessive-compulsive disorder (OCD), phobic disorders, generalized anxiety disorders, and post-traumatic stress disorder (PTSD).

If you have generalized anxiety disorder, you have a pervasive feeling of fear and worry that persists even though nothing seems "wrong." It's a feeling that something is off, but you can't quite put your finger on what that is. If you suffer from panic disorder, you may feel sudden intense anxiety (10 on a scale of 1 to 10) for no reason that you can identify. You may have a panic attack, with heart palpitations, shortness of breath, and dizziness.

If you have OCD, you tend to have obsessive thoughts or actions—for example, you may check to see whether the stove is turned off five times before you leave the house, or you may repeatedly wash your hands, all to keep bad things from happening. Or you might be phobic of heights, snakes, plane flights, or elevators. Post-traumatic stress disorder (PTSD) means you relive traumatic events in your thoughts or dreams. This can leave you as hypervigilant as an air-traffic controller—and this stress may lead to chronic illness. Stress feeds anxiety, and anxiety can be stressful. It's a catch-22 that can make life miserable.

Stress-Buster Diet

If you have an anxiety disorder, the best diet for you is one that keeps your blood sugar at a steady level all day long. That's because your symptoms may worsen when your blood sugar takes a nosedive. This means choosing lean proteins, whole grains, veggies, and fruit, and nixing refined sugars and starches. You may do best "grazing" all day long, with small meals and snacks, never letting yourself get too hungry.

Eliminate coffee, tea, and energy drinks if you suspect caffeine may be making you anxious. You can slowly reintroduce them to see if there is any effect on your symptoms.

natural news

Want a natural destressor? Include coldwater fish in your diet, to lower the stress response and levels of cortisol, the stress hormone. "Research shows that fish oil has a beneficial effect probably at the adrenal gland level," says Alan C. Logan, N.D., FRSH, author of *The Brain Diet* and an invited faculty member of the Harvard Medical School's Mind-Body Institute. "New research shows that omega-3 fatty acids are good for anxiety as well as depression." Add salmon, mackerel, sardines, and anchovies to your diet, or use a fish oil supplement to get your omega-3 fatty acids.

Great GABA

You'll find GABA (gamma-aminobutyric acid) in your central nervous system—specifically, in your brain. It's a neurotransmitter, which means it affects the way neurons "talk" to each other. GABA puts the brakes on the activity of nerve cells in the brain, which means it eases overstimulation and generally slows us down, including our heart and lungs. If you feel anxious, it could mean you don't have sufficient levels of this important amino acid.

Folk remedies like passion flower can help correct this imbalance. Like the drugs that treat anxiety, including Valium and Xanax, it targets GABA in the brain and increases it. A small study published in the *Journal of Clinical Pharmacy and Therapeutics* in 2001 showed that passion flower was as effective as oxazepam (a medication used to ease anxiety disorders—brand name Serax) for generalized anxiety disorder, without any of the side effects.

Thanks to Japanese researchers, we also know that GABA tea is a natural way to balance your mood. In Japan, GABA is added to soft drinks, chocolate, bread, and even noodles! Talk about a Happy Meal!

natural news

"Letting go of worry is like putting down a big boulder that you're carrying," says Jacob Teitelbaum, M.D., a board-certified internist and the medical director of the national Fibromyalgia and Fatigue Centers in Annapolis Maryland, and author of *From Fatigued to Fantastic!* "You're going to feel charged up. Most of the things you're worrying about never happen. Let go by asking yourself, 'Am I in imminent danger?' This will put your worries and obsession in perspective and goes a long way to settling your adrenal glands down." Dr. Teitelbaum also recommends a handy anxiety helper known as L-theanine, an amino acid found in green tea. As a bonus, it boosts mental focus, so your thinking will be sharper. You can find it in green tea, gum, and capsule form. One brand of it is called Suntheanine, made by Taiyo.

Homeopathic Help

One of the simplest ways to ease anxiety or nervous tension is to use the homeopathic remedy known as Calms Forte. Its combination of homeopathic ingredients, including passiflora, chamomila, and avena sativa, work together to calm the nervous system and also ease insomnia. You can find it at your neighborhood health food store or by visiting www.1800homeopathy.com.

Ah, Aromatherapy!

Aromatherapy can be incredibly helpful during periods of anxiety, according to holistic aromatherapist Jade Shutes, B.A., Diploma AT, founder of the East West School for Herbal and Aromatic Studies in Willow Spring, North Carolina. "Because of the link between our sense of smell and the limbic or emotional center of the brain, aromatherapy has the ability to soothe and reduce feelings of anxiety," Shutes says. Studies show that if you smell something soothing, like lavender, jasmine, or peppermint, it has the potential to influence mood states, including anxiety. "Aromatherapy won't take you out of a #10 panic state, but it can be helpful with stress management and as a preventive, which is key with anxiety," says Dr. Logan.

Shutes recommends these natural remedies as anti-anxiety antidotes:

The Soothing Bath

> 5 drops lavender oil (Lavandula angustifolia)
>
> 2 drops neroli oil (Citrus aurantium)
>
> 3 drops mandarin oil (Citrus reticulata)

Place essential oils in either 1 cup of milk or 2 tablespoons of honey, and then add to the bath once you are in it.

The Anxiety Inhaler

Another easy way to utilize essential oils for anxiety is to make up smelling salts you can carry with you throughout the day. Think of it as an "anxiety inhaler," Shutes says.

> 4 drops ylang ylang oil (Cananga odorata)
>
> 7 drops mandarin oil (Citrus reticulata)
>
> 2 drops vetiver oil (Vetiveria zizanioides)

Put all the oils in a 5 mL or 10 mL amber bottle and, with the cap on, shake for two to three minutes. Remove cap and fill with sea salt. Replace cap and shake again.

When needed, simply remove the cap from the bottle, place the bottle under your nose, and take a few deep breaths (breathing in through the nose).

Flower Power

Bach Flower Remedies (www.bachremedystore.com) can work wonders for anxiety. They are made from a "sun tea" (a sun and boiling method) of specific wildflowers or trees known for their healing properties, then diluted (similar to homeopathic remedies, in that regard). They work to balance negative emotions, freeing the body's energy to heal itself. In 2007, a study in the medical journal *Complimentary Health Practice Review* showed that Bach Rescue Remedy was effective in reducing anxiety.

You can benefit from Bach Flower Remedies in several ways. You may want to use the dropper and put several drops under your tongue so it's absorbed quickly. You can add a few drops of the remedy to a glass of water and sip it slowly. Nancy Buono, a Bach Foundation Registered Practitioner (BFRP) and the director of Bach Flower Education, also recommends the following remedies for anxiety.

You can place two drops of any applicable remedy into a 1-ounce dropper bottle filled with three quarters of spring water. (Use four drops if you are using Rescue Remedy). Take this personal formula by mouth a minimum of four times each day, four drops each time, especially in the morning and before retiring. If you are unable to swallow this or are sensitive to alcohol (which they contain), simply apply the remedies externally to the wrists and/or temples, or use them in an atomizer or tub of water.

Behavior	Bach Flower Remedy
Generally anxious and stressed	**Rescue Remedy,** to reduce stress and tension
Worried or fearful about life problems: finances, travel, terrorism, illness, and so on	**Mimulus,** to put fears into perspective
Anxious for no apparent reason; something feels wrong	**Aspen,** to restore a sense of calm and security

For more information, visit www.bachcentre.com, www.bachflowereducation.com, and www.bachremedystore.com.

The Relaxation Response

Learning to use the "Relaxation Response" pioneered by Dr. Herbert Benson of the Benson-Henry Institute for Mind-Body Medicine at Massachusetts General Hospital in Boston can be very helpful when it comes to dealing with anxiety. "Research shows it is a very effective tool for anxiety and stress management, especially in any medical condition where anxiety is a factor, such as irritable bowel syndrome and migraines," says Dr. Logan.

Dr. Benson's Relaxation Response is, in simplest terms, a form of meditation that reduces stimulation in the limbic or emotional center of the brain. When you repeat a simple phrase, it helps stop the train of worrisome thoughts and reduces your body's production of stress hormones like cortisol and epinephrine. Practice the Relaxation Response as follows:

1. Find a nice quiet place where you won't be disturbed.

2. Relax all the muscles of your body.

3. Focus on repeating a word, phrase, or image silently to yourself.

4. When unwanted thoughts arise, let them pass.

5. Spend 10 to 20 minutes in this state once or twice a day.

The key is consistency. The more you use the Relaxation Response, the more effective it becomes. With practice and commitment, the payoffs can be reduced anxiety and more peace of mind. Practice does make perfect, so relax and meditate as regularly as possible. For more information, visit the Benson-Henry Institute for Mind-Body Medicine website at www.mbmi.org.

The Power of Breathing

Another method for reducing your stress is a technique developed by Dennis Lewis, author of *The Breath of Presence: Awakening to Who You Really Are* (www.authentic-breathing.com). Lewis says the belly is one of the major areas that get tight and tense when we are under stress: "This greatly affects our internal organs, our breath, our energy, and our overall health." Lewis's belly breathing exercise is also an excellent practice for whenever you are anxious or tense, since it will help relax you and center your energy. It's easiest lying down, but you can also do it while sitting, standing, or walking; over time, it will help slow your breathing and make it more natural. Practice Dr. Lewis's breathing technique as follows:

1. First, get comfortable. Lie down on your back on your bed, a mat, or the carpet. Put your feet flat on the floor and bend your knees.

2. Simply pay attention to your breathing for a minute or two. See if you can sense which parts of your body your breath touches.

3. Stay with your breathing and begin to rub your hands together until you can feel them becoming very warm.

4. Place your hands on top of each other on the stomach, with the center of your lower hand touching your belly button. Continue to notice your breathing. Without forcing it, see if your belly wants to expand as you inhale and retract as you exhale.

5. If your belly seems tight, rub your hands together again until they are warm again and then massage your belly, especially right around the outside edge of your belly button. Notice how your belly begins to soften and relax.

6. Now rub your hands together again until they are warm and put them on your belly again. Notice how this influences your breathing. Don't try to do anything. Simply watch and enjoy as your belly begins to come to life, expanding as you inhale and retracting as you exhale.

7. If your belly still seems overly tight and does not want to move as you breathe, press down with your hands on your belly as you exhale. Then as you inhale, gradually release the tension. Try this several times. Notice how your belly begins to open more on inhalation.

8. When you are ready to stop, be sure to sense your entire abdominal area, noting any special sensations of warmth, comfort, and energy. Spend a few minutes allowing these sensations to spread into all the cells of your belly all the way back to your spine.

A revised version of this practice, as well as many more safe, powerful exercises and practices, is included in Dennis Lewis's book *Free Your Breath, Free Your Life*. The Belly Breathing Practice and all quotations are taken from Dennis Lewis's website www. authentic-breathing.com and used with his permission. Dennis Lewis is the author of *The Tao of Natural Breathing, Free Your Breath, Free Your Life*, and the audio program *Natural Breathing*.

dial your doc

It's time to see your health practitioner if you feel that anxiety is significantly affecting your day-to-day living and functioning. These supplements, dietary changes, and breathing techniques are not a substitute for proper medical care.

Biofeedback

Using biofeedback on a regular basis can help reduce anxiety. A new do-it-yourself biofeedback program, created by Deepak Chopra and Andrew Weil, M.D., is called Healing Rhythms. You can find it at www.wilddivine.com.

Natural R$_x$

Calms Forte: As directed.

Gamma-aminobutyric acid (GABA): 100 mg.

L-theanine: 200 mg of green tea. A good brand is Suntheanine.

Omega-3 essential fatty acids: 1,000 mg EPA/DHA.

Passion flower: ½ tsp., 40 drops, or 2.5 mL three times daily.

Selenium: 200 mcg.

St. John's wort: 900 mg daily. Preliminary research supports usefulness in OCD and generalized anxiety disorder. Never mix St. John's wort with antidepressants.

Arthritis

Oh, your aching joints. If you have osteoarthritis (OA) or rheumatoid arthritis (RA), you know how this condition can affect your life, causing pain and stiffness in the joints (*arthritis* means "joint inflammation"). Osteoarthritis, the most common form of arthritis, happens when the cartilage that cushions our joints degenerates over time, but you don't necessarily have to be "old" to get it. In fact, knee OA is more common than ever for 30- and 40-year-olds. If your mom and dad developed OA when they were 40, odds are you'll develop it early, too, although it may not be in the same joint. Rheumatoid arthritis can also be inherited. RA is an autoimmune condition, which means the body's immune system attacks the cell lining inside the joint, resulting in inflammation and pain.

The 411 on Joints

When joints are working the way they should, they help you move through life with ease. Each of our bones is covered with a smooth, hard cartilage tissue that allows them to glide at the joint so it doesn't hurt when we move our legs to walk or dig in the garden or ride a bike. Cartilage gets its strength because of tiny, interlocking collagen fibers. We also have another built-in buffer known as *synovial fluid*, which is found in the synovial membrane between the bones. This acts as a lubricator and absorbs shocks to the system like shock absorbers in your car. To help stabilize the joint, there are ligaments on either side of the bone as well.

Things go wrong when collagen fibers are disrupted and lost, and cartilage becomes weak. If you are 20 percent over your ideal body weight, for example, this puts significant stress and pressure on your joints. Eventually, cartilage breaks down. At this point, without our built-in natural cushioning, pain is the result.

Is It Osteoarthritis?

How do you know if you have osteoarthritis? One of the first symptoms is stiffness in the morning, usually in the hips or knees. These are common places to have OA, as they are weight-bearing joints. If you've been active, you'll also feel the after effects, especially if you've had a particularly busy day. If you hear creaking noises, it doesn't mean your house is haunted—this is another symptom of OA. You may also find that you are not able to move as easily (and without pain) as you once did.

If you have a physical job, like building houses or roads, or if you're a professional jock, you're more likely to experience OA. But desk jockeys are not exempt. You may feel OA in your hands, elbows, shoulders, and neck. Unfortunately, you can feel OA in different parts of your body at the same time!

Is It Rheumatoid Arthritis?

As we've said, rheumatoid arthritis is an autoimmune disease. If you have RA, you know that it is a chronic inflammatory condition (your skin may also look pinkish-red) that can also feature low-grade fever, a feeling of being bone tired (pun intended!), and weakness. RA causes joints in the hands, knees, elbows, and shoulders to become swollen, painful, stiff, and tender. In severe cases, joints may become disfigured, like a gnarly tree. It's common to experience periods of remission when you have no symptoms and "flares," when tissues are inflamed. Recently, scientists have discovered that smoking can increase the risk of RA. Yet another good reason to quit.

The Role Food Plays

When it comes to keeping the symptoms of OA and RA under control, consider the role of the diet. Phyllis D. Light, R.H., director of herbal studies at Clayton College of Natural Health in Birmingham, Alabama, and a nutritional consultant at her private practice in Huntsville, recommends removing processed sugar, white-flour products, dairy, artificial sweeteners, and alcohol, and reducing caffeine and red meat consumption from the diet. In its place, add whole grains, fresh fruits, and veggies. If you've been thinking of going vegetarian and you have OA, go for it. This type of diet has been shown in studies to improve your symptoms.

It's also important to discover whether you have any food allergies. "Many people today have gluten sensitivity, which can contribute to joint pain and stiffness," says Light. "Keeping a food diary can help you determine whether you are sensitive to certain foods."

Identifying foods that can trigger allergic reactions can be very important when it comes to RA. Foods like wheat, corn, milk, other dairy products like cheese, and beef are common culprits. If you have a history of allergies especially, you may want to speak to your rheumatologist about food allergy testing.

natural news

Agatha M. Thrash, M.D., the co-founder of the Uchee Pines Lifestyle Center in Seale, Alabama, says that some folks with rheumatoid arthritis respond well to a diet entirely free of foods in the nightshade family, including tomatoes, potatoes, eggplant, and peppers. Nightshade refers to approximately 2,600 plant species, including poisonous ones. Plants bear flowers with five sepals, petals and stamens, and one pistil that often ripens into a berry. You'll need to follow the diet strictly for three months to adequately test whether you are sensitive to the toxic alkaloids found in nightshades.

The "Go To" Herbal Supplements

Herbs can help you feel better naturally if you have arthritis by reducing inflammation and pain. This can also be a good choice if you want a remedy to use consistently without the side effects of some medicines like NSAIDs (nonsteroidal anti-inflammatory drugs) such as aspirin and ibuprofen, which can cause stomach upset. NSAIDs can further degenerate cartilage, too, and we don't want that! Two effective herbs with evidence-based support for help with arthritis are ginger and turmeric.

Ginger

Ginger is known as the "warming herb," and its active compound, zingibain, eases the pain and inflammation of OA and RA, while boosting circulation. It's definitely worth trying, to help you feel better. Research in the medical journal *Medical Hypothesis* showed that when patients took 500 to 1,000 mg a day of powdered ginger, 75 percent experienced relief in pain or swelling. In another study at the University of Miami, Florida, patients with knee OA took a standardized extract of two ginger species (Zingiber officinale and Alpinia galanga). After six weeks, they noted a marked improvement in the pain they experienced. While ginger capsules are effective, ginger tea is a simple and delicious way to add this soothing herb to your diet. Ginger is also great for an upset stomach and nausea.

Turmeric

Curcumin is the active compound that gives turmeric its distinctive yellow color. This phyto or plant chemical is a powerful anti-inflammatory herb and is often used in ayurvedic medicine in India. Research in India shows it is effectiveness in improving morning stiffness and joint swelling when 1,200 mg is taken each day. In fact, it was comparable to the prescription medication phenylbutazone, but without the side effects.

risky remedy!
Check with your doctor if you are taking prescription medications. Turmeric and ginger are very mild blood thinners.

Boswellia

Preparations such as pills and creams made from the Boswellia serrata tree bark's gummy resin, called salai guggal, contain active anti-inflammatory ingredients known as boswellic acids. This OA and RA remedy also defends against free-radical damage and the migration of inflammation-producing cells to the inflamed body area. You can either take it as a supplement or apply it directly to the joints.

Stinging Nettles

Suffering from RA? You may benefit from stinging nettles, a flowering plant used for centuries to treat rheumatism and arthritis. This handy herb helps support healthy histamine response and reduces pain and swelling. "When my clients stop using nettles, they miss it," says Phyllis Light. "The effect is pretty immediate when it comes to pain relief." You can take nettles in tea, tinctures, and capsules.

Capsaicin

You may like it in chili peppers, but this fiery herb can also be a soothing balm for OA symptoms. We're talking about cayenne, or more specifically, its active ingredient, capsaicin, a plant compound that helps to trigger the release of feel-good endorphins, helping to ease pain. In addition, cayenne increases circulation to areas such as the extremities (feet, knees, hands, head). It also helps to move toxins out of the body. You can use it as a salve or cream, or take it as a supplement.

natural news

Selenium may be an important nutrient when it comes to cutting the risk of OA, according to new research presented at the American College of Rheuma-tology Annual Scientific Meeting. Further studies need to be done to determine whether selenium supplements can help prevent OA.

Why You Need Glucosamine Sulfate and Chrondroitin Sulfate

You may also find that glucosamine sulfate and chrondroitin sulfate can help relieve your OA symptoms. You'll find glucosamine in your joints. Its number one job is to stimulate cartilage and help joint repair. It's also anti-inflammatory. Chrondroitin sulfate is found in cartilage and stimulates cartilage repair. Together they work to keep joints healthy.

In fact, a 2006 study by the National Institutes of Health, published in the *New England Journal of Medicine*, that involved 1,500 volunteers compared the effectiveness of glucosamine and chrondroitin to Celebrex, a prescription anti-inflammatory. The results? The dynamic duo of glucosamine (1,500 mg) and chrondroitin (1,200 mg) was shown to be statistically significant when it came to effectively relieving moderate to severe knee pain due to OA. Of the people in this subgroup, 79 percent experienced 20 percent or greater pain reduction.

natural news

Essential fatty acids are a natural remedy for arthritis. Researchers at Cardiff University in Wales, United Kingdom, have proven that the omega-3 fatty can help reduce the pain and inflammation of arthritis. The participants in the study took 1,000 mg of extra-high-strength cod liver oil capsules daily.

Bust a Yoga Move

For those who suffer with arthritis, try this simple yoga exercise from Stephen Hartman, the director of professional training and association at the Kripalu Center for Yoga & Health in Stockbridge, Massachusetts. It requires only a few minutes and results in improved flexibility and movement.

1. Before getting out of bed in the morning, bring your attention to the area where you feel the arthritis.

2. Start moving the area or joints, in slow motion, in small circular movements and then back-and-forth movements, called micromovements. This stimulates that area of the body to produce synovial fluid and reduces the amount of friction on the bones before you get out of bed.

3. Instead of cursing the area that is afflicted, spend this time visualizing healing light and kindness to that part of your body and all that it does for you.

Alternative Arthritis Therapies

Like yoga, meditation and acupuncture can help manage pain. Meditation can put you more in touch with your body and help you be less judgmental of where you are now with your OA and RA. For meditation tapes, visit Jon Kabat-Zinn's website, www.mindfulnesstapes.com.

With acupuncture, you'll be able to move the joint more and do the activities you want to do. Depending on the person, acupuncture treatments can reduce pain and stiffness and improve daily functioning. See Appendix B to find an alternative therapy practitioner.

Ah, Aromatherapy!

Holistic aromatherapist Jade Shutes, B.A., Diploma AT, recommends this topical pain relief blend for OA:

> 1 oz. vegetable oil (apricot kernel or sunflower)
>
> 7 drops black pepper
>
> 4 drops lemongrass
>
> 4 drops helichrysum (everlasting)

Massage on painful joints as needed.

Shutes recommends this foot or hand bath or compress for RA:

> 2 drops German chamomile
>
> 2 drops helichysum (everlasting)
>
> 2 drops lavender

Fill basin with water at the desired temperature and add chosen essential oils and/or hydrosols. A dispersant such as vegetable oil or milk may be used but is not necessary in a hand or foot bath. Place feet or hands in the basin and soak for 5 to 10 minutes. Add ½ cup of Epsom or sea salts for enhanced benefits.

To make a compress, fill a sink or large bowl with approximately 1 liter of hot or cold water, as desired. Place 5 to 10 drops of selected essential oils along with a dispersant (if desired) in the water. Place a cotton or flannel cloth in the water and swish around the water. Wring out the cloth to the desired amount of moisture and place on the area to be treated. At this point, if indicated, you can drop an additional one to three drops of your chosen combination of essential oils directly to the compress; then apply the compress to the pained area. A hot compress should be left on until it has cooled to body temperature; then repeat and reapply. Repeat three to four times. A cold compress can be refreshed every five to seven minutes.

You can find essential oils at www.leydenhouse.com.

Natural R$_x$

Alfalfa (Medicago sativa): 1 TB. of leaves per cup of water, 3 cups daily. Has vitamin K to help in calcium absorption; reduces inflammation.

Boswellia (Boswellia serrata): A typical dose of Boswellia is 300 to 400 mg 3 times a day of an extract standardized to contain 37.5 percent boswellic acids. Anti-inflammatory; pain reliever.

Cayenne (Capsicum annuum): Tincture, 5 drops or 0.33 mL three times daily; topical cream, 0.5 percent capsaicin three times daily. Reduces the pain and inflammation of OA; increases circulation.

Condroitin sulfate: As directed.

Devil's claw (Harpagophytum procumbens): One 100–300 mL capsule twice daily. Reduces pain and inflammation of OA.

Ginger (Zingiber officinale): Roscoe tea, 1 TB. per cup of hot water, 3 cups daily. Hot compresses of ginger tea can also be beneficial. Capsules, 500–1,500 mg one to three times daily with meals. Anti-inflammatory.

Glucosamine sulfate: As directed.

MSM (Methyl sulfonyl methane): As directed. Strengthens connective tissue and "feeds" the joint; good for OA and RA; good sulfur adjunct—arthritis sufferers tend to be sulfur deficient.

Omega-3 fatty acids: 1,000 mg as a fish oil. For a certified mercury-free pure product, visit www.nordicnaturals.com—you can even get it lemon flavored!

Stinging nettles (Urtica dioica): Capsules and tablets: 200 mg three times daily. Anti-inflammatory; reduces pain and swelling of RA.

Turmeric (Curcuma longa): L. 500 mg two to three times daily; take with flaxseed oil or lecithin for best absorption. Antioxidant; good for OA and RA.

Asthma

If you are one of the growing number of people with asthma, oxygen is one thing you can't count on when you need it most. Asthma is a chronic disease. It causes the bronchial tubes, the airways that help move air into and out of your lungs, to swell, making it more difficult for you to breathe. You may wheeze, cough, or have tightness in your chest, too. When your symptoms are really awful, you have what is known as an asthma attack. When this happens, your airway muscles tighten, your cells produce more mucus, and as a result, your airways become even more narrow and inflamed, like a clogged pipe, so very little air can get through. According to the Asthma and Allergy Foundation of American, 20 million Americans suffer from asthma.

Asthma can run in families, and it can be triggered by many things, including respiratory infections like colds and pneumonia, exposure to cold weather, exercise, emotional upset, and anxiety. If you take certain medications like beta-blockers, aspirin, and NSAIDs (nonsteroidal anti-inflammatories), they may worsen your asthma. So can preservatives like sulfites, found in red wine. If you've got tummy problems like gastroesophageal reflux disease (GERD), when stomach acid backs up into the esophagus, this can aggravate asthma, too.

Allergies can often be a contributing factor when it comes to asthma. In the spring, especially, allergies to pollen from trees and grass can trigger allergies and asthma. But year-round, asthma can be aggravated by other allergens, including mold, dust mites, and animal dander. Your asthma might also be triggered by irritants like pollution, cigarette smoke, paint fumes, and even scented products, like perfume.

The Allergy-Asthma Connection

An allergy occurs when the immune system in the body, our defense against viruses and bacteria, goes into overdrive and reacts to a normally innocuous substance as if it were a foreign invader. The allergen binds onto an immune system cell, or what is known as a *mast cell*, and releases chemicals called histamines that cause inflammation in our bodies. (This is why we take antihistamines.) According to a small study done in the United Kingdom and reported in the *New England Journal of Medicine* in 2002, it seems those who have asthma have more mast cells in the smooth muscle of their airways than those who don't.

def•i•ni•tion

As part of your immune system, you'll find **mast cells** in the bronchial tubes. When a mast cell comes in contact with an allergen, it binds to it like a key in a lock and releases chemicals called histamines and cytokines, which cause inflammation and lead to the symptoms of allergies and asthma.

Allergens can be environmental (as we've seen before) or in the foods we eat. Kids often outgrow their allergies to eggs, milk, soy, and wheat. But unfortunately, it's not happening as quickly as it did before. According to Johns Hopkins researchers in the *Journal of Allergy and Clinical Immunology* in 2007, less than half (only 42 percent) of kids had outgrown milk allergies by age 8. For adults, once allergies are developed, they're here to stay. Sensitivities can include seafood, including lobster, shrimp, and crab. Peanuts can be a big trigger for both kids and adults. Another study by Johns Hopkins researchers in the same medical journal two years earlier revealed that 9 percent of kids will outgrow allergies to tree nuts such as almonds, pecans, and cashews.

Whether or not you outgrow your allergies, elimination diets are effective in helping identify allergens and treating asthma. You'll need to be off all offending foods (include those with artificial dyes and preservatives, if you can) for two weeks to see a difference. If you'd like some guidance, you may want to be tested by a board-certified allergist to determine what foods you are allergic to. Once you know what they are, avoid those allergens.

Increase Your Antioxidant Intake

In addition to decreasing exposure to allergens, it's smart to increase your intake of antioxidants. Antioxidants can improve asthma symptoms and strengthen overall immunity. In fact, experts think the increase in the rate of asthma can be partly attributed to the fact that we don't get enough of these powerful nutrients, including beta carotene; vitamins A, C, and E; and mineral co-factors that assist in antioxidant defense mechanisms, such as zinc, selenium, and copper. Antioxidants protect cells from oxidative damage that occurs when tissues become inflamed and mucus is produced as well.

Vitamins and Minerals

If you're an asthmatic, you'll want to take vitamin C every day. Vitamin C is found in the lining of the airways that lead to the lungs, and if you don't have enough, your lungs may not work as well as they should. This is called pulmonary (which means it has to do with the lungs) dysfunction. In fact, a study in the *American Journal of Epidemiology* in 1998 based on research done in China showed that vitamin C from the diet can help protect against the loss of pulmonary function. Vitamin C also stabilizes those mast cells we were just talking about and, as a result, inhibits histamine release by white blood cells. In addition, Vitamin C is anti-inflammatory and gives our immune system a boost.

Remember when we said that exercise can trigger an asthma attack? Well, interestingly, a double-blind, crossover study conducted at the Rabin Medical Centre in Israel found that persons with exercise-induced asthma who took vitamin C saw a dramatic decrease in asthmatic attacks, coughing attacks, and lung discomfort. Supplementing with high doses of vitamin C (3,000 mg) before exercise may help prevent an asthma attack.

Research also shows that vitamin E is important when it comes to how well the lungs function. A study at the University of Buffalo in 2001 that appeared in the *American Journal of Respiratory and Critical Care Medicine* showed that vitamin E improved lung function.

Mighty Magnesium

Mighty magnesium is another important nutrient for asthmatics. That's because it relaxes bronchial smooth muscle tissue and helps to reduce bronchial spasms. Its anti-inflammatory effects also help to modulate histamine release. Kids with asthma showed improvement after two months of supplementing with 300 mg of magnesium daily, according to a 2006 study in the *European Journal of Clinical Nutrition*. Not only did they have few episodes, but they also needed to reach for their rescue inhalers less. This doesn't mean that magnesium is a replacement for medicine your child might be taking, but it might be a useful adjunct. Talk to your pediatrician to see if this is right for your child.

Essential Asthma Nutrients

You'll want to take advantage of several nutrients, too. Quercetin, for example, is a natural antihistamine, the first choice for many naturopaths when it comes to treating allergies, and it can be helpful for asthma as well. Quercetin stabilizes mast cells, which helps to block the release of histamines. An extra bonus? It's an antioxidant, which means it helps scavenge toxins that can damage our cells. You'll find this nutrient in many fruits and veggies—specifically, the skin of red apples, red grapes, red onions, and green tea.

Margot Longenecker, N.D., a naturopathic physician who practices in Branford and Wallingford, Connecticut, recommends a formula from Vital Nutrients called BCQ that contains quercetin along with Boswellia serrata, Bromelain, and Curcuma longa extract to decrease inflammation and mucus production. "I've found this to be a great combination," says Dr. Longenecker.

 risky remedy! ⎯⎯⎯⎯⎯⎯⎯⎯⎯⎯⎯⎯⎯⎯⎯⎯⎯

Yes, quercetin is beneficial, but according to Suzy Cohen, the author of *The 24-Hour Pharmacist*, it's important not to combine quercetin with the heart medication digoxin. "There could be a dangerous spike in digoxin levels, increasing the risk of side effects. Quercetin supplements may also render certain 'quinolone' antibiotics such as Cipro or Levaquin less active so you stay sick."

Go Tropical!

Think pineapples when it comes to asthma relief. That's because taking Bromelain, a nutrient that comes from the enzymes in pineapple stems, helps the body absorb quercetin better. Bromelain is also a powerful anti-inflammatory. Together, they turn down the volume on the immune system, reducing inflammation. Ideally, you can munch on fresh pineapples, but if not, supplements can also help.

Omega-3 Fatty Acids

Think fish—specifically, what's inside: essential omega-3 fatty acids. These compounds are found in coldwater fish like cod, mackerel, and herring (or in tasty supplements as well), and in flax seeds and flax-seed oil. They work as natural anti-inflammatory agents, improving the *forced expiratory volume* (FEV) for asthmatics. This couldn't be more important; it's difficult for people with asthma to totally clear their lungs when they breathe out; as a result, they breathe in less air. Improve your FEV, and you breathe easier. Make sense?

def•i•ni•tion

Forced expiratory volume (FEV) is how much air you can exhale after taking a deep breath. Doctors use this to measure your pulmonary (lung) function.

natural news

Because caffeine is similar chemically to the asthma drug theophylline (brand names are Bronkodyl and Slo-bid, among others), it also improves airway function. The reason? It's a weak bronchodilator.

Herbal Help

Herbal remedies like licorice with anti-inflammatory properties can help ease asthma, too. An animal study in the medical journal *International Immunopharmacology* showed that glycyrrhizin, the active ingredient in licorice, helps alleviate asthmatic symptoms in mice. Licorice is a decongestant and an expectorant, both helpful when it comes to asthma symptoms. Keep in mind that licorice can increase blood pressure, so be careful with this remedy if you have hypertension.

Garlic and Onion

It may sound strange, but what happens in your gut can affect your breathing. Asthma can be affected by bowel flora, like when different strains of the bacteria in the gut have been disrupted by antibiotics and poor diet. Garlic, a member of the allium family, is excellent in helping to normalize flora. It also has sulphur compounds that tone tissue, specifically in the lungs.

We've already seen the benefits of quercetin. Onions, another member of the allium family, also contain quercetin, so you may want to add this food to your diet as well.

Ginkgo Biloba

Ginkgo biloba, known for improving mental acuity, has also been found to reduce the symptoms of asthma, including wheezing, coughing, and shortness of breath, as well as their frequency.

Lobelia

Native Americans often smoked the herb lobelia, a natural bronchodilator, as a remedy for asthma. It's also an expectorant, which means it acts like cough syrup does, to clear out mucus from the lungs. You should use it only under the guidance of your health practitioner, as it can be toxic in high doses.

Pycnogenol

A plant extract from the bark of a French maritime pine tree has also yielded a possible solution to asthma. A proprietary extract called Pycnogenol, which is rich in bioflavonoids, has been shown in a study in the *Journal of Asthma* in 2004 to help ease mild to moderate asthma in kids ages 6 to 18. This may be due to its antioxidant and anti-inflammatory properties. It also helps to vasodilate blood vessels.

natural news

Help may be on the way for millions of asthma sufferers, thanks to the natural ozone scavengers found in aromatic plants like lemon, rose, and pine trees. Exposure to ozone, especially in polluted environments, can cause airway inflammation and lung injury. Antibodies also produce ozone in inflammatory tissues as a defense against asthma. The presence of this ozone activates more antibodies, creating a vicious cycle. Ozone scavengers help break the cycle and make treating asthma easier. Researchers have found that inhaling limonene, the main component found in the essential oil of citrus, is most effective in preventing asthma symptoms in animals. Anecdotal evidence shows that people who suffer from asthma and other related diseases also experience very positive effects when using limonene.

The Ayurvedic Perspective

Hilary Garavaltis, an ayurvedic practitioner and the dean of curriculum for the Kripalu School of Ayurveda at the Kripalu Center for Yoga & Health in Stockbridge, Massachusetts, recommends these ayurvedic practices for keeping the nasal passages clear and gently lubricated. This allows them to maintain their own strength and integrity against pathogens and pollutants.

◆ Use a neti pot to cleanse your sinuses with warm saltwater. This is especially helpful during challenging allergy seasons or when you feel you have been exposed to pollution or pathogens, Garavaltis says.

◆ After nasal rinsing, always follow up with an oil lubricant. This can be just simple sesame oil or a blended "nasya" oil prepared with herbs that you can get from an ayurvedic practitioner.

◆ Regular breathing exercises can help keep the channels clear and open, and can strengthen the lungs.

In addition, you may want to try an ayurvedic remedy for asthma, the leaves of the Tylophora asthmatica plant. This natural solution eases symptoms because it contains compounds called alkaloids that act as natural antihistamines. This puts the brakes on mast cell release of histamines that cause inflammation.

Homeopathic Remedies

More than 50 homeopathic remedies for asthma are available, depending on your symptoms. But a good place to start is one of the most generally used, called Grindelia. You can also take it as an herbal tincture. "It helps to break up the mucus and helps with breathing, especially during sleep, shortness of breath, and bronchitis," says Dr. Wiancek. "It's especially good for asthma in older people or people with emphysema."

Another homeopathic remedy for asthma that Dr. Wiancek recommends is Gelsemium. "It works for the anxiety that accompanies asthma. Often people become fearful that they won't be able to breathe."

You'll find a combination remedy for breathing problems associated with asthma at www.1800homeopathy.com. Asthma remedy #83 contains three ingredients: arsenicum alb, which helps with respiration; ipecac, which alleviates tightness in the chest; and Kali phos, which settles nerves. Use it only after you consult with your health practitioner.

Flower Power

According to an Asthma U.K. research study, 69 percent of people with asthma say stress triggers their symptoms. To address the emotional components of asthma, Bach Flower Remedies can be very helpful. Nancy Buono, a Bach Foundation Registered Practitioner (BFRP) and the director of Bach Flower Education, recommends the following remedies to help manage the emotions that accompany asthma.

Behavior	Bach Flower Remedy
Overwhelming feeling of too much to do	Elm
General stress or the effects of extreme emotions (fear, anger, excitement) that may stress the body	Rescue Remedy
General anxiety and stress	Rescue Remedy to reduce stress and tension
Worry or fear about life problems: finances, travel, terrorism, illness, and so on	Mimulus to put fears into perspective and restore courage
Anxiety for no apparent reason, something feels wrong	Aspen to restore sense of calm and security
Environmentally sensitive	Crab Apple to cleanse and purify

You can take Bach Flower Remedies sublingually (under the tongue) or place two drops in a glass of water and sip it. You can also combine these remedies by placing two drops of each into a 1-ounce bottle with a dropper top filled three quarters with spring water. (If you choose Rescue Remedy as part of your formula, it counts as one remedy and you would use four drops.) If desired, you may add a teaspoon of brandy, apple cider vinegar, or vegetable glycerin as a preservative.

natural news _____

A SUNY Buffalo study found that children with asthma who blamed themselves for a family disturbance were at increased risk for an asthma attack. A Bach remedy that may offer relief is Pine, which relieves guilt, helping those who feel that things are always their fault.

This personal formula should be taken by mouth a minimum of four times daily, four drops each time, especially in the morning and before retiring. If you can't swallow or are alcohol sensitive, just apply the remedies externally by moistening the lips, wrists, and/or temples, or use in an atomizer or tub of water. You can find more information at www. bachcentre.com, www.bachremedies.com, and www.bachremedystore. com.

Bust a Yoga Move

Hitting the yoga mat may be a way to alleviate asthma symptoms, certain studies show. In one study in the British medical journal *Clinical Research Education*, 53 volunteers learned how to do yoga, including postures and meditation, and practiced it for 65 minutes very day. This practice helped them to manage their bronchial asthma more effectively than the control group, lessening the number of weekly asthma attacks.

The volunteers also learned pranayama breathing. Practicing the dirgha pranayama, or the Yogic three-part breath, can reduce some of the effects and fear associated with asthma, says Stephen Hartman, the director of professional training and association at the Kripalu Center for Yoga & Health in Stockbridge, Massachusetts. "How many of us were ever taught how to breathe? Many people breathe from their chest. Many breathe from their stomach. Learning how to breathe consciously and fully can retrain repetitive breath patterns and strengthen the diaphragm and lungs to work more efficiently. Being able to learn how to operate the lungs properly and how to relax the lungs at will can reduce the symptoms of asthma attacks."

Here's how to practice the dirgha pranayama:

1. Sit erect and relax your abdomen.

2. Place your palms on your belly and breathe into your lower lungs, feeling your diaphragm drop and your belly expand into your palms. Repeat several times.

3. Shift your palms to the sides of your rib cage, and breathe into your chest, feeling your rib cage expand to the sides. Repeat several times.

4. Place your fingertips on the front of your chest just below the collarbones. Breathe into the upper part of your chest and feel your hands lifting. Repeat several times.

5. Combine all three in-breaths to make what is called a dirgha pranayama inhalation.

6. Exhale completely, gently contracting the abdomen to squeeze out residual air.

7. Repeat this cycle several times, moving your hands to the different parts of your body. Focus on filling and emptying your lungs completely.

8. Rest your hands in your lap and continue this breathing pattern for several minutes.

dial your doc

If you ever suffer from an acute asthma attack, consult your physician or an emergency room immediately.

For more breathing exercises that can help asthma, visit www. breathing.com.

Natural R_x

Asthma Remedy #83 (www.1800homeopathy.com): As directed.

Asthma tincture: As directed.

Bach Flower Remedies (Elm, Rescue Remedy, Pine, Mimulus, Aspen): As directed.

BCQ: Take between meals as directed. Available at www.vitalnutrients. com.

Bromelain: 500–750 mg; 3 times a day between meals on an empty stomach.

Cayenne pepper: Capsicum frutescens. Tincture: 5 drops three times daily.

Gelsenium homeopathic remedy: As directed.

Ginger tea: 1 TB. per cup of water, 3 cups daily. Good for circulation; anti-inflammatory.

Ginkgo biloba tincture: ¼ tsp., 20 drops, or 1.3 mL three times daily. Standardized extract: one 40–80 mg capsule containing 24 percent glycosides and 6 percent lactones three times daily.

Grendelia homeopathic remedy: As directed.

Hesperidin: As directed. Like quercetin, an antioxidant.

Licorice root extracts: ¼ to ½ tsp. Can be liquid form, either tincture or licorice solid extract.

Lobelia tincture: ¼ tsp., 20 drops, or 1.3 mL three times daily.

Lungwort: Pulmonaria officinalis. As directed.

Magnesium: 1,000 mg in divided doses. If loose stools, cut back dose.

Multivitamin and mineral: As directed.

Omega-3 fatty acids from flaxseed oil or cod liver oil: 3,000 mg.

Quercetin: Up to 1,000 mg twice daily; take 20 minutes before meals.

Tylophora asthmatica: As directed.

Vitamin C: 3,000 mg daily in divided doses. Usual dose is 200–500 mg daily; higher doses before exercise can actually stop an attack from happening.

Vitamin E: 400–800 IU daily.

Autism

This baffling and often heartbreaking condition is the fastest-growing developmental disability in the United States. According to the Centers for Disease Control, as of 2007, 1 in 150 children is now autistic. Autism is more common in boys than in girls; boys are four times as likely to be autistic.

To date, no one knows the exact cause of autism, but many experts believe there is most likely a genetic predisposition. One theory is that when this is compounded by other environmental factors, like vaccines, autism can develop. Until 1992, childhood vaccines contained the heavy metal thimerosal as a preservative. Thimerosal is a form of mercury, a neurotoxin that is harmful to the brain.

According to the National Autism Association, which analyzed data from the U.S. Department of Education, from 1992–1993 to 2000–2001, there was an average increase of 644 percent among all U.S. children. This was at the same time that the number of childhood vaccines containing thimerosal grew threefold. Animal studies have shown a direct link between mercury toxicity and autism. Thimerosal is still used as a preservative in some flu vaccines that are given to infants and pregnant moms-to-be. So ask for a mercury-free shot if you get one.

 risky remedy! _____

Vaccines also contain other toxic substances, including antifreeze, dyes, disinfectants, formaldehyde, and aluminum, which has been associated with Parkinson's and Alzheimer's diseases.

What Is Happening to My Child?

According to Mary Ann Block, D.O., of the Block Center in the Dallas, Texas, area, autistic children often develop symptoms after receiving a series of vaccines on or about the age of 2. "You don't notice a child becoming autistic at 5. You notice it when the nervous system is still fragile and developing and putting down the nervous system pathways for speech," Dr. Block says.

Parents may start to notice speech delay or regression. Often a child is developing normally, and then after a vaccination series, parents have videotapes that show this reversal in speech and development. Other symptoms include engaging in hand slapping, being in their own world, and not making eye contact.

Bryan Jepson, M.D., a physician at Thoughtful House, in Austin, Texas, and author of *Changing the Course of Autism*, says he often hears from parents that they thought their child was deaf because he didn't respond to his name.

natural news

Parents need to understand their rights when it comes to vaccines, according to Dr. Block. "Pediatricians and schools tell parents that they have to vaccinate their children, but they may not have to—at least, not immediately." Educate yourself about vaccinations from sources other than your pediatrician. If you can, put off vaccinations and let children develop a strong immune and nervous system before you vaccinate. A good place to learn about vaccinating your child safely is Generation Rescue. Visit www.generationrescue.com.

Don't Wait to Take Action

Whatever the reason a child becomes autistic, parents often wait too long to take action after they notice a problem with their child. But it may be because they are getting the wrong advice. According to Dr. Jepson, often parents take their child to the pediatrician and hear, "He's a boy. Some boys talk late. Let's wait for a while and see what happens." Says Dr. Jepson, "They put it off until things become more readily apparent. This is the wrong answer. The right answer is, 'Let's check it out immediately and start treatment.' Early intervention is key because the brain is still pretty malleable. If you can get rid of some of the toxicity and support children's immune systems, they are more likely to recover more quickly. They don't have as far to catch up if you can get to them early."

Along with medical treatments, Dr. Block recommends putting children in a program for auditory, visual, and sensory integration to "retrain the brain" and help autistic kids function at a higher level.

"The sooner they get started in a program, the better," says Dr. Block. Getting children started in the appropriate educational environment is also highly important.

What's in the Gut

Traditional medicine now uses antipsychotic medications to treat autism, since it still views autism as a psychiatric disorder. But this doesn't fix autism, and risk factors include heart problems and diabetes. "Drugs, at best, cover up symptoms," says Dr. Block. "They don't fix the problem. In my practice, we have many patients we have brought back to recovery." There, and with other nutritionally oriented doctors, one of the first things they do is address the child's gut.

That's because what happens in the gut, or the colon, or the large intestine, doesn't stay there; it affects what happens in the child's brain. According to Alan Logan, N.D., author of *The Brain Diet* and an invited faculty member at Harvard's Mind-Body Institute, research shows that bad bacteria are "setting up camp" in the guts of autistic kids. When kids have less desirable bacteria in the gut, it provokes the response of immune chemicals, cytokines, which causes an inflammatory response throughout the body, including the brain. The end result is autism and other cognitive difficulties, including anxiety and depressive symptoms. "The gut is like Grand Central Station of the nervous system," says Dr. Logan. "Ninety percent of serotonin, for example, a mood-regulating neurotransmitter, operates outside of the brain, predominately in the gut."

natural news

One technique that is used to try to remove heavy metals, including mercury, from the bodies of autistic children is *chelation therapy*. This process involves using chelating agents like dimercaptosuccinic acid (DMSA) and alpha lipoic acid to bind and remove heavy metals like lead, arsenic, and mercury from the body. But it shouldn't be done if your child has mercury amalgam fillings. (These should also be avoided. Ask your dentist to use composite fillings instead.)

The Help of Friendly Bacteria

Autistic kids tend to have a lot of ear infections, and this often means a lot of antibiotics. Antibiotic treatment can kill the good bacteria in the intestinal tract, throwing off the delicate balance needed in the gut to ensure proper function. Because of this, there is often an overgrowth of yeast, bacteria, or parasites in the gut. It's like something out of an old western when it comes to bad versus good bacteria in the gut. Both are fighting for space, and you want to make sure the good guys win. Taking a nutritional supplement of this good bacteria can help re-establish the normal levels in the intestinal tract of your child.

Probiotics, or friendly bacteria, not only help to inhibit less desirable bacteria, but they also help to dampen the inflammatory response in the bodies and brains of autistic kids. Supplements with live cultures of "friendly bacteria" can be especially helpful if your child is sensitive to dairy products like yogurt. "I've had several children who were diagnosed autistic, but when we treated their yeast, they completely recovered," says Dr. Block. Often yeast in the gut is also responsive to caprylic acid.

A comprehensive stool analysis can also help determine whether treatment is needed for hidden problems in the gut such as yeast overgrowth, parasites, and any bacteria that should not be there. Dr. Block says that at her center, about 25 percent of the patients have parasites, about 50 percent have bacteria, and about 90 percent have yeast overgrowth.

Eliminating Offenders

It's very common for autistic kids to have a reaction to casein or dairy products and gluten, a protein that is found in wheat, rye, and cereals. These must be eliminated, although it won't be easy at first. "Parents often find it a challenge to eliminate these foods because they are often the only ones their children will eat," says Dr. Block. "But the good news is, getting them out of the diet will also make a big difference." That's because allergies to foods and inhalants can cause symptoms such as anger, temper tantrums, attention problems, hyperactivity, lethargy, stomach distress, headaches, and a decrease in cognitive function.

You can also identify food allergies through a food elimination challenge, by removing foods that are suspect for a period of two weeks to see if symptoms improve. A test for gluten and casein urinary peptides can determine whether there are problems digesting gluten, found in wheat and other grains, and casein, from dairy products. New research indicates that if these foods are not broken down properly, they can mimic the effects of opiate drugs (those derived from the opium plant) such as heroin and morphine, and affect opiate receptors in the brain involved with speech and auditory processing.

Low blood sugar affects the nervous system of autistic kids, too, so it's important to avoid sugars and focus on giving them protein-rich foods five to six times a day.

Necessary Nutrients

Most autistic kids are deficient in nervous system vitamins like vitamin B_{12} and other B vitamins, so it's important to supplement with these nutrients. Dr. Block says in a double-blind crossover study published in *Biological Psychiatry*, vitamin B_6 was found to be more effective than methylphenidate (Ritalin) in a group of hyperactive children.

Magnesium is also very beneficial for the nervous system. When kids don't have enough, they can be fidgety, anxious, and restless, and have learning difficulties. Zinc deficiency may make children irritable, tearful, and sullen. DMAE (dimethylaminoethanol), a neurotransmitter precursor, helps to improve behaviors, mental concentration, puzzle-solving ability, and organization.

Since children's weight varies, it's important to see a nutritionally oriented doctor for the right dosages. Certain nutrients work better for some children than others, too.

Finding a Doctor to Work with You

It's important to find a specially trained doctor to work with you as you move forward with treatment. A doctor can guide you with dietary restrictions as well. Unfortunately, one of the most difficult and frustrating things about being the parent of an autistic child is finding the right doctor to work with you. Conventional doctors often do not understand the complexities of autism, so it's important to do your research and find a specialist who can help your child. Here are some places to start:

> **National Autism Association:** www.nationalautismassociation. org. Look for the list of Defeat Autism Now (DAN) doctors.

> **Thoughtful House:** www.thoughtfulhouse.org

> **Autism Research Institute:** www.autism.com

> **Generation Rescue:** www.generationrescue.org

Natural R$_x$

Caprylic acid: As directed by your doctor.

DMAE: As directed by your doctor.

Essential fatty acids: 500 mg EPA, 300 mg DHA. Autistic children have increased oxidative stress, so they have greater need for omega-3 fatty acids than a normally developing child—cod liver oil has been shown to help.

Folic acid: Dose to be set by body weight.

Magnesium: Dose to be set by body weight.

Multivitamin and mineral supplement: A good brand is Learner's Edge Child Essence. Take it in divided dosages.

Probiotics: 30 billion colony-forming units of Lactobacillus GG (Culturelle), 5 billion CFU of Lactobacillus plantarum 299V, 1 billion CFU of Life Start (Natren), 4 mg of Bifidobacterium infantis 35624 (Align).

Vitamin B$_6$: Dose to be set by body weight.

Vitamin B$_{12}$: Dose to be set by body weight.

Vitamin C: Dose to be set by body weight.

Zinc: Dose to be set by body weight.

Backache

Picked up more than you can carry? Slept on the wrong side of the bed? Not standing up straight? Overdid that workout? For all these reasons and more, when you strain the muscles around the spine, you could end up with a backache—and, according to the National Institutes of Health, 8 out of 10 of us do at some time. One of the theories is that although we are designed to walk and run (and carry things, work out, and so on), we do spend a good amount of our time—you guessed it—sitting down, whether it's working on the computer, talking on the phone, taking in that meeting, or commuting to and from work. Although moving is better than being stationary, standing also puts pressure on the spine.

Yes, you can take over-the-counter medicines for back pain, like aspirin and ibuprofen, or what are known as NSAIDs (nonsteroidal anti-inflammatories), but long-term use can lead to problems like stomach ulcers. You might want to focus on natural remedies, such as improving the diet by eliminating alcohol, dairy, caffeine, sugar, and high-fat foods; eating whole foods and fruits and veggies; and adding nutrients like glucosamine, MSM (methyl sulfonyl methane), and omega-3 fatty acids. When you take these steps together, it can help the body regenerate and repair itself.

Supplemental Aid

One nutrient many natural experts recommend for lower-back pain is glucosamine sulfate. That's because it is effective for disc and cartilage degeneration and connective tissue repair. It's also one of the primary building blocks of the substances that make up both cartilage and synovial (joint) fluid. The body uses glucosamine to make glycosaminoglycan (GAG) compounds that act like tiny sponges, in the sense that they are responsible for maintaining the right water content in the cartilage matrix. More moisture means more resilience. Sound good?

Chondroitin sulfate is another handy nutrient for your back pain tool-kit. When taken as a supplement, methyl sulfonyl methane (MSM), an organic sulfur compound found in food and in our bodies, is an extremely absorbable nutrient. It feeds the joint in the same ways that glucosamine does, helping in the formation of connective tissue.

natural news

A natural shrinking of the spongy discs in our backs between verte-bral bones happens when we hit our 40s and 50s. This is also a classic time for back pain. Coincidence? Maybe not. Hydration, drinking enough water, is associated with normal shrinkage instead of exacer-bated shrinkage. So aim for eight cups a day minimum, not including coffee and soda. Drink more if you exercise.

Natural Painkillers

Want to ease pain with fewer side effects? Choose herbal painkillers. Unlike NSAIDs, these herbs don't upset the stomach, but they do pro-vide relief.

Devil's Claw

Devil's claw (harpagophytum procumbens) is found in south and southwestern Africa, and it's packed with anti-inflammatory and pain-relieving properties. In fact, a recent study in the medical journal *Spine* (2007) showed that devil's claw provides pain relief comparable to the prescription brand Vioxx.

Turmeric

If you like Indian food like curry, you've got a head start on the pain-relieving benefits of turmeric. The active ingredient in turmeric is the yellow pigment known as curcumin, which gives curry its distinctive look. Turmeric has both antioxidant and anti-inflammatory benefits, which help it relieve your back pain. This may be due to its ability to block what is known as substance P, a pain neurotransmitter in the body. In animal studies, research shows that it's as effective as cortisone or phenylbutazone, which is used to reduce pain and inflammation.

Unlike these two drugs, which are associated with toxicity, turmeric has no known side effects.

Bromelain and Boswellia

Bromelain (from pineapples) and Boswellia, an ayurvedic herb that comes from India, both possess anti-inflammatory properties that ease back pain. Research shows that Boswellia extract produced a significant reduction in joint pain, swelling, and morning stiffness, while improving general health and well-being. Boswellic acid also improves blood supply to joint tissues.

You can also take boswellia, salicin, and cherry (Prunus cerasus), all anti-inflammatory compounds (as well as high in antioxidants) in a formula called End Pain. Begin with two capsules three times daily. After six weeks, you can often lower the dose to one capsule three times daily or take it as needed. It should start to work within one week, but it can take two to six weeks for you to experience the full benefits. Visit www.vitality101.com for more information.

Willow Bark

Since the early 1800s, willow bark has been used as a kind of "natural aspirin." The active ingredient in willow bark is salicin, a compound similar to salicylic acid, which is found in aspirin and has anti-inflammatory effects. Since it's a natural form, though, it's safer and much more gentle on the stomach. (Don't use willow bark if you are allergic to aspirin.) Studies show that willow bark is effective in relieving lower-back pain. When participants in a study published in the medical journal *Rheumatology* (2001) took 240 mg of willow bark (brand name Assalix), they gained just as much symptom relief as those that took rofecoxib, an NSAID for lower-back pain.

natural news

Jacob Teitelbaum, M.D., the author of *Pain 1-2-3: A Proven Program for Eliminating Chronic Pain Now*, recommends fresh ginger for back pain. Just cut up ginger into slices about ⅓ inch thick and place them in a bag in the refrigerator to dry. When you'd like a cup of tea, take out a slice, dice it up, pour hot water on it, and add stevia (a natural sweetener, which is better than loading up on sugar), and enjoy!

The B Vitamins

Dr. Teitelbaum also recommends vitamins B_1, B_2, B_6, and B_{12} to help chronic back pain. These vitamins may have the ability to help muscles relax, and may also decrease neuropathic pain.

Go Fish!

The back loves omega-3 essential fatty acids. Why? Because omega-3s help reduce inflammation and, as a result, back pain. A study in the medical journal *Surgical Neurology* showed that when 250 participants with nonsurgical neck and back pain took 1,200 mg of omega-3 essential fatty acids, 80 percent were satisfied with the results. Like willow bark, it provides benefits without side effects like stomach ulcers. To get your omega-3s, eat coldwater fish like cod, salmon, mackerel, or halibut, or take a fish oil or flaxseed oil supplement.

When a Chiropractor Can Help

Chiropractic treatments can be an important way to help the back and the body as a whole heal itself. The chiropractor uses gentle force to realign misaligned vertebrae, freeing pinched nerves and sending proper nerve flow from the spine throughout the body. "Chiropractic is not just for neck and back pain, but it's to balance out the whole system," says holistic chiropractor Lisa Cowley, D.C., whose practice, Alternative Healthcare, is in Southold, New York. "It's another way of turning on the light switch of energy." Holistic chiropractors like Dr. Cowley incorporate exercise, strength training, stress reduction, nutrition, and stretching into their treatment programs.

Some of the many benefits of chiropractic include these:

◆ Relief from acute and chronic neck and lower-back pain

◆ Enhanced immune system function

◆ Improved respiratory function

◆ Greater nerve supply to the heart and coronary arteries

◆ Improved circulation

Ah, Aromatherapy!

Aromatherapist Jade Shutes, B.A., Diploma AT, says the essential oil of peppermint is widely used in various over-the-counter remedies for muscle aches and pain. You can create your own massage oil to reduce back pain as follows:

Backache Relief Oil

> ½ oz. sunflower or apricot kernel vegetable oil
>
> ½ oz. St. John's wort herbal oil (Hypericum perforatum)
>
> 7 drops peppermint oil (Mentha x piperita)
>
> 2 drops rosemary oil (Rosmarinus officinalis)
>
> 4 drops lavender oil (Lavandula angustifolia)

Mix together in a 1-ounce glass bottle. Shake for a few minutes and then apply to the back.

Using Alternative Therapies

Studies show massage can be effective in treating persistent back pain, which is no surprise to anyone who's had a massage. Researchers at the University of Toronto compared comprehensive massage therapy to components of massage therapy (soft tissue manipulation, remedial exercise, and posture education) and placebo in the treatment of subacute lower-back pain. At the one-month follow-up, 63 percent of subjects in the comprehensive massage-therapy group reported no pain, as compared with 27 percent of the soft-tissue manipulation group, 14 percent of the remedial exercise group, and 0 percent of the placebo (laser therapy) group.

Acupuncture is also widely used by people who have chronic lower-back pain, and studies show it can bring relief as well. A high-tech version of acupuncture called transcutaneous electrical nerve stimulation (TENS) has been helpful to some people. In this practice, small electrodes are placed on the skin where it hurts. The electrodes then transmit a mild electrical current to the tissue, which can help boost the level of endorphins, the body's natural painkillers.

The Healing Touch of Craniosacral Therapy

Craniosacral therapy is used for a wide range of problems, including chronic back pain. Developed in the 1970s by osteopathic physician and surgeon John E. Upledger, craniosacral therapy is designed to release restrictions in the membranes and cerebrospinal fluid that surround and protect the brain and spinal cord so the central nervous system can perform at optimum efficiency.

"It's a light-touch, hands-on manual therapy that primarily targets the central nervous system and the membranes surrounding it," says Roy Desjarlais, L.M.T., CST-D, vice president of clinical services at the Upledger Institute, who has practiced craniosacral therapy for 20 years and now teaches the techniques around the world. "We see the whole body as being connected. If the nervous system is operating optimally, the rest of the body has a better chance to operate optimally. Your immune system works better and your neurological pathways are more relaxed and efficient."

If you choose to have a session(s) of craniosacral therapy, you'll just need to lie on a table for between 15 minutes to one hour. (You'll probably want to take off your shoes.) Using a feather-light touch ("starting with the weight of a nickel," as they say at the Upledger Institute), your therapist will work to release any restrictions you may have in your body by monitoring the rhythm of the cerebrospinal fluid as it flows through the system.

In this way, the practitioner works with the body to help it heal itself. "Your body always knows where the greater balance is," says Desjarlais. "When we put our hands on, we are actually following tissues to find holding patterns so we can release the tissue again. By using light pressure and working our way in more slowly, the body sees us as more of a helper than a threat, which makes us more efficient."

Physical, mental, and emotional stresses can be reflected in the body and will show up in the tissue for practitioners to evaluate. Because of this, craniosacral therapy can also help restore emotional balance.

To date, the Upledger Institute has trained more than 90,000 health care practitioners in over 56 countries in the use of craniosacral therapy. It's practiced by a variety of health care professionals, including osteopathic, allopathic, and naturopathic physicians; doctors of chiropractic medicine; physical therapists; psychologists; acupuncturists; dentists; and massage therapists. It's safe for children, infants, and even newborns. "Craniosacral therapy helps remove restrictions on a neurological level," says Desjarlais. "It works with your body's innate desire to get back to balance." To find a craniosacral practitioner and for more information, visit www.upledger.com.

Bust a Yoga Move!

Two yoga positions (asanas), the Bridge and the Supine Twist, are particularly good for low-back pain, says Stephen Hartman, the director of professional training and association at the Kripalu Center for Yoga & Health in Stockbridge, Massachusetts.

The Bridge strengthens the muscles of the back, shoulders, buttocks, thighs, and legs; stretches and tones abdominal muscles and all internal organs; expands the chest; strengthens lungs and brings awareness to depth of breath; and brings elasticity to the spinal column.

Perform the Bridge as follows:

1. Lie on your back with your knees bent, feet close to the buttocks, and palms down close to your sides, with your feet and knees hip width apart.

2. Exhale and press down through the soles of the feet. Press the feet firmly and evenly into the floor, and engage the abdominal muscles, quadriceps (thighs), and gluteus maximus (buttocks). Inhale and lift the pelvis toward the ceiling.

3. Breathe deeply and feel the weight shift toward the shoulders.

4. Press down into the heels and lift the hips higher. Walk the shoulder blades together. Press your sternum toward your chin.

5. Interlace your fingers and press your knuckles toward your heels, straightening the arms. Press down through the arms and shoulders.

6. To release, inhale and release the hands, and open the space between the shoulder blades. Exhale and roll down slowly. Extend the legs and relax.

The Supine Twist removes stiffness from the hips, spine, shoulders, and neck, and rotates and aligns the spine while maintaining spinal flexibility and hydrating the spinal discs. It also increases the circulation of blood and oxygen to the spine; slims the hips, thighs, and waistline; and provides a massage to the abdomen, stimulating digestion. Another benefit? It simulates peristalsis (muscle contractions in the digestive tract that move food along), improves digestion, and helps relieve constipation.

Perform the Supine Twist as follows:

1. Lie on your back with your arms at shoulder height in a T position, with the palms facing down. Press out through the fingertips, feet, and crown.

2. Place the right foot on the left leg slightly above the knee.

3. Exhale and engage the abdominal muscles, and press out through the left foot. Lift the right hip and bring the right knee across the body toward the floor on the left side. Keep the arms and shoulders on the floor. Flex the left foot and press out through the heel. Turn your head to the right.

4. Breathe deeply and inhale; lengthen and exhale. Twist a little farther. Alternate between pressing the knee down and pressing the shoulder down.

5. To release, exhale and lift the knee and torso back to the center. Return the right leg to the floor. Relax. Repeat on the other side.

Natural Rx

B complex vitamin: 50 to 100 mg daily.

Boswellia: 333 mg three times daily.

Bromelain: 500 mg three times daily between meals.

Capsicum back plaster: As directed.

Chondrotin sulfate: 200–400 mg two to three times daily.

Devil's claw extract: 50–100 mg.

End Pain: 1–2 capsules three times daily as needed. Contains willow, boswellia, and cherry in optimal dosing. www.vitality101.com.

Glucosamine sulfate: 750 mg twice daily.

MSM (methyl sulfonyl methane): 750 mg three times daily.

Omega-3 essential fatty acids: 1,000–5,000 mg.

Turmeric: One 400–600 mg capsule: 100 percent curcumin three times daily.

Willow bark: 120–240 mg of salicin extract three times daily.

Bad Breath (Halitosis)

Bad breath is often a combination of things, like a buildup of bacteria in the mouth and a digestive tract that isn't functioning the way it should. Unfortunately, you may not know if you have bad breath, because you really can't rely on the "blow on your hand" test. A better way to tell is if you have a metallic taste in your mouth, or the taste of mucous in the back of your throat, says Phyllis D. Light, R.H., a professional member of the American Herbalist Guild and director of Herbal Studies at Clayton College of Natural Health in Birmingham, Alabama.

Improve Digestion

As we said, if you aren't digesting food the way you should, it can affect your breath. Betaine HCl, a natural hydrochloric acid, can change all this by making the digestive process work better. Probiotics, or friendly bacteria, can also help digestion. If someone has a really ill colon, Pamela Hannaman, N.D., a naturopathic physician who trained at Bastyr University, starts with a combination of friendly bacteria, acidophilus bifidus, and saccharomyces boulardii, a friendly fungus, to seed the gut and help crowd out pathogenic bacteria and fungus. Fiber, more fruits and vegetables, fermented foods of some sort (like yogurt), plenty of water, and exercise also help keep digestion humming along.

Go for the Greens

Chlorophyll can sweeten the digestive tract and, in turn, your breath. Why? First, chlorophyll binds toxins, which is why it's often used to remove heavy metals from the body through a process that is known as *chelation therapy*. Second, chlorophyll is green. This means it has a basic pH, so it's *alkaline*—this helps support the friendlier bacterial strains that we're likely to see in the gut.

def•i•ni•tion

> **Chelation** is a process that uses a synthetic amino acid, EDTA (ethylene diamine tetra acetic acid), to bind and remove heavy metals like lead and mercury from the body. One theory is that this can stop excessive free-radical production, which can allow the body to heal itself.
>
> **Alkaline** is a pH above 7 on the pH scale 0 to 14. A pH of 7 is neutral. Eating a "green" or plant-based diet can help you have a more alkaline pH, from 7.0 to 7.5, which is thought to be more conducive to good health. You can find simple kits to test your saliva at your health food store.

Both wheat and barley grass have high chlorophyll content. You can buy wheatgrass or barley grass as a loose powder and put 2 teaspoons in water or vegetable juice. You can also grow your own wheatgrass, snip it, and put it through your juicer. Or you can get chlorophyll with mint flavoring at your local health food store.

Scrape That Tongue!

Besides brushing after every meal and flossing every day, using a tongue scraper, a U-shaped instrument that can get your tongue really clean, is a great tool for your clean-mouth arsenal. That's because you use it to scrape bacteria and mucous off your tongue. Yuck, right? But it's better than bad breath.

First, brush your teeth, tongue, and palette with a toothbrush. Next, scrape your tongue from back to front with a tongue scraper. According to Dr. Hannaman-Pittman, because the taste buds are little projectiles, it's like getting down into the pile of the carpet: "With a tongue scraper, you're able to get bacteria that are down in between the taste buds at the base, so it makes your breath fresher."

Natural Rx

Acidophilus bifidus multi-layer pearls: 1-25 billion They don't need to be refrigerated and deliver the bacteria intact and alive. Find them at www.consumerlab.com and www.enzy.com.

Barley grass: 2 tsp. in water or vegetable juice.

Betaine HCl: As directed by your holistic health practitioner.

Saccharomyces boulardii (a strain of yeast): 5 billion; take between meals with cool water.

Wheatgrass: 2 tsp. in water or vegetable juice.

Bladder Infection (Cystitis)

If you're a woman, you may have had a bladder infection; up to 20 percent of women have. And if you've had one, you're not likely to forget it. Not only do you feel like you have to go to the bathroom all the time, but it's not much fun once you get there! Although you may not urinate much, you will still suffer from pain and burning—and this won't be relieved by "going."

You'll find that bladder infections, or what is known as cystitis, are often caused by bacterial infections caused by Escherichia coli or E. coli. Your doctor will likely discover these bacteria and white blood cells in your urine when doing a urine culture.

When It Hurts to Go

Ask any man about bladder infections, and you'll probably get a blank stare. That's because, as women, our anatomy works against us. This means we're the ones who are most prone to this condition. Why? It's because our urethras are much shorter than a man's is (it makes sense if you look at an anatomy chart), and this means that bacteria have a very short trip from the anus to the vagina.

It doesn't take much to trigger an infection. Maybe you overuse antibiotics, which can destroy the "friendly bacteria" we need to stay well. An infection can also be triggered by that romantic getaway, a diaphragm, spermicides, and douches.

Supplements and Remedies

Herbs can be tremendously soothing when it comes to bladder infections. This can be good news if you're suffering. Try herbs like uva-ursi and dandelion, marshmallow, juniper, horsetail, and Oregon grape, for starters. You also have a choice. You can either make up a nice pot of, say, marshmallow tea, or use a tincture if you're on the go, to get relief from your symptoms.

Studies show that using dandelion and uva-ursi together can help reduce the recurrence rate of bladder infections. This is thought to be because uva-ursi has antibacterial properties and dandelion, a diuretic, increases urination. Research still isn't definitive about long-term use of this combination, however, so check with your health care practitioner.

You may also want to take 3,000 mg of vitamin C in divided doses (cut back on the total if you experience diarrhea) and 10,000 IU of vitamin A daily to help build up the immune system to fight infections.

If you have chronic bladder infections, the homeopathic remedy Staphysagria may do the trick, says Beverly Yates, N.D., a naturopathic physician and director of the Naturopathic Family Health Clinic in Mill Valley, CA. "It can be really helpful—particularly if it's a chronic case and it's really a burning, stabbing kind of pain when you urinate." Staphysagria eases inflammation of the urethra in men and women. It can also help balance emotions.

Helpful Practices

As we've said, it's wise to avoid sugar and refined carbohydrates, such as white flour, because bacteria feed on them and this promotes bacterial growth.

But using proper hygiene practices can help as well, says Dr. Yates. "Sometimes women don't know that they should always wipe from the front to the back so they don't infect the urethra with bacteria. Often that solves the problem all by itself."

dial your doc

If not treated correctly, a bladder infection can affect the kidneys. If symptoms are not resolved within 24 hours, see your health care practitioner.

Women should also wear cotton underwear, says Dr. Yates. This means no synthetics, no nylon, and no lycra spandex. If you have a chronic history of bladder infections, consider going commando when you go to bed at night. It just might help.

Natural Rx

Cranberry: 4–8 glasses daily.

Dandelion (Taraxacum officinale): Tincture, ½ tsp., 40 drops, or 2.5 mL in water three times daily; tea, 1 TB. per cup of water, 3 cups daily.

Homeopathic remedy—staphysagria: Three or four 30C pellets every two to three hours until symptoms improve.

Horsetail (Equisetum arvense): Tincture, ½ tsp., 40 drops, or 2.5 mL in water twice daily; tea, 1 TB. per cup of water, 2–3 cups daily.

Juniper (Juniperus communis): Tincture, ½ tsp., 40 drops, or 2.5 mL in water three times daily; tea, 1 TB. per cup of water, 3 cups daily.

Marshmallow (Althaea officinalis): Tincture, ¼ tsp., 20 drops, or 1.3 mL in water three times daily; tea, 1 TB. per cup of water, 3–5 cups a day. Capsules: 100–200 mg twice daily.

Oregon grape (Mahonia aquifolium): Tincture, ½ tsp., 40 drops, or 2.5 mL three times daily; tea, 1 TB. per cup of water, 2–3 cups daily; capsules, 100 mg three times daily. Because of the alkaloid content, Oregon grape shouldn't be used if you have liver problems or you are pregnant.

Uva-ursi (Arctostaphylos uva-ursi) tincture: ½ tsp., 40 drops, or 2.5 mL in water three times daily. Capsules and tablets: 300–400 mg daily.

Vitamin A: 10,000 mg.

Vitamin C: 3,000 mg in divided doses.

Bronchitis

If you have bronchitis, your *bronchi* are inflamed, which makes it painful and difficult to breathe. You may also have a deep, hacking cough. (You know the one.) Chronic bronchitis lasts for weeks, if not months. Acute bronchitis lasts for a shorter period, maybe for a week or so.

If you're a smoker, you're more likely to develop bronchitis, especially when you get a cold. But as the skies in cities become more filled with pollution, nonsmokers are affected by bronchitis, too. Secondhand smoke is also a big factor. Quitting smoking, working in a smoke-free environment, and avoiding secondhand smoke can all make a big difference when it comes to whether you'll be affected by bronchitis. If you do have bronchitis, natural remedies like foods, supplements, and herbs can help.

def•i•ni•tion

The trachea, or windpipe, splits into two branches called the **bronchi,** which carry air to and from the lungs.

Reach for Warm Foods and Supplements

Courtney Gilardi, a naturopath who practices at the Kripalu Center for Yoga & Health in Stockbridge, Massachusetts, suggests using the principles of warming when it comes to bronchitis. Instead of reaching for a cold glass of juice, grab a hot licorice tea or a hot slippery elm tea. If you have a dry throat and are coughing, try cherry bark tea. Ginger is anti-inflammatory, so a hot cup of ginger tea will decrease the inflammation of the bronchi.

Warm foods, soups, stews, veggie soups, and chicken broths also help you breathe easier, decrease the inflammation, and thin secretions. Choose broths that are high in potassium, which means lots of green leafy vegetables. This helps keep and replenish fluids by neutralizing acidity (which tends to happen when we are sick and there is inflammation) and alkalizing the system, which is the ideal state for the body to operate in.

You may also want to go for the greens—a green food supplement, that is. Choosing a green food supplement that contains spirulina, a micro-algae rich in beta carotene, iron, B12, gamma linolenic acid (GLA, an essential fatty acid), and chlorophyll can help you breathe easier. That's because the diuretic properties of these nutrients help clear the lungs, and chlorophyll brings oxygen to cells. A good brand of green food is Garden of Life. You can find it in your health food store or at www. gardenoflife.com.

Other foods to choose are red and orange veggies like squash, yams, and carrots so you're guaranteed to get beta carotene. This nutrient is important for lung health and can help boost the immune system by providing powerful antioxidants to your diet. So pick a peck or two!

Vitamin E is also important in fighting bronchitis, but it can be tough to get enough from diet alone. (You will find this fat-soluble nutrient in nuts.) Instead, you might want to get a good multivitamin with the antioxidants A, C, and E; zinc, an excellent antiviral nutrient; and selenium, an immune booster. All of these can help defend you against viruses and bacteria. Bronchitis can be caused by either of these.

natural news

With nonsmokers, food allergies may play a role. Foods that produce mucous, like dairy, citrus, and soy products, can lead to bronchitis by causing fluid buildup in the lungs, so it's important to avoid these foods. Stay away from sugar, too, because it just generates more inflammation in the body. Although you may want to reach for orange juice, it's loaded with natural sugars. So reach for a good vitamin C supplement instead.

Tap the Healing Power of Herbs

When bronchitis begins, usually you have a dry, painful cough. Next comes tightness in the chest, wheezing, and fever. Since there is very little expectoration and phlegm (mucous produced by the respiratory system expelled by coughing) in the beginning (this happens later), Dr. Gilardi recommends mucilaginous herbs like marshmallow, licorice, and slippery elm to keep everything soft and open.

Licorice and marshmallow are also herbal demulcents. This means they coat and soothe mucous membranes. This is just what you need when you have bronchitis. These handy herbs also help cool the fires of inflammation and break up congestion. Dr. Gilardi also likes to use the herb mullein. "It has anti-inflammatory and immune-stimulant effects, but it has a really good affinity with the lungs and the chest, so it works for any kind of infection."

Break Up Congestion with a Poultice

It sounds old-fashioned, but a *poultice* can be a bronchitis sufferer's best friend. "Your kitchen is your best pharmacy," says Dr. Gilardi. "I've had amazing success with garlic and onion poultices. It works as a circulatory stimulant to bring more blood to the area and more circulation. Since the medicine is absorbed through the skin, if you do it before bed, you'll actually be able to taste the garlic and onion in your mouth." Talk about morning breath!

def•i•ni•tion

A **poultice** is a warm, mediated compress that's applied to the skin to ease inflammation.

Here's how to make a garlic and onion poultice:

1. Cut up a couple of onions and put them in an oven-safe bowl. Crush a few cloves of garlic and put them on top. Add a few tablespoons of apple cider vinegar.

2. Put the bowl in the oven at 350°F for an hour until the onions and garlic are soft and syrupy.

3. Let cool. Press the mixture through a strainer, and rub all the liquid (which makes a paste) on your chest.

4. Place plastic wrap on top to hold it in place. Warm a microwaveable heat pack for a couple minutes or so, to your preference (you can make one yourself with a tube sock and rice or flaxseed and lavender), and place it on top of the plastic wrap and poultice on your chest. Leave it on overnight.

When you take off the poultice in the morning, lie on your forearms with your chest down. Ask your partner or a friend to make a loose fist, as if he or she were holding an egg lightly, and have him or her gently tap on the back to stimulate the thymus and the immune system. Tapping on the back over the lungs can help expectorate what's in the lungs. (This is from a practice called "Do In," which is from the yogic and Japanese Do In tradition.)

dial your doc

If you have a fever of 101°F to 102°F for more than two days, see your doctor, to rule out pneumonia.

Homeopathic Help

Homeopathic remedies can offer relief for the dry coughs and irritation that come with bronchitis. One homeopathic combination called Bronchial Irritation #3 contains aconite, which eases inflammation and anxiety, and bryonia, causticum, and phosphorus, which help ease those coughing fits. You can find it at www.1800homeopathy.com.

Give Yourself Some Breathing Space

Holistic aromatherapist Jade Shutes, the founder of the East West School for Herbal and Aromatic Studies (www.TheIDA.com) in Willow Spring, North Carolina, recommends the following herbal breathing salve to soothe the discomfort of bronchitis through its expectorating, immune-enhancing, and antimicrobial essential oils.

1. Place ½ cup apricot kernel oil (or use a combination of vegetable or herbal oils) with ½ ounce beeswax.

2. Melt this in a double boiler at medium temperature. Stir often to ensure the merging of oils with the beeswax.

3. Place the following essential oils together in a 2-ounce glass jar:

   10 drops eucalyptus oil
   7 drops rosemary oil
   5 drops tea tree oil
   5 drops lemon oil
   4 drops peppermint oil

4. When the oil and beeswax has melted, remove from heat and pour the salve into the jar with the essential oils. Shake and let stand until hardened. Once hardened, the salve is ready for use. Apply to chest area and under nose as needed.

risky remedy!

Because echinacea stimulates the immune system, you shouldn't take it if you have any autoimmune disease like Hashimoto's thyroiditis, Graves' disease, rheumatoid arthritis, type 1 diabetes, or multiple sclerosis. Autoimmune diseases occur when the immune system overacts to substances and tissues normally present in the body. You also shouldn't use echinacea if you have tuberculosis, leukemia, HIV or AIDS, or liver disorders, or if you are taking immunosuppressant medications.

Natural Rx

Echinacea: 200 mg twice daily, capsules and tablets. Builds immunity.

Ginger: 300 mg twice daily, tea for cough and congestion three times daily. Builds immunity.

Licorice tincture: ½ tsp., 40 drops, or 2.5 mL three times daily.

Marshmallow tincture: Tea: 1 TB. per cup of water, 3–5 cups daily; ¼ tsp., 20 drops, or 1.3 mL three times daily.

Mullein tea, infusion of leaves: 1 TB. per cup of water, 3 cups daily.

Multivitamin and mineral supplement containing vitamins A, C, and E, and zinc.

N-acetylcysteine (NAC): 1,000 mg daily; amino acids to break up mucous.

Omega-3 essential fatty acids: 1,000 mg daily.

Slippery elm tincture: ½ tsp., 40 drops, or 2.5 mL three times daily.

Cancer Prevention

The Big "C." Scary stuff. Why does it happen and what can we do to stop it? Although the exact cause of cancer remains unknown, the American Cancer Society estimates that up to 75 percent of cancer cases are caused by environmental factors (which means we may have some control over them), things like exposure to the sun, toxins, radiation, smoking, alcohol, and diet. In fact, a full one third of all cancer deaths can be traced to dietary factors and a lack of exercise.

Raising the bar when it comes to preventing cancers can be as simple as making a few lifestyle choices, such as eating a healthy diet, supplementing nutrients as needed, exercising regularly, and limiting exposure to toxins. First, let's learn more about why diet is such a big factor when it comes to cancer risk.

Why Diet Matters So Much

Eating right can dramatically impact the likelihood of developing cancer. If you aren't getting the right nutrients in your diet and through supplementation (see Chapter 3 on just why everyone needs this), especially antioxidants (more about these later) to repair cellular damage caused by highly reactive and toxic free radicals, your risk for cancer rises. "We all get DNA hits over our lifetimes," says Bradley Willcox, M.D., a clinical scientist and geriatrician at the Pacific Health Research Institute at the University of Hawaii in Honolulu and co-author of *The Okinawa Program: How the World's Longest-Lived People Achieve Everlasting Health—And How You Can Too.* "The more hits we get, the more we're at risk for cancer." The big question is, are you getting the necessary nutrients to help fix and repair the body when it is in need?

Simple Changes, Big Results

Many Americans don't eat the way they should. But with simple changes, you can turn this around. Experts like Karen Collins, M.S., R.D., an advisor to the American Institute for Cancer Research, say a plant-based diet is the overall formula that shows the most protection. The Okinawans in Japan, some of the most longest-lived people in the world, eat primarily a plant-based diet. So there must be something to this! Dr. Willcox found that, in Okinawa, people use the three fourths rule. This means you fill your plate with three fourths of plant foods (vegetables, fruits, whole grains, and beans), and one fourth animal food, such as meat, poultry, or seafood. You can go all out and become a vegetarian, but that's not really necessary unless that's something you feel strongly about. Good substitutes for animal protein include legumes, whole grains, and beans.

Go Hormones and Antibiotic Free

When you do eat meat—and also chicken and eggs—choose free-range products without hormones and antibiotics. This is especially impor-tant for children. The longer hormones are in the body, the greater the risk is for cancers, specifically breast cancer.

Go Fish!

You'll also want to include fish—but do monitor your fish intake to avoid mercury, another toxin. The bigger the fish, like tuna and halibut, the more mercury it's going to have. Instead, choose smaller salmons, like sockeye and Chinook. Salmon from Alaska is preferable because the water is cleaner there.

Pack in the Phytochemicals by Picking a Rainbow

Fill your shopping cart with fruits and vegetables—a rainbow of color in red, orange, yellow, green, purple, and blue—and you'll be sure to get a wide array of cancer-fighting nutrients called phyto or plant chemicals that act as antioxidants to help prevent free radicals from damaging our cells, says Timothy Birdsall, N.D., the vice president of integrative medicine for the Cancer Treatment Centers of America. (If you have kids, you can make a game out of how many different colors you can get in your shopping cart!)

When you choose a variety of fruits and vegetables, you'll be picking up important nutrients like glutathione, one of the biggest phytochemical players we have when it comes to fighting cancer. We have glutathione in every cell in our bodies, and it plays an important role as an anti-oxidant, an immune-system booster, and a detoxifier. We get the most nutrient value from raw fruits and veggies because cooking destroys this important compound.

Mix It Up!

In other cases, cooking releases nutrient value (tomato sauce is the best way to get the nutrient lycopene, for example), so make it a point to include both raw and cooked veggies in your diet. Switch back and forth between soups and salads, raw veggies and cooked veggies. "When you choose healthy sources of protein, a low-fat diet, and healthy carbohydrates, and add a broad spectrum of fresh fruits and vegetables, then you've got the core of a really healthy cancer-prevention diet," says Dr. Birdsall.

Versatile Antioxidants

As we've seen, antioxidants are the cornerstone of healthy eating when it comes to lowering cancer risk. Different antioxidants work in different parts of the body to help prevent illness. When it comes to the arteries, for example, antioxidants in *flavonoids* or bioflavonoids like blueberries can help keep cholesterol from getting oxidized and forming plaque so the arteries can't dilate as well.

Certain antioxidants are also specific for different kinds of tissue. Hawthorne berry, for example, has very good antioxidant effects on blood vessels. Milk thistle and rose hips are good for the liver, while green tea is beneficial for the esophagus, pancreas, and, yes, even the skin. Black raspberries, which contain plant compounds called anthocyanins that act as antioxidants, can help prevent esophageal cancer and keep precancerous growths from

def•i•ni•tion

Flavonoids are compounds found in most plants that have potent antioxidant benefits. You can find them in fruits and beverages such as green and black tea, blueberries, raspberries, apples, and citrus fruits.

becoming malignant, preliminary study findings suggest. Apricots and non-dairy-based dark, bittersweet chocolate (both contain flavonoids) are also loaded with anticancer agents. Dark chocolate is higher in antioxidants even than wine.

natural news

If you don't get much sun exposure and don't choose the right foods, you may not be getting enough vitamin D, which is important for bone strength and may also help lower the risk of colorectal, breast, lung, and prostate cancer. "Vitamin D plays a role in keeping cells in a normal or noncancerous form and controlling their growth and reproduction," says Karen Collins. To get vitamin D safely from the sun, aim for 15 minutes with the hands, arms, and legs exposed three times a week. (Apply sunscreen to protect your face from skin cancer—it's especially vulnerable.) You'll also find vitamin D in foods like salmon, mackerel, egg yolks, milk and fortified juices, breakfast cereals, and soy milk. If your diet totals less than the recommended amount, or you're fair skinned and shun the sun, or you live in northern climes and it's winter, take 1,000 IU a day to close the gap.

Top Cancer-Fighting Foods

You can see why eating a variety of fruits and vegetables is important to provide the widest range of cancer protection. Keeping this in mind, when you go to the grocery store the next time, fill your cart with some of these key cancer fighters. (You'll also find more foods to choose in Chapter 2.) The next time you go to the store, choose a few different fruits and veggies. Make it a habit to rotate what you eat from now on, for maximum cancer prevention.

Cruciferous vegetables: Broccoli, cauliflower, spinach, Brussels sprouts, turnips, kale, bok choy, and the entire cabbage family supply phytochemicals called isothiocyanates that stimulate enzymes in the body that detoxify carcinogens before they can damage the DNA. In some preliminary human studies, people who eat cruciferous vegetables report lower than average risks for bladder cancer. Indole-3-carbinol, a potent antioxidant, is found naturally in these type of veggies, too. Studies indicate that dietary sources of Indole-3-carbinol may help prevent estrogen-related cancers like breast, endometrial, and cervical cancer. Cruciferous veggies also supply fiber, which most folks need more of on a daily basis.

Onions and garlic: These foods contain another group of phytochemicals called allyl sulfides, which are antioxidants and also stimulate carcinogen-detoxifying enzymes.

Dark green leafy vegetables: Cruciferous vegetables like spinach, romaine lettuce, collard greens, and mustard greens supply beta carotene, lutein (another antioxidant carotenoid), and folate (a B vitamin needed for healthy DNA).

Citrus fruit: Fruits such as oranges and grapefruit contain vitamin C (an antioxidant) as well as certain flavonoids (also antioxidants). Red and pink grapefruit also supply lycopene, the antioxidant carotenoid famously found in cooked tomatoes.

Berries: Blueberries, blackberries, and strawberries are chock-full of vitamin C and anthocyanins (powerful antioxidant phytochemicals in the flavonoid family). Raspberries contain a substance called ellagic acid that has been shown to reduce the incidence of colon cancer and can help keep precancerous colon polyps from turning malignant.

Tomatoes: Along with other red produce such as red grapefruit, sweet red pepper, watermelon, and guava, tomatoes may help reduce cancer risk because they contain lycopene. In laboratory studies, lycopene seems to protect cells' DNA with its strong antioxidant power and its ability to stimulate enzymes that deactivate carcinogens before they can get cancer started. In some research, lycopene seems to be even more effective working synergistically with other phytochemicals found in other vegetables and fruits. Evidence of tomato consumption's protective effect is strongest for cancers of the prostate, lung, and stomach, and, to a lesser degree, the pancreas, colon, rectum, esophagus (throat), mouth, breast, and cervix.

Deep orange vegetables: Carrots, apricots, yams, sweet potatoes, and winter squash contain beta carotene, a form of vitamin A and a powerful antioxidant. Vitamin A can prevent cancer cell formation by inhibiting the binding of carcinogens to the cell wall, while beta carotene may protect DNA. Legumes, grains, seeds, bell peppers, and cantaloupe also contain these nutrients, along with greens such as spinach, seaweed, blue-green algae, broccoli, and other cruciferous vegetables.

Whole grains: Whole-wheat bread and pasta, bulgur, brown rice, and oatmeal provide dietary fiber, which acts in a variety of ways to reduce risk of cancer. How? Whole grains contain fiber, which slows the release of carbohydrates and prevents the overproduction of insulin. This protects us against cancer, because too much insulin can "feed" hormone-dependent cancers, such as breast, prostate, ovarian, and colon cancers. Whole grains also contain phytochemicals (plant chemicals) that can reduce the cancer-causing effects of free radicals. Whole grains even help lower blood cholesterol and remove toxins from the body.

Dried beans: Kidney, navy, and black beans (the darker the better, since the darker the bean, the higher the content of antioxidant phytochemicals), but also garbanzo beans and lentils, are the most concentrated sources of dietary fiber. They're also a source of phytochemicals that are antioxidants (such as phytic acid), saponins (which reduce the ability of cancer cells to grow and spread), and others that may help control some hormone levels. "Beans are also a good source of the iron and protein we need," says Karen Collins. "When you eat less meat, it makes adding these nutrients even more important."

Coldwater fish: Salmon, tuna, and mackerel all contain omega-3 fatty acids and should be included in a healthy diet as well. Omega-3 fatty acids have been associated with a lower risk for a number of hormone-associated cancers, like breast cancer. Aim, too, for a high intake of healthy monounsaturated fats like canola and olive oil.

Mighty mushrooms: When it comes to adding nutrients to your diet, you'd be wise to consider adding immune-stimulating maitaike, reishi, and shiitake mushrooms. That's because mushrooms contain a category of substances called beta glucan. In simplest terms, it "wakes up the immune system" so it's ready for invaders, says Dr. Birdsall. The immune system does that by recognizing self versus nonself. Interestingly, all of our cells have markers on them that identify each of us uniquely.

Green tea: Green tea has important cancer-fighting abilities. It helps cells repair damage or, if they cannot be repaired, self-destruct so they don't get replicated. Green tea may also have an anti-angiogenic effect, which means it helps to prevent the proliferation of blood vessels to supply tumors with an increased blood supply. "I would it rank up there with fruits and vegetables as probably one of the easiest, most effective things that people can do for cancer prevention," says Dr. Birdsall. "It appears to have a linear affect. The more you drink, the greater the effect. For cancer treatment, we recommend high doses, such as 8 to 10 cups a day, which is more than what people can drink, so we use a green tea supplement for those patients. But probably 4 cups a day from a cancer prevention standpoint has a pretty powerful effect."

natural news

It's easier than you think to limit (or eliminate) the amount of toxic chemicals, pesticides, and herbicides around the house that can increase your risk of cancer. To go natural, for example, when you clean windows, add ⅓ cup of white vinegar to a liter of water. Use baking soda and water for scrubbing tasks all over the house. To clean clothes, add a cup per load. Instead of using an air freshener with toxic chemicals, use boxes of baking soda to absorb odors in the kitchen and bathroom. For wood, pure lemon oil brings out the natural stain and is nontoxic. When it's laundry time, choose laundry products that are hypoallergenic and free of both preservatives and dye. Skin rashes on young children are often due to harsh laundry detergents. Skip antibacterial soaps because they can also make you antibiotic resistant, as can meat, poultry, and dairy that is not antibiotic free. Use plain old-fashioned soap and water instead.

What Foods and Practices to Avoid

Remember these no-no's when it comes to cancer prevention:

Too much weight. Weight gain during adulthood (recommended limit is an 11-pound gain), especially weight centered on the waist, is a definite no-no. It increases the risk of cancers of the colon, breast (after menopause), endometrium (uterus), kidney, esophagus, probably prostate, and more. Up to 20 percent of cancer deaths are due to excess poundage.

Too much red meat. Eat no more than 3 ounces a day. Amounts beyond that are linked to an increased risk of colon and stomach cancer, and perhaps breast cancer as well. Another reason to limit the red meat you eat? A high intake of saturated fat from food like red meat contributes to the risk of prostate cancer for men.

Too much saturated fat from high-fat meats and rich dairy products. This seems to promote insulin resistance (resulting in high levels of insulin in the blood, which may promote cancer growth).

Too much alcohol. Women should have no more than one standard drink per day, and men should have no more than two per day.

Too much couch time. A sedentary lifestyle means trouble for weight control. Being proactive and getting moving can directly lower your cancer risk. Aim for at least 40 minutes of cumulative activity each day; if you have to break it up into periods of, say, 10 minutes, that's okay. If you're feeling ambitious, new research in the medical journal *Archives of Internal Medicine* shows that a 60-minute strenuous workout (aerobics, running, swimming) more than 5 days a week (over 10 years) can lower the risk of invasive breast cancer by 20 percent and early-stage breast cancer by 31 percent.

natural news _____

Invest in a good, small particulate carbon filter or buy filtered water. Read the label first. Eight out of 10 bottled waters are not filtered. Make sure it's filtered for pesticides, chlorine, lead, mercury, and parasites. Keep a pitcher of cold water in the refrigerator, along with individual glass bottles for every family member. You'll drink more water and less soda. Give your pets filtered water, too, and a daily teaspoon of ground flaxseed or oil on their food. It's great for their coat and makes it shiny. Choose a high-quality pet food. If you find a word on a label that you don't understand, it's probably a chemical.

Specific Nutrients for Specific Conditions

Research shows that certain nutrients, supplements, and lifestyle recommendations can help prevent certain types of cancer. Some recommendations work for more than one type. Here we give you the big picture about the most common kinds of cancer and what you can do to begin to boost health and well-being right now.

Lung Cancer

To avoid lung cancer, there's no substitute for avoiding tobacco and secondhand smoke. (According to the American Cancer Society, smoking also ups the risk of mouth, larynx, throat, esophagus, bladder, kidney, pancreas, cervix, and stomach cancer, and some leukemias.) It's also smart to follow recommended precautions regarding radon and airborne asbestos. When it comes to diet, a recent World Health Organization (WHO) report states that eating the equivalent of at least 4 cups of fruits and vegetables daily could reduce worldwide lung cancer 12 percent. A variety of natural phytochemicals act as antioxidants to protect cells from DNA damage that can lead to cancer.

Slashing Risk

When it comes to cutting lung cancer risk, grab those eye-catching fruits and veggies. Carotenoids, which are natural compounds rich in beta carotene (which provide a source of vitamin A), lutein, lycopene, zeaxanthin, and so on. are found in red, yellow, orange, and dark green fruits and vegetables. A Chinese study that looked at the diet of more than 18,000 men aged 45 to 64 found that smokers who ate the most vegetables rich in carotenoids like carrots, oranges, papayas, tangerines, peaches, and red peppers cut their risk of lung cancer by a whopping one third. (Nix high-dose supplements of vitamin A, though, as they may increase risk.)

When you quit smoking, it's even more important to up your folate consumption. In one study, ex-smokers who ate the most foods that contain folate, including dark green vegetables such as spinach, broccoli, and asparagus, cut their risk of lung cancer by 40 percent. We know that regular physical activity and weight control may also help reduce risk.

The Power of Vitamin E

Vitamin E is well named—and the "E" is for *excellent*. Gamma-tocopherol, the form of vitamin E that occurs naturally in walnuts, pecans, and sesame seeds, and in corn, soybean, and sesame oils, may help stop the growth of prostate and lung cancer cells, according to a new Purdue University study. Gamma-tocopherol inhibits several enzymes that regulate cell growth and induce cancer-cell death, but leaves healthy cells alone. For this reason, it's best to take mixed forms of vitamin E supplements, those that contain gamma-tocopherol and alpha-tocopherol.

Vitamin D and Lung Health

Vitamin D may also play a role in keeping the lungs healthy, with greater concentrations of vitamin D resulting in greater lung health benefits. A study in a recent issue of *CHEST*, the peer-reviewed journal of the American College of Chest Physicians (ACCP), showed that patients with higher concentrations of vitamin D had significantly better lung function, compared with patients with lower concentrations of vitamin D. It could be because vitamin D affects the growth of many cell types and may promote repair and growth of the lung.

Breast Cancer

For post-menopausal women, controlling weight, getting regular physical activity, and limiting alcohol are three of the best ways to prevent breast cancer. Other steps that can improve health include limiting saturated fat, getting adequate dietary fiber, and adding lignans to the diet.

In fact, lignans, plant compounds found in fruits and veggies—specifically, flaxseed (grind it up and put it in yogurt or smoothies), dark whole-grain bread, peaches, broccoli, oranges, winter squash, and strawberries—can help postmenopausal women with breast cancer live longer, according to a study presented at the 2008 annual meeting of the American Association for Cancer Research. Researchers evaluated the dietary lignan intakes of 1,122 women diagnosed with breast cancer who participated in the Western New York Exposures and Breast

Cancer Study between 1996 and 2001. In postmenopausal women, those with a high lignan intake were 70 percent less likely to die from breast cancer. Lab studies showed that lignans impacted hormone levels and tumor growth.

The Benefits of Fiber

As we said before, evidence suggests that fiber can be helpful in preventing cancer by reducing blood sugar elevations and resulting surges in insulin levels. This is especially important when it comes to breast cancer. Nifty fiber also helps by binding estrogen in the gut, which results in lower circulating estrogen levels.

Fabulous Folate

Research in the *American Journal of Clinical Nutrition* in 2007 showed that high folate intake (a B vitamin that occurs naturally in food) from diet and supplements reduced the risk of post-menopausal breast cancer. Folate may also help reduce colon cancer. Fill your plate with leafy green veggies and boost your protection.

A Note on Soy

Soy is fine to include as part of a healthy diet, but it is now considered unlikely to offer breast cancer protection to women who did not grow up eating it before puberty. That's because, when women are younger, soy seems to be able to change the structure of ducts within breast tissue to make them less vulnerable to cancer-causing damage later. This is something to keep in mind if you are raising girls.

natural news

An apple a day keeps breast cancer away? Well, yes! Cornell researchers recently found that rats that were fed the equivalent of one, three, or six apples a day had a breast cancer tumor incidence that was reduced by 17, 39, and 44 percent, and the number of tumors was reduced by up to 61 percent. The reason? Powerful phytochemicals that act as antioxidants stop cell-damaging free radicals. So get munchin'.

Prostate Cancer

It's not only women who need to watch the scale. When it comes to prostate cancer, it's especially important for men to watch their weight as well. "According to one study obese men diagnosed with prostate cancer are more than twice as likely to die of the disease than leaner men, and face more than three times the risk that the cancer will spread beyond their prostate," says Karen Collins. Previous studies suggest that obese men who get prostate cancer may be more likely to have recurrence of cancer after treatment, but it is not known whether weight reduction could change that tendency.

Drink Green Tea

In Asia, men have a lower incidence of prostate cancer. Researchers think this may have something to do with their intake of green tea. In a new study in the American *Journal of Epidemiology*, men who drank five or more cups of green tea a day had less risk of developing advanced prostate cancer. The natural phytochemicals in green tea, which are known as catechins, seem to increase the enzymes that deactivate carcinogens that could otherwise begin the process of cancer development. Green tea's polyphenol phytochemicals can also block prostate cancer tumors from growing larger and spreading, and even promote prostate cancer cell self-destruction.

Choose Soy-Based Foods

In addition to drinking more green tea, Asian men eat more soy-based foods than Western men do, which may help explain the lower prostate cancer rate there. New research in the medical journal *Cancer Research* shows the power of the soybean when it comes to helping prevent the spread of human prostate cancer in mice. This is thanks to the antioxidant isoflavone compound found in soybeans known as genistein.

Pick a Pomegranate or Two

Two new studies show pomegranate juice, from the fruit of the Punica granatum tree, may help fight prostate cancer, reports the *Harvard Men's Health Watch*. When scientists at the University of Wisconsin grew cells from highly aggressive cases of human prostate cancer in tissue cultures, pomegranate fruit extracts slowed the growth of the cultured cancer cells and promoted cell death by *apoptosis*, or cell suicide. Pomegranate components can also retard *angiogenesis*, a process that supplies tumors with the new blood vessels that they need to grow.

In a preliminary study of men with prostate cancer, pomegranate juice lengthened patients' *PSA* doubling time (the longer the doubling time of PSA or prostate-specific antigen, a protein produced by the cells of the prostate gland, the slower the tumor is growing) from 15 months before treatment to 54 months when on the juice.

def•i•ni•tion

PSA, or **Prostate-Specific Antigen**, is a protein produced by the cells of the prostate gland. A PSA test measures the level of PSA in the blood. Prostate cancer can be found early by testing the amount of PSA in the blood.

Let the Sun Shine

Recently, researchers at the Comprehensive Cancer Center of Wake Forest University found that men with high sun exposure had half the risk of prostate cancer as men with low sun exposure. The risk reduction, researchers theorize, is due to vitamin D manufactured from sun exposure. Calcitriol, the most active metabolite of vitamin D, has been shown in laboratory experiments to slow prostate cells from dividing, slow the growth of prostate cancer cells, inhibit the spread of prostate cancer cells, and cause the death of prostate cancer cells. Studies suggest the same may be true in humans.

Colorectal Cancer

It's no surprise that fiber tops the list of to-do's when it comes to the prevention of colorectal cancer. Dietary fiber helps lower the risk of colorectal cancer by moving waste through the gut more rapidly, while normal bacteria in the gut ferment the fiber to form substances that protect the colon cells. As we've seen, fiber also helps reduce the risk of hormone-related cancers by tying up hormones like estrogen in the gut, reducing blood levels.

Fruit is also your friend. A study in the medical journal *Cancer Research* in 2006 showed that women in a study at Brigham and Women's Hospital in Boston who ate fruit reduced their risk by almost half for cancerous colon polyps. How did they do it? They ate fruit five or more times a day. See Chapter 2 in Part 1 for different antioxidant-packed fruits that might appeal to you that can help add up to that five or more a day. To prevent colon cancer, it's also important to limit red meat, saturated fat, and excess alcohol.

Bladder Cancer

Multitasking green tea is also good as a preventative to bladder cancer. A new study in the *Journal of Clinical Cancer Research* reveals the potential of green tea extract to work as a potential anticancer agent by targeting cancer cells in the bladder while leaving healthy cells alone. The study showed that green tea extract inhibits cancer cell growth and has additional anticancer effects.

In simplest terms, green tea extract affects cell skeletal proteins so that the cells become more mature, more adhesive to one another, and less mobile. It interrupts the invasive process of the cancer. In other words, for cancer to grow and spread, malignant cells must be able to move. Green tea extract inhibits that mobility, keeping cancer cells confined and localized, where they are easier to treat. Researchers concluded from this study that at least three cups would be beneficial. More research is in the works.

Skin Cancer

Chronic damage to the skin can damage the DNA of skin cells, which can promote various types of skin cancer, so it's important to be sun smart. Some sunscreens now even contain green tea. Farmers in Asia don't have the skin cancer rate we have in the United States, and the thinking is that this is because they drink a lot of green tea. Studies show that the nutrients in green tea actually protect us from skin cancer, so it's a good idea to add some to your diet, too.

Choose a waterproof sunscreen with a minimum of 30 SPF (preferably 50 SPF), with both UVA and UVB block, and apply it generously

30 minutes before sun exposure. Pay special attention to your face, nose, ears, and shoulders. Reapply every hour or after you go in the water. Use a sunscreen on a regular basis, including cloudy days, since 80 percent of the sun's UV rays pass through the clouds. It's extremely important to choose a sunscreen that is PABA, or paraben, free because parabens are known carcinogens.

To lessen your risk of skin cancer, avoid the sun when the rays are the strongest, from 11 A.M. to 4 P.M. (The sun's rays are also stronger at higher altitudes and closer to the tropics.) Wear a hat and sunglasses, especially at high altitudes, because the sun can burn your retina. (You can actually get a melanoma of the eye.) Use a natural lip balm (no petroleum products, please) with sun protection so you don't develop cold sores from too much sun exposure. Nix tanning parlors. See the section on sunburn for more information about natural remedies for it.

The Role of the Mind and Body

Besides choosing good-for-you foods, choose good-for-you practices, like relaxation, yoga, meditation, massage therapy, or qigong, to melt the stress away. A branch of science called psychoneuroimmunology explores the relationship between the mind and the body related to post-neurologic functioning and immune system functioning. "It does appear that there are a whole variety of signaling pathways that can be affected by doing things like tai chi or yoga or other means of relaxation, exercises that can dramatically improve immune functions," says Dr. Birdsall. "Partly this is because we tend to live in a stressful environment, and when we are under stress, the body produces stress hormones like cortisol. I think there is some truth to the fact that when you deal effectively with stress, are able to enjoy life, set positive goals, learn to be optimistic, and enjoy your life, it can be dramatic in terms of that whole-emotion component that feeds into the immune system."

The Importance of Exercise

Studies show that exercise is vital to weight control—not only to weight loss (which almost always requires significant changes in food choices and/or amounts), but especially to the ability to maintain a healthy weight. "Exercise seems to reduce cancer risk even when weight does not change, possibly due to reducing levels of insulin and insulinlike growth factors," says Karen Collins. It's also an excellent way to reduce stress and decrease mood swings, and it's much healthier than turning to a box of cookies or a quart of ice cream! If you need guidance, ask your health practitioner how to identify your healthy weight range. (Don't be shy!) You can also ask for help in finding and moving toward the physical activity level that is right for you.

Working With Your Doctor

Be sure to discuss and follow your doctor's advice about cancer screenings in terms of what is right for you based on your individual family history and other risk factors. "Healthy lifestyles don't replace the need for screenings," says Collins. "Even a perfect lifestyle can't 100 percent protect you from cancer, and cancers detected early are treated with far greater success than those caught late in their development."

Natural Rx

Choose these foods for their cancer prevention properties. You'll find more about functional foods that can improve your health in Chapters 3 and 4 in Part 1:

Acidophilus bifidus (probiotic): Use this friendly bacteria for immune health that starts in the gut. Four billion to 10 billion daily.

Berries: Blueberries, blackberries, strawberries, and raspberries.

Calcium: A new study from the American Cancer Society shows that calcium can help reduce the risk of colon cancer by 30 percent. Take 1,000 mg; those over 50 should take 1,200 mg.

Calcium D-glucarate: A form of this natural compound known as glucaric acid can be found in apples, broccoli, cabbage, and bean sprouts; it helps remove toxins and carcinogens from the body. Take 400 mg daily.

Carotenoids: Concentrated sources include oranges, papayas, tangerines, and peaches, as well as red peppers and carrots.

Citrus fruits: Oranges, red and pink grapefruit.

Cruciferous vegetables: Broccoli, cauliflower, spinach, Brussels sprouts, turnips, kale, bok choy, and the entire cabbage family.

Dark green leafy vegetables: Spinach, romaine lettuce, collard greens, and mustard greens.

Deep orange vegetables: Carrots, apricots, yams, sweet potatoes, and winter squash contain beta carotene, a form of vitamin A and a powerful antioxidant.

Dried beans: Kidney, navy, and black beans (the darker the better, since the darker the bean, the higher the content of antioxidant phytochemicals), but also garbanzo beans and lentils, since they are the most concentrated sources of dietary fiber.

Flaxseed: Good source of lignans. Protective against breast cancer. Keep ground flaxseed refrigerated. Don't use if you have estrogen receptor positive breast cancer, since it acts as a weak estrogen in the body. 30–50 g per day.

Folic Acid: 400 mcg a day.

Green Foods: A good brand is Garden of Life Perfect Food Original Super Green Formula (www.gardenoflife.com), with 46 phytonutrient-dense superfoods, 13 sprouted ingredients, probiotics, and digestive enzymes. www.gardenoflifeusa.com. Take as directed.

Green tea: Green tea has important cancer-fighting abilities. It helps cells repair damage or, if they cannot be repaired, self-destruct so they don't get replicated. Can also take as a supplement.

Indole-3-carbinol: This antioxidant is found naturally in cruciferous vegetables like broccoli and cabbage. Take 400 mg daily as a supplement.

Maitake mushrooms: Active ingredient is beta-glucan polysaccharide. Immune booster. Take 3–5 g a day as capsules, extract tablets, or food.

Multivitamin and mineral: www.gardenoflifeusa.com. A simple insurance policy for immune health.

Omega-3 essential fatty acids. Found in coldwater fish—salmon, tuna, and mackerel. Associated with a lower risk for hormone-associated cancers, including breast and prostate cancer. May also prevent colon cancer. Take as a supplement 1,000 mg of DHA and EPA.

Onions and garlic: These foods contain another group of phytochemicals called allyl sulfides that are antioxidants and that also stimulate carcinogen-detoxifying enzymes.

Pomegranate juice: From the fruit of the Punica granatum tree; may help fight prostate cancer.

Selenium: Antioxidant; may help prevent breast cancer. 55 mcg a day.

Tomatoes: The lycopene found in cooked tomatoes acts as an antioxidant.

Vitamin D: 1,000 IU daily.

Vitamin E: Mixed tocopherols with Gamma-tocopherol and alpha tocopherol. 400 IU daily.

Whole grains: Whole-wheat bread and pasta, bulgur, brown rice, and oatmeal provide dietary fiber, which acts in a variety of ways to reduce the risk of colon cancer (and probably several other types, too).

Carpal Tunnel Syndrome (CTS)

Whether you're pounding your keyboard or pounding the pavement with a jackhammer, if your hands ache, tingle, or feel numb, you may have carpal tunnel syndrome, or CTS. You get CTS when you do one action too much of the time, over and over again. Any kind of repetitive motion can do it, most commonly typing on your computer, BlackBerry, or all-in-one cell phone. You can also get it from working on a machine or from a hobby, like knitting. It happens when the median nerve, which runs from the forearm into the hand, becomes compressed at the wrist where the carpal tunnel is located, a slender area that contains the median nerve and tendons.

Ten percent of the population has CTS, and up to 50 percent of industrial workers do. People who have Reynaud's disease (in which the small blood vessels go into spasm and people get cold hands and feet) are at higher risk for CTS. Some studies show that women are even more predisposed to CTS than men because hormones can influence CTS. So you may find that your CTS is worse around PMS and/or when you enter menopause. With PMS, CTS is aggravated because there is swelling and fluid retention, so be particularly careful when it comes to diet, especially sodium intake.

natural news

"Carpal tunnel syndrome is a lot more common today," says Courtney Gilardi, N.D., a naturopathic doctor who practices at the Kripalu Center for Yoga & Health in Stockbridge, Massachusetts. "You used to see it just with factory workers like machinists and seamstresses, but with the advent of personal computers and laptops, that has all changed." However, she says awareness about the need for proper ergonomics and body dynamics and posture has also grown. "People are better educated about it now."

Anti-Inflammatory Supplements

Get fruity! To reduce inflammation, think pineapples—specifically, bromelain, an enzyme derived from pineapple stems that relieves pain and swelling. You can get it in a supplement or go for the real thing and chop up a pineapple from your grocery store or local farmer's market. Many naturopaths such as Dr. Gilardi are advocates of food as medicine. "There's a big benefit in eating raw food with live enzymes. You're just so much closer to the source." Another of her favorite anti-inflammatory remedies is the ayurvedic herb boswellia, which is effective for both CTS and arthritis. (Devil's claw also works well for both conditions to reduce inflammation.)

Taking 500 mg of the plant-based chemical or phytochemical quercetin, which has anti-inflammatory properties, and bromelain capsules twice daily between meals can also help reduce the inflammation of the median nerve. Flaxseed oil and omega-3 essential fatty oils can also work anti-inflammatory magic. To boost circulation, which can be a related issue, try ginger and ginkgo biloba. Drinking lots of water (up to eight glasses a day) helps with circulation and helps get rid of waste products from metabolism.

natural news

Eating a lot of Indian food can help carpal tunnel syndrome, too. Why? The turmeric (curcumin) in Indian foods is a natural anti-inflammatory, and this means it can reduce the inflammation of the median nerve in your wrist.

Another simple way to find relief, according to Jacob Teitelbaum, M.D., author of *Pain Free 1-2-3*, is to take 250 mg of vitamin B_6 a day. Birth-control pills can cause a B_6 deficiency, so if you are taking them, it may be even more important to supplement your intake of B_6.

Get the Support You Need

If you do a lot of typing, take a break from it once an hour. Specially designed keyboards and mouse devices can help take pressure off your wrist. Yoga stretches like Downward Dog can also help give your fingers a nice stretch.

You may also want to wear a wrist brace. Dr. Teitelbaum suggests wearing a "cock-up" wrist splint so your hand stays in a neutral position. This can help take the pressure off that median nerve. A new clinical study in *The Journal of Hand Therapy* in 2007 shows that using a hand-traction device called C-TRAC can help relieve pressure on the median nerve by stretching what is known as the transverse carpal ligament. A group of 19 patients used C-TRAC for 5 minutes three times daily for four weeks. Pain, tingling, and numbness all decreased. You may find it useful too. For more information, visit www.ctracforcts.com.

natural news

Why not give yourself a nice hand massage? Dr. Gilardi recommends using wintergreen oil and Tiger Balm for relief. You can find them in Asian Food Shops and health food stores.

If you're a marathon text messenger, you may have "BlackBerry Thumb," another form of repetitive stress injury. Thumb tendonitis happens when the tendons along the thumb side of the wrist swell or get irritated from overuse. You can get a wrist brace with what is known as a Thumb Spica to immobilize the thumb (www.medsupports.com). You may also find relief with the pain gels and creams that help, at www.vitality101.com. Give them several weeks to work. But you may want to consider giving your thumbs a rest, too!

Natural Rx

Boswellia serrata: 300 mg three times a day.

Bromelain: As directed.

Burdock: 200 mg, in capsules.

Devil's claw tincture: ¼ tsp., 20 drops, or 1.3 mL three times daily.

Flaxseed oil: 2,000 mg daily.

Ginger: 300 mg twice daily.

Gingko biloba: 300 mg twice daily.

Omega-3 essential fatty acids: 1,000 mg.

Quercetin: 500 mg twice daily between meals.

Tiger Balm salve: Apply topically.

Turmeric: One 400–600 mg capsule [100 percent curcumin] three times daily.

Wintergreen essential oil: Apply topically.

Cataracts

Sight is priceless, perhaps never more so than when you have problems with it. That's what happens when you get a cataract. You may find that you have a spot on the lens of your eye that blocks your vision, or you may "see" things in a hazy way, like through a fog. The size and location of a cataract determines how it impacts your sight.

Often you'll experience a reduction in vision at first. You may need more light to read by or have difficulty reading street signs when you're driving. You may get a cataract in one eye and not the other, and this will affect your depth perception. This is not what you want when you're navigating; it can lead to missed steps and accidents.

How Cataracts Form

As we've seen in other conditions, free radicals, a byproduct of our metabolism when we convert food into energy, can be a main cause of disease. It's no different when it comes to cataracts. Up to 20 percent of folks who get cataracts are cigarette smokers. No surprise, since smoking increases the free radicals the body must contend with. Are you a sun worshipper? This can cause photo oxidation, which can degrade the lens of the eye. Oxidation can also cause eye aging.

In a healthy eye, the body removes these free radicals by delivering "free radical scavengers" to the eyes in the form of antioxidant nutrients like vitamin C and glutathione. But people who have senile cataracts have been shown to be low in vitamin C and glutathione, says Marc Grossman, O.D., L.Ac., lead author of *Natural Eye Care: Your Guide to Healthy Vision*. In addition, as the lens of the eye ages, it hardens and loses its ability to focus. This process is similar to hardening of the arteries.

Cataracts get worse over time and are the major cause of blindness. Over 40 million people in the United States suffer from cataracts. After age 75, 50 percent of people have cataracts. The standard treatment for cataracts is to remove the lens using a technique called phacoemulsi-fication. A surgeon uses an ultrasonic beam to break up the hardened lens and then vacuums up the pieces from the eye with a suction device. Pretty cool, huh? Afterward, an artificial lens called an intraocular lens (IOL) is inserted to replace the cataract lens.

Although surgery can be an excellent option for those with severe vision loss, Dr. Grossman believes the cataract is a symptom of an underlying condition. "It signals that the natural processes of your body are breaking down on some level and that the normal flow of nutrients into the eyes and waste products out of the eyes has been compromised. So treating the underlying condition that causes the cataract is vital. Because cataracts progress slowly over many years, there is often time for preventive measures to work quite successfully." In fact, in the early stages of a cataract, surgery may not be necessary. "Through nutritional and other complementary medical treatments, it is possible to slow and even reverse the growth of cataracts," Dr. Grossman says.

Foods and Nutrients to Focus On

Since free radicals play such a large role in the formation of cataracts, you'll want to include plenty of foods packed with antioxidants. This includes carotenoids, which are in orange and red veggies like squash and carrots. (Yes, Bugs Bunny did have it right!) It's important to pick foods that are high in vitamin C and bioflavonoids (also high in antioxidants), too, like citrus fruits, berries, green tea, onions, and dark chocolate. You can also take a bioflavonoid supplement that contains quercetin, the most effective bioflavonoid in the prevention of cataracts. All of these nutrients help prevent cataracts by quenching free radicals.

Focus on Dark Green Leafy Veggies

Research in the *Journal of Nutrition* shows that lutein and zeaxanthin, antioxidants found in dark green leafy vegetables like kale, spinach, collard and turnip greens, and broccoli, help protect the eye lens cells from exposure to ultraviolet light—one of the leading causes of cataracts. "Lutein and zeaxanthin reduced UVB-induced damage by 50 to 60 percent and provided protection against oxidative damage that can contribute to age-related cataract development," says Joshua Bomser, a study co-author and associate professor of nutrition at Ohio State University. To reap the benefits, aim for the recommended nine servings (or 4.5 cups) of a variety of fruits and vegetables a day. Says Bomser, "Proper nutrition is important in maintaining ocular health."

Foods to Lose

To eliminate even more free radicals, try to cut out fried and processed foods and saturated and hydrogenated oils. Avoid caffeine (green teas are the exception) and products that contain artificial colors, flavors, and preservatives.

Ease up on your sugar habit, too, including refined carbohydrates, like white flour and pasta that quickly raise blood glucose levels. Nix "good-for-you" natural drinks that contain loads of sugar, like fruit juices. "Even milk sugar, or lactose, found in dairy products can contribute to cataract formation because it destroys vitamin C and glutathione in the lens," says Dr. Grossman, whose website is www.naturaleyecare.com.

natural news

Go organic, if you can, to avoid pesticides and herbicides, as this just adds to the toxic load that your body (and your eyes) must handle. This is especially true when it comes to things you eat often, like milk, eggs, yogurt, fruits, and veggies.

Try an Elimination Diet

Sensitivity to dairy foods can also make eye problems worse by causing sinus congestion, which can impair lymph and blood drainage from the area around the eyes. This means nutrients don't reach the eyes, and toxins and metabolic wastes can't be eliminated as efficiently. To see if dairy products are an issue for you, try doing a food-elimination diet for two weeks to see if you become less congested. Gradually reintroduce dairy products one at a time to identify your specific problem foods.

An Eye to Supplements

Vitamin C is especially important when it comes to preventing cataracts. "The normal, healthy lens contains a higher level of vitamin C than any other body organ except for the adrenal glands," says Dr. Grossman. When cataracts are forming, the vitamin C level in the lens is very low. Similarly, the vitamin C level in the aqueous humor, fluid that gives nutrition to the lens, is low when cataracts are forming.

Glutathione

Both glutathione and alpha lipoic acid are also important to eye health. Glutathione is the most important antioxidant the body makes (it consists of three amino acids: cysteine, glycine, and glutamic acid) and is essential to maintaining good vision—but taken directly, it is poorly absorbed. Several nutrients can help increase your glutathione levels. The main nutrients are n-acetyl-cysteine (NAC), alpha lipoic acid, vitamin C, vitamin B_2, vitamin B_6, selenium, and zinc.

Alpha Lipoic Acid

Alpha lipoic acid has incredible benefits for healthy eye function. Dr. Lester Packer of the University of California at Berkeley has published important research on this antioxidant's ability to halt complications resulting from blood sugar imbalances and hardening of the lens. Dr. Packer's research has confirmed that oxidative damage results in cataract formation and that increasing antioxidants, like alpha lipoic acid, in particular, can help prevent or stop cataract formation.

Bilberry and Vitamin E

When it comes to herbal help, research has shown that bilberry, or the European blueberry, taken with vitamin E may help prevent the formation of cataracts. The active compound in bilberry is called anthocyanidin, and vitamin E is a powerful antioxidant. Together they can help protect your eyeballs. Take 80 to 160 mg of a bilberry extract that is standardized for an anthocyanidin content of 25 percent three times a day, for best results.

natural news _____

Wear 100 percent UV-blocking wraparound brown or amber sunglasses and a wide-brim hat to protect your eyes from sun damage.

Natural Rx

Alpha lipoic acid: 120–300 mg daily.

Bilberry extract with vitamin E: Standardized to contain an anthocyanidin content of 25 percent. 80 mg to 160 mg three times a day.

Eye drops: Containing N-Acetyl-Cysteine (NAC) 1.0 percent. www.
naturaleyecare.com. Ocularvet eye drops for cataracts in pets.

Glutathione: 250–900 mg daily.

Homeopathic eye drops: Cineraria maritima, shown to reduce early
cataracts in 22.5 percent of cases. www.naturaleyecare.com.

Lutein: 6 mg daily.

Quercetin and rutin with vitamin C: 1,000 mg daily. Quercetin seems
to be the most effective bioflavonoid in the prevention of cataracts.

Vitamin C: 92,000 mg daily.

Zeaxanthin: 1–5 mg daily.

Chronic Fatigue Syndrome/Fibromyalgia

Imagine being so tired that you don't have the energy to do the simplest tasks, like make a meal, take a shower, or even brush your teeth. If you have chronic fatigue syndrome (CFS) or fibromyalgia, and over six million folks in the United States or 1 in 50 do, you don't have to imagine it—you live it, every day. Unfortunately, when you have chronic fatigue syndrome or fibromyalgia, taking a nap, a break, or a rest doesn't make it go away. When you have chronic fatigue syndrome, besides being bone-tired, you may experience headaches, muscle and joint pain, and insomnia and other symptoms. Typical symptoms of fibromyalgia include achy joints, fatigue, insomnia, and difficulty concentrating. The overlap between chronic fatigue syndrome and fibromyalgia is so high that they are often considered the same complaint.

Factors to Consider

Like CFS sufferers, fibromyalgia sufferers are often women in their 40s and 50s. We're not exactly sure what causes CFS and fibromyalgia. A virus or microbe may set up a cascade of symptoms that become chronic. Think of it like tripping a row of dominoes that just won't stop. If you think you have CFS or fibromyalgia, you are diagnosed according to your symptoms, not lab testing. Once you have your diagnosis, your treatment needs to be tailored to you, since everyone is different.

Still, the areas of treatment fall under the general categories of addressing sleep, hormonal support, infections, nutritional support, and exercise—what Jacob Teitelbaum, M.D., medical director of the Fibromyalgia and Fatigue Centers and author of *From Fatigued to Fantastic!* calls the SHINE Protocol. You can learn more about it at www.Vitality101.com, including seeing the placebo controlled study showing that 91 percent of patients improve, often dramatically (matiotendfatigue.com). The overall concept is that optimizing energy production is critical, and managing diet and using supplements can often bring relief naturally.

natural news

For more information on this condition, see *The Complete Idiot's Guide to Fibromyalgia, Second Edition,* by Lynne Matallana; Laurence A. Bradley, M.D.; Stuart Silverman, M.D., and Muhammad Yunus.

Foods That Help and Hinder

A healthy diet is critical in managing CFS and fibromyalgia, and dietary antioxidants are of paramount importance. When you have CFS and fibromyalgia, the body is under increased oxidative stress, which means it is manufacturing more free radicals that can damage healthy cells. To fight free radicals better, stock up on a rainbow of deeply colored fruits and vegetables that are bursting with antioxidants. (Chapter 2 has more detailed information about antioxidants.)

If you don't feel up to cooking because of low energy and aches and pains, try to prepare one meal that you can eat several times. Cook foods that balance blood sugar, like whole grains and lean protein and vegetables, for antioxidants and fiber—this can lower inflammation in the body. If you are just too tired to don the chef's hat, why not choose healthy frozen options like Amy's or Kashi foods? You can find more choices than ever before in your grocery store. Your health food store has even more choices. It's worth taking a shopping trip for healthy frozen foods!

Keep in mind, too, that avoiding certain things in your diet is just as important. "Removal of monosodium glutamate (MSG) and aspartame has been shown to dramatically improve symptoms of fibromyalgia," says Dr. Logan. "They may be gaining access to the brain more readily." It's also critical to remove artificial food dyes and preservatives like benzoates to avoid provoking symptoms. "That's an absolute must." It's important to investigate food intolerances as well, such as those to dairy and wheat.

natural news _____

If you've ever thought about going vegetarian, here's another reason to do so. "Studies show that a vegetarian or vegan (no dairy or eggs) diet with lots of fruits, veggies, nuts, seeds, sprouts, and berries with dark pigments like cranberries, blueberries, and black currants may improve the symptoms of fibromyalgia," says Dr. Logan. "Sufferers had decreased pain and joint stiffness, and improved sleep quality, physical performance, mental health, and overall well-being." Even if you make moderate changes by incorporating some of these nutrients in the diet, you will benefit.

Reviving Supplements

It tastes like sugar, but it does a whole lot more. It's a handy little nutrient known as *D-ribose*, and research proves it's very beneficial for people who suffer from an energy crisis. Dr. Teitelbaum's study showed that D-ribose boosts energy almost 50 percent, while at the same time easing symptoms of fibromyalgia like insomnia, pain, and brain fog.

def•i•ni•tion _____

D-ribose is a naturally occurring carbohydrate found in all living cells.

For best results, he recommends taking 5 g of D-ribose three times a day for one month and, after that, twice a day. You can find it on line at www.Vitality101.com or at your health food store.

Yes, you can go fish, but you can also keep a handy bottle of lemon-flavored cod liver oil in your fridge. Cod liver oil is loaded with anti-inflammatory omega-3 fatty acids. In fact, research shows that it's one of the most powerful nutrients to help with inflammation and mood in CFS and fibromyalgia. Omega-3 fatty acids dampen the inflammatory cytokines that can otherwise influence mood, energy levels, and cognitive functions. This is important because brain fog, or "fibro fog," is a common complaint among those who suffer from CFS and fibromyalgia.

Fish oils also can help with the growth of nerve cells in those who have chronic fatigue, says Alan Logan, N.D., author of *The Brain Diet* and an invited faculty member at Harvard Medical School's Mind-Body Institute. Folks who have these conditions are also often depressed, mainly because they are used to being on the move. "People with CFS and fibromyalgia are used to being very active before they got ill, and so their whole lives have been turned upside down," says Dr. Logan. Research shows that omega-3 essential fatty acids can help. A good brand is Nordic Naturals (www.nordicnaturals.com).

Fighting Fatigue and Pain

Naturally, sleep is of tremendous importance if you suffer from fibromyalgia. Unfortunately, it's not so easy to get those zzz's, since the hypothalamus in the brain regulates how we sleep and fibromyalgia suppresses its function. The hypothalamus also regulates a lot of other body functions, like body temperature, hormone function, and blood pressure. To get your sack time—ideally, eight to nine hours a night—you may want to try a natural compound called the Revitalizing Sleep Formula (www.vitality101.com).

To address common nutritional deficiencies related to fibromyalgia, Dr. Teitelbaum recommends taking an NAC supplement (N-acetylcysteine), coenzyme Q10 (CoQ10), and acetyl-l-carnitine. You may also want to take a supplement of DHEA (dehydroepiandrosterone), a hormone made by the adrenal cortex in the brain to help with hypothalamic suppression. It's a good idea to have a holistic practitioner guide you with the dosage. You can also visit www.vitality101.com, where you will find a free online program which will analyze your symptoms and tailor a treatment protocol just for you. Often having fibromyalgia and CFS puts the immune system at less than tip-top shape. This means you can get sick more often than you should. To help turn things around, start with your digestive system because its health largely determines overall immunity. One of the easiest ways to give your digestive system a boost is to add probiotics, or friendly bacteria, to your supplement routine in the form of acidophilus pearls, says Dr. Teitelbaum. You may need prescription antifungals as well.

Research shows that qigong can help relieve the pain of fibromyalgia and improve functioning. In a recent acupuncture study involving people with fibromyalgia, participants experienced significant improvement after eight weeks of treatment. Check the credentials of an acupuncturist, along with treatment cost and procedures, before you have a treatment. To find a practitioner, visit the website of the National Certification Commission for Acupuncture and Oriental Medicine at www.nccaom.org.

natural news _____

Research shows that biofeedback can help ease the pain of fibromyalgia. Biofeedback teaches you to alter your brain activity, blood pressure, muscle tension, heart rate, and other critical bodily functions. Deepak Chopra, M.D.; Dean Ornish, M.D.; Andrew Weil, M.D.; and other medical experts have created a do-it-yourself biofeedback program called Healing Rhythms (www.wilddivine.com). It provides breathing, relaxation, and meditation techniques to improve physical and mental health.

Working with Your Doctor

For best results, it's very important to look for a nutritionally oriented doctor. The average time spent from initially going to the doctor with these symptoms to actually getting a formal diagnosis is seven years, says Dr. Logan. "It's important to exclude other known and often treatable conditions before a diagnosis of CFS is made, and some doctors don't have the time or patience to work with you to come to a satisfactory conclusion," Dr. Logan says. "It's very important to find a doctor that you have a good relationship with." The Fibromyalgia and Fatigue Centers nationally (www.FibroandFatigue.com) specialize in treating CFS and fibromyalgia.

natural news _____

Preliminary research by the University of Virginia shows that magnet therapy can be useful for fibromyalgia pain. The type of magnet is important, says Dr. Teitelbaum, because the strength and field configuration can be critical. He says the Nikkan Company magnets seem to be fairly reliable (www.relievepain.com).

Natural Rx

Acetyl l-carnitine: 1,000 mg daily for three or four months. Helps energy and weight loss.

Acidophilus pearls: 2 pearls twice daily for five months.

CoQ10: 200 mg daily for three to six months. Vitalineformulas.com.

D-ribose: 5 g three times daily. Corvalen, www.corvalen.com.

Omega-3 fatty acids: EPA/DHA 1,000–2,000 mg daily—take a mercury-free brand. Fish oil has been shown to improve symptoms in patients with both CFS and fibromyalgia.

Energy Revitalization System Vitamin Powder: 1/2 to 1 scoop a day. www.vitality101.com.

Evening primrose oil: Take with a total of 1,000–2,000 mg of EPA/ DHA daily. Especially important if you have PMS—research shows that combining omega-3 fatty acids with evening primrose oil (gamma linoleic acid), which also has its own anti-inflammatory effect, is beneficial.

Magnesium citrate: 500 mg daily, less if having diarrhea. Reduces inflammation and also is important for cellular energy; shown to be helpful in alleviating fatigue.

N-acetylcysteine (NAC): 500–650 mg daily for three to six months.

Revitalizing Sleep Formula:: 1–4 caps at bedtime. www.vitality101.com.

Colds

If you've got a cold (infectious nasopharyngitis), you've got an infection of the upper respiratory tract. About 35 percent of colds are caused by rhinoviruses, from the Greek word *rhin*, meaning "nose." When the immune system battles this type of viral infection, it produces the all-too-familiar symptoms of sore throat, nasal congestion, runny nose, watery eyes, hacking cough, and sometimes fever. The average American adult suffers two to three colds a year; the average young child has as many as nine. Unlike colds, flu symptoms begin abruptly and may include headache, chills, muscle aches, fatigue, high fever, cough, and runny nose.

The traditional prescription for colds and flu involves rest, fluids, and aspirin or acetaminophen. Antibiotics are of little use, since they target bacteria. Antibiotics also often lower susceptibility and your immune response because they also kill the healthy bacteria. Often, though, doctors prescribe an antibiotic before knowing whether it's a viral or bacterial infection. Natural remedies like herbs and vitamins, though, can help a cold.

Immune-Boosting Herbs

Herbs that boost your immune system, like echinacea or purple coneflower (you may have this lovely flower in your garden), can be a boon when you have the sniffles. Used at the first sign of a cold, echinacea taken in tea or dried herb form may help you get over a cold faster, make the symptoms milder, or stop a cold before it starts. One way we think echinacea works is by boosting levels of a naturally occurring chemical in the body known as properdin, which helps our cells resist infection. A 2002 study in the medical journal *Alternative Medical Review* showed that certain echinachea extracts of E. purpurea and E. angustifolia, and larch arabinogalactan extracted from Larix occidentalis, increased properdin production by 21 percent. Echinacea may also stimulate the immune system into increased actions, perhaps by acting as a threat. For this reason, echinacea is not recommended for those with autoimmune diseases such as Hashimoto's Thyroiditis, Graves' disease, type 1 diabetes, and multiple sclerosis.

natural news

Taking echinacea at the first sign of a cold can help reduce symptoms, say University of Alberta researchers in a study published in the *Journal of Clinical Pharmalogical Therapy* in 2004. A group of 282 volunteers, aged 18–65, who usually had two or more colds a year took echinacea at the first sign of a cold for a total of seven days. Researchers tracked symptoms through a scoring system. The results? Volunteers who took echinacea experienced 23 percent lower symptom scores that those who did not.

Goldenseal

Often echinacea and goldenseal are taken together, giving your immune system a jump-start and making it stronger to battle infection. What makes goldenseal so special? Thanks to the alkaloid berberine, this member of the buttercup family is an immune system booster, with natural antibacterial and antiviral properties. Berberine from the stems or roots of the goldenseal plant "wakes up" or activates white blood cells known as macrophages so they can destroy viruses like those found in the common cold. Goldenseal's properties can also be soothing to mucous membranes, which is just the ticket when you have the sniffles. Several studies have also shown it can be effective in treating diarrhea. For best effect, take a standardized goldenseal extract. You'll find this at your favorite health food store.

natural news

Native American tribes such as the Iroquois and Cherokee first showed American settlers how to use goldenseal to treat skin diseases and ulcers. Goldenseal also made a fashion statement way back when. Native Americans used it as a dye for clothing. Look out, *Project Runway!*

Astragalus

When you want to get good mojo going, think astragalus or, in Chinese, *huang qi*, for "yellow energy." Practitioners of traditional Chinese medicine use it to balance the vital energy, or qi, thought to flow through all beings. So it makes sense that astragalus is often used to shorten the duration of a cold and flu. Studies in China have shown it to be effective when used as a preventive measure against the common cold.

Garlic

Sure, garlic is great when you're cooking, but did you know it's also antiviral, antibacterial, and antimicrobial? Garlic contains allicin, which helps support your immune system and relieve cold woes, too. It's an expectorant, so it helps to bring up mucous. It's also a diaphoretic, so when you have a cold, it increases the sweating process. It does thin the blood, so if you're taking a blood thinner, check with your health practitioner first.

Ginseng

Native to China and Korea, Asian ginseng (Panex Ginseng) is packed with natural chemical compounds with medicinal properties known as ginsenosides that boost and strengthen immunity. A key herb in Chinese medicine for over 2,000 years, ginseng is also called "man root" because of its shape. Research shows that ginseng can improve concentration, as well as enable you to think more clearly. If you have type 2 diabetes, ginseng may also help by lowering blood sugar levels. Check with your doctor before using it.

Elderberry

You may know about elderberry wine, but did you know that the blue-black berries of the elderberry shrub have been used for centuries in Europe for treating colds and flu? That's because elderberries provide nutritional support for the immune system. Specifically, elderberries are chock-full of natural compounds called flavonoids, including quercetin, which are high in vitamin C and help strengthen the immune and respiratory systems. Since they have antiviral, antibiotic, and antibacterial qualities, when taken at the first sign of a cold, elderberry supplements may help reduce its length so you feel better faster.

Ginger

Ginger is known as the warming herb. And if you've ever chewed on spicy candied ginger from the health food store, you know why! Its gentle warming sensation is soothing for digestive upset like nausea, but it also is a go-to herb for cold relief. That's because ginger root is immune boosting and antiviral. It also contains natural compounds known as gingerols and shogaols that can help ease coughing and relax you—just the thing to encourage healing. Traditional practitioners of Chinese medicine believe the warming effects of ginger can help sweat out the cold virus. Try a nice cup of ginger tea and see how much better it makes you feel.

Vitamin C

In the 1960s, vitamins were widely thought to be good for only preventing vitamin-deficiency diseases like scurvy. In 1970, Nobel Prize winner Dr. Linus Pauling, a chemist and biochemist, wrote the book *Vitamin C and the Common Cold*, advancing the view that vitamin C could help prevent and treat cold and flu. Since then, there has been much controversy over whether vitamin C works to prevent or shorten a cold. But a meta-analysis (a statistical way of combining results) of 30 studies done by the Cochrane Database Systematic Review in 2004 found that vitamin C supplementation decreased the duration of colds by 8 percent in adults and 14 percent in children. Most of the studies used a dose of 1 g a day.

How does vitamin C work? When it comes to colds, it helps reduce the amount of histamines that are released in the body, which can lead to symptoms like sneezing and that runny nose. Vitamin C is also a powerful antioxidant, which means it battles free radicals, a byproduct of our metabolism that can damage healthy cells. We don't make our own vitamin C, and we can't store it in our bodies, either. You need to replenish it on a daily basis. Fortunately, you can find vitamin C in some of your favorite foods, like oranges, grapefruit, sweet red peppers (yes, you heard that right!), those leafy greens, and strawberries. Avoid orange juices when you have a cold, though, as they are filled with natural sugars that can contribute to mucous production.

Ah, Aromatherapy!

Holistic aromatherapist Jade Shutes, B.A., Diploma AT, and founder of the East West School for Herbal and Aromatic Studies in Willow Spring, North Carolina, recommends these soothing treatments for colds:

Sea salt bath for colds:

1. In a glass bowl, combine 2 cups fine sea salt or Epsom salts with 5 drops rosemary, 4 drops eucalyptus globulus or radiata (E. radiata for children or adolescents), and 2 drops lemon.

2. Fill a bath with warm or hot water, add the sea salt blend, and immediately get into the bath.

3. Swish water to break down salts and move essential oils around.

Massage oil for colds:

1 oz. sunflower or apricot kernel vegetable oil

6 drops rosemary oil

4 drops peppermint oil

3 drops ginger oil

4 drops lemon oil

Mix all oils and rub on the chest, upper back, neck, and shoulders. Apply in the morning and evening or as needed throughout the day.

Steam inhalation:

1. Bring 4 cups water to a boil. Remove from stove and place 2 drops eucalyptus, 1 drop rosemary, and 1 drop lemon into the water.

2. Place a towel over your head and stand over a bowl of steaming water.

3. Breathe in through the nose and out through the mouth. Be sure to close your eyes while doing this, to avoid eye irritation.

Natural R$_x$

Astragalus: For prevention; 300 mg twice daily.

Echinacea tea: 1 TB. per cup of water, 3 cups a day. Capsules and tablets: 200 mg twice daily for a maximum of two weeks.

Elderberry tonic/tea: 1 TB. per cup of water, 3 cups daily. High in vitamin C; stops spread of the cold virus; acts as a diaphoretic, increasing the sweating process; also decreases inflammation and sinus congestion.

Garlic: Eat two or three cloves daily. An antioxidant; contains allicin, an antibiotic, antiviral, antibacterial, and antimicrobial; an expectorant and diaphoretic; increases the sweating process.

Ginger: 300 mg twice daily, in capsule form. An antioxidant and antiviral; relieves cold symptoms, reduces pain and fever, and suppresses coughing; has a mild sedative effect.

Ginseng: 100 mg daily. Improves overall health and vitality; boosts energy; combats the physical effects of stress; empowers the immune system.

Goldenseal: 100 mg three times daily for a maximum of two weeks, in capsule and tablet form. Immune stimulating; works well with echinacea.

Selenium: 200 mcg daily. An antioxidant; deficiency results in depressed immune function.

Vitamin C: 200–3,000 mg daily in divided doses. An antioxidant; preventive for colds and flu; reduces histamine release.

Zinc: 15–50 mg daily. Important trace element for immune function; inhibits the cold virus.

Constipation

When you can't go when you need to go, you're constipated. Being constipated means the body isn't able rid itself of the end products of digestion. This can lead to toxins building up in your system and leave you feeling tired, headachy, and gassy. For women, constipation can even be a risk factor for breast cancer. According to a study published in the medical journal *Lancet*, women who were severely constipated and had fewer than two bowel movements a week had 4.5 times the risk of precancerous breast changes, compared to women who had one or more bowel movements per day.

Why You Can't Go

From a natural perspective, the health of the digestive tract in large measure determines the health of the body as a whole. Let's face it, if you aren't digesting, absorbing, and eliminating correctly, something is off. This can affect your overall immunity and health in the long run, and in the short run leave you with constipation. One of the reasons you may be constipated is a lack of fiber. If you don't have enough fiber in your diet, you don't "go" as often as you should, and waste products and residual toxins begin to build up in the body. Slow transit time also reduces the body's ability to absorb valuable nutrients it needs.

Constipation can also be caused by eating too many processed foods, junk foods, and foods with preservatives, additives, hormones, and artificial flavors and colors. When we consume alcohol, caffeine, and smoke, it also increases the toxic load in the body.

What's Normal?

At the very least, you should be visiting the bathroom one time a day to—well, you know. But ideally, say naturopathic doctors, you should go two to three times a day. (Many traditional doctors use three times a week as a goal for patients!) But if you've been going only two to three times a week, any improvement is a step in the right direction.

Typical Causes of Constipation

Constipation can be caused by a poor diet, not enough water, certain meds, or a lifestyle as a couch potato. As we've said, one of the biggest reasons people have difficulty having bowel movements is a lack of fiber, so one of the simplest ways to "move things along" is to increase your intake. The minimum you need is 25 g a day of fiber, but most Americans get 10 to 12 g, says Brenda Watson, a naturopathic doctor, Certified Nutritional Consultant, and author of *The Fiber 35 Diet*. "Often people equate frequency going to the bathroom with having enough fiber, and it doesn't necessarily mean that. Typically, they go in for their colonoscopy and find they have *diverticulosis*."

def•i•ni•tion

Diverticulosis occurs when you have small pouches that bulge outward through weak spots in the colon wall. Each pouch is called a diverticulum. Pouches (plural) are called diverticula. Most people with diverticulosis do not have any discomfort or symptoms. However, symptoms may include mild cramps, bloating, and constipation.

Other things, like travel, can disrupt bathroom schedules. "Typically we block it out mentally because we don't have time to go," says Dr. Watson. "So a lot of it is psychological or mental."

Improve Transit Time with Fiber

When we eat enough fiber, it improves the amount of time it takes for food to go from point A to point B in the body. "Fiber pushes undigested food through the large intestine," says Robert S. Harris, N.D., a naturopathic doctor who practices in Frankfort, New York, is also a member of the adjunct faculty in biological science at Herkimer County Community College in Herkimer, New York. "A meal should never stay in the digestive system more than 24 hours."

How does fiber work? In the simplest terms, it acts as a bulking agent that gets the ball rolling so to speak, a process known as peristalsis. When this happens, waste products and toxins are moved out of the body.

To improve your fiber intake, aim for 25 g to start and work up to 35, says Dr. Watson. "Start reading labels. As a rule of thumb, don't eat any whole grain like bread or a wrap that doesn't have more than 3 g of fiber." Wheat and oat bran are also both helpful forms of fiber. But start with small amounts so you don't overwhelm your system. You'll want to drink more fluids, too, because fiber absorbs water.

Cooked and raw cruciferous vegetables like broccoli, cabbage, and cauliflower contain fiber, too. Just recently, New Zealand researchers found that broccoli sprout extracts help prevent bladder cancer in animals (*Cancer Research*, 2008). Apples contain pectin, a type of fiber that can also help get things moving. For more information, visit www.fiber35.com.

Fiber Supplements

Often psyllium is the bulk-forming laxative of choice when it comes to constipation. According to a study in the medical journal *Phytomedicine* (2008), psyllium husks are also therapeutic for mild to moderately elevated cholesterol. Psyllium's soluble fiber or mucilage accounts for its medicinal action; just add water and psyllium seeds swell to more than 10 times their original size, become gelatinous, and help move things along more easily. (Think of those toys that say "just add water"!) A study in the medical journal *Gut* proved psyllium's effectiveness, with over 82 percent of respondents who had irritable bowel syndrome finding significant relief.

But for some, over-the-counter fiber supplements that contain psyllium are too harsh. Beverly Yates, N.D., founder of the Naturopathic Family Health Clinic in Mill Valley, California, suggests a more gentle approach, like flax seeds. "They're much less irritating," says Dr. Yates. "Not only do they act as a bulking agent as they pass through the intestine and absorb water, but flax seeds also contain nutritive oils that nourish the lining of the gut from the mouth to the anus, and help lubricate the stool and make it easier to pass. You have a much better chance of getting into a normal bowel-elimination pattern three or four times a day."

You can purchase fresh flax seeds and a grinder for $15 to $20 at most health food stores. Put the seeds in the grinder, push the button, and count to 10. When you lift the top, you'll have nice, fluffy flax seeds that smell great. Then go wild! You can put them on anything—toast, salads, vegetables—or mix them up with salad dressing.

Herbal Help and Other Handy Remedies

One of the most common herbal laxatives, cascara sagrada helps ease constipation and restore bowel tone, thanks to compounds called anthraquinones, which have laxative effects. Cascara sagrada has a long history of use by Native Americans. Commission E, the expert panel that evaluates herbal medicines for the German counterpart of the FDA, endorses it as a safe, effective laxative.

Senna: The leaves and pods of the senna plant, like cascara sagrada, also contain anthraquinones. Senna is an FDA-approved nonprescription drug for adults and children ages 2 and older. You can take it as a capsule, tablet, or liquid extract.

Aloe: Taking aloe latex orally can help, too. Aloe is soothing for the skin on the outside as well as on the inside, says Dr. Yates, because the effects of the anthraquinones (you'll also find them in cascara sagrada and senna) in the aloe. You can take a teaspoon of aloe juice with water.

risky remedy!

Don't use cascara sagrada for more than two weeks. Also don't use it if you have an ulcer, ulcerative colitis, Crohn's disease, irritable bowel syndrome, hemorrhoids, or other gastrointestinal conditions, or if you are pregnant.

Apple cider vinegar: Dr. Yates also often has her older patients take a teaspoon or two of apple cider vinegar in water or lemon, orange, or grapefruit juice—anything acidic—because they often lack enough stomach acid for proper digestion.

Fennel and vervain: Fennel can be helpful for indigestion, gas pains, irritable bowel syndrome, and infant colic. The herb vervain also has a mild laxative effect, but if you have heart disease, high blood pressure, diabetes, or asthma, consult a physician before using it.

Omega-3 essential fatty acids: People don't typically think of essential fatty acids for constipation, but they can be a boon if you suffer from it. High-quality fish oil such as cod liver oil (a good brand is Nordic Naturals) and flaxseed oil supplements can be excellent additions to your regimen. You can add flaxseed oil to yogurt, a smoothie, or salad dressing.

Magnesium: Magnesium can be a real help, says Dr. Yates. "Both cardiac tissue and the smooth muscle of the intestine need magnesium to be able to relax." People who have a spastic colon or who pass spaghetti-like feces (and don't have colon cancer) do not have relaxed intestines. "The stool should look like an imprint of the colon," says Dr. Yates.

Water: Drink lots of water, all day, every day, and when you eat flax seeds, drink extra glasses, please. Most people who are chronically constipated just don't drink enough water, says Dr. Yates. Aim for a half-ounce of water per pound of weight. To make it simple, cut your weight in half; that's how many ounces of water you need to drink every day.

natural news

When you have a bowel movement, use a step to bring your knees up so you are in more of a squatting position. A specially designed stepstool called the Life Step fits under the toilet. When you sit on the toilet, you just pull it out and put your feet on it, to get into a squatting position. For more information, visit www.renewlife.com.

Detoxify the Body

If you tend to be constipated, Dr. Watson suggests you try a whole-body herbal cleanse two times a year to help your system detoxify by stimulating the liver to release toxins into the gallbladder and then into the gut. The cleanse lasts 15 to 30 days. During this time, cut back on processed foods and up your intake of fruits and vegetables and fiber, too, like flax and oats. Be sure to drink plenty of water as well. You can also try a daily multicleanse to support the channels of elimination, or dandelion, ginger, and chamomile detoxifying teas. You'll find whole-body cleanses, daily multicleanses, detoxifying teas, and fiber supplements at the health food store. Another idea? Take a sauna to help flush out toxins.

natural news

Exercise is one of the best ways to relieve and prevent constipation. "We are a society that still does not exercise as much as we should," says Dr. Harris. "A lack of exercise leads to constipation. Movement of the abdominal muscles helps to cause the rhythmic peristalsis that is responsible for moving food through the intestinal tract." Exercise also helps reduce stress. This is important because when the body is under stress, one of the systems it shuts down to handle what it perceives as an emergency is the gastrointestinal system.

Natural R_x

Aloe vera: 1 tsp. with water.

Apple cider vinegar: 1–2 tsp. in water.

Cascara sagrada: As directed.

Daily multicleanse: As directed. www.renewlife.com.

Flaxseed: Sprinkle on foods you like.

Magnesium: 300–700 mg.

Omega-3 essential fatty acids: 1,000 mg EPA/DHA.

Psyllium: As directed.

Senna: As directed.

Whole-body cleanse: As directed. www.renewlife.com or WBCleanse. com

Depression

Being depressed is a lot more than just having an occasional bad day. It's like a rain cloud is following you around all the time, and the sun seems like a distant memory. Depression not only affects your mood; it also affects the thoughts you have in your head, the way you act, and even how well you feel physically. You may have trouble sleeping or getting out of bed in the morning. You may overeat or not feel like eating. For the one million Americans who suffer from depression, it can also mean that the things that used to interest you and elevate you from the mundane no longer bring you joy.

When depression is really severe, it can lead to thoughts of suicide because you just want "out." But this is never a solution, because depression will pass with the proper course of treatment. Sometimes natural remedies can be a helpful adjunct. In fact, according to a study done at Harvard Medical School and published in *Understanding Depression*, more than half of people who have depression or anxiety use alternative medicine therapies.

Reasons You May Be Blue

Depression can be caused by many things, often by major life changes. Perhaps you lost a loved one, a job, or your house. Maybe your finances are in turmoil. It's important to keep in mind that everyone is different. This means that what may cause you to be depressed may not affect someone else. *This is okay.*

Do you have a relative who suffers from depression? This wouldn't be unusual, as depression tends to run in families. If you have an undiagnosed medical condition like hypothyroidism (not enough thyroid hormone—see the chapter on thyroid disorders), this can cause depression. So can chronic fatigue syndrome and fibromyalgia, because you can't be as active as you used to be. You have to look closely on the medical circulars that come with certain prescription medicines but many of these, particularly beta blockers, can cause depression.

Also, if you aren't eating right and don't have enough vitamin B_{12} or omega-3 essential fatty acids, this can totally affect how you feel. "Nutrition influences the structure and the function of the brain, and often we lack the vitamins and minerals we need to operate the machinery of the brain effectively," says Alan Logan, N.D., author of *The Brain Diet* and an invited faculty member of Harvard Medical School's Mind-Body Institute. "Depending on your genetic susceptibilities, it can present itself as depression now, and later in life as conditions like Alzheimer's disease. Science is now showing that nutrition can influence whether you get a condition and the degree to which you get a condition."

Getting Happier: Nutrients You Need

We know that good fats are important for the brain. This is because the brain, command central for everything we think, see, and do, is more than 50 percent fat. This is why omega-3 fatty acids are so important: they enable the neurons to operate at tip-top shape, helping them to communicate so we can think clearly and feel well. When we don't have enough omega-3 fatty acids, this can lead to depression.

Eating fish and seafood can help banish the blues because they are naturally chock-full of omega-3 essential fatty acids. Go for coldwater fish like cod, salmon, and mackerel for the best benefit. Or you can take fish oil supplements, particularly eicosapentaenoic acid (EPA), to improve the effectiveness of antidepressant medications. A good brand is Nordic Naturals. You should include other nutrients as well, says Dr. Logan, "Folic acid, B_{12}, selenium, and zinc are linked with depression, and all of them influence omega-3, so they're probably the most important nutrients someone should consider taking in dealing with depressive symptoms, from a nutritional standpoint."

St. John's Wort

You'll find it in every health food store. That's because one of the most popular natural remedies for depression is the herb St. John's wort (Hypericum perforatum). Many find that it can be helpful, especially if they don't experience relief from their depression or don't like the side effects from their prescription meds (like dry mouth, nausea, headache, or effects on sexual function or sleep). St. John's wort also costs less than many antidepressant medications, and you can get it without a prescription. You can take St. John's wort in capsules, teas, and extracts.

St. John's wort has been studied extensively in Germany and is widely used in Europe for mild to moderate depression. One of its mechanisms is thought to be similar to selective serotonin reuptake inhibitor antidepressant drugs, or SSRIs, such as Prozac. St. John's wort helps prevent nerve cells in the brain from reabsorbing serotonin, a brain chemical that helps us feel happier. In one German clinical study, 66.6 percent of patients with mild to moderate depression found relief when taking a 300 mg dosage of standardized St. John's wort extract (0.125 percent hypericin content) three times daily (Fortschr Med 1993). New research now suggests that a St. John's wort supplement taken once a day may be as effective as the prescription drug sertraline (Zoloft) for people with mild to moderate depression. Unlike sertraline, St. John's wort didn't affect sleep or sexual function.

dial your doc

If you are taking any prescribed medications, check with your doctor before switching to St. John's wort, to avoid the risk that the depression will worsen. (Suicide is always a risk when it comes to depression.) Another important reason is that, when you take St. John's wort, half of all prescribed medications, including birth-control pills, will be eliminated in your body much more quickly because it speeds up your metabolism. Also, don't take St. John's wort with other antidepressants. Furthermore, St. John's wort interacts with certain drugs used to control HIV infection, anticancer drugs, and drugs that help prevent organ rejection, and it can also make you more sensitive to sunlight.

SAM-e

Give S-adenosylmethionine, or SAM-e ("sammy"), a gold star when it comes to treating depression. "SAM-e is arguably the supplement with the highest level of evidence to support its use in the treatment of depressive symptoms," says Dr. Logan. "A number of controlled trials have shown that both oral and intravenous SAM-e is of value in the treatment of depression."

We can find SAME-e in every cell. This clever compound helps alleviate the blues by increasing our stockpile of the feel-good brain chemical serotonin and dopamine, a hormone-like substance that affects our ability to experience the good (pleasure) and the bad (pain). When you take SAM-e as a supplement, you boost the levels of both of these substances, and this helps to ease depression.

Ginkgo Biloba

If you have an AARP card, check out ginkgo biloba for depression. Used in combination with other herbs, it may give you the lift you need. That's because ginkgo biloba improves circulation—blood flow to the brain—which can help to elevate mood (it may help improve memory, too). Ginkgo biloba also assists in preserving omega-3 fatty acid levels, which we know is beneficial. You can easily take it in supplement form.

Folic Acid

As we've seen before, the nutrient folic acid can influence your mood. If you don't have enough, you're more likely to be depressed. "People who have the lowest levels of folic acid are the least likely to do well with talk therapy or prescription antidepressant drug therapy. The same thing is true for B$_{12}$," says Dr. Logan. "Studies show that folic acid improves the effectiveness and lowers the side effects of antidepressant medications."

Ah, Aromatherapy!

Holistic aromatherapist Jade Shutes, B.A., Diploma AT, recommends these remedies to soothe mild depression:

Uplifting massage blend:

> 1 oz. sunflower or apricot kernel vegetable oil

> 6 drops bergamot oil (Citrus bergamia)

4 drops clary sage oil (Salvia sclarea)

2 drops neroli oil (Citrus aurantium)

Blend all ingredients and use as a massage oil.

Rejuvenating bath:

3 drops ylang ylang oil

2 drops clary sage oil

5 drops sweet orange oil

Combine ingredients with ½ cup milk or 1 tablespoon of honey. Add to the water once you are in the bath. Relax and enjoy.

natural news

When researchers at Boston University School of Medicine and McLean Hospital asked volunteers to hit their yoga mats, they found that practicing yoga produced increased GABA (gamma-aminobutyric) levels, which can help ease depression and anxiety. The effect for volunteers was similar to treatment with antidepressants. This doesn't mean you should throw away your pills or cancel that therapy appointment, but yoga might be a useful adjunct to what you are using now.

Flower Power

Bach Flower Remedies are made from a "sun tea" of specific wildflowers or trees known for their healing properties, then diluted (similar to homeopathic remedies, in that regard). Nancy Buono, a Bach Foundation Registered Practitioner (BFRP) and the director of Bach Flower Education, suggests adding two drops of the chosen remedy to a glass of water or juice and sipping it at intervals. You can also place two drops of each remedy into a 1-oz. dropper bottle filled three quarters with spring water. You can combine up to six or seven remedies in your treatment bottle. (If you choose Rescue Remedy as part of your formula, it counts as one remedy and you would use four drops.) If desired, you may add a teaspoon of brandy, apple cider vinegar, or vegetable glycerin as a preservative.

The personal formula should be taken by mouth a minimum of four times daily, four drops each time, especially in the morning and before retiring. If a person is unable to swallow or is alcohol-sensitive, apply the remedies externally by moistening the lips, wrists, and/or temples, or use in an atomizer or tub of water. The remedies are available at local health food shops and online at www.bachremedystory.com. The following indications for each of these remedies will give you a better idea of which one might be best for you.

Behavior	Bach Flower Remedy
Have recently lost a loved one, been in an accident, had surgery, or received some very bad news, and, as a result, have lost interest in life	**Star of Bethlehem,** to console and comfort
Feel hopeless, as if there is nothing that can be done to change or improve the situation (an illness, a bad relationship, a job, and so on)	**Gorse,** to restore hope and brightness
Feel self-hatred or self-disgust	**Crab Apple,** to relieve embarrassment and boost self-esteem
Discouraged when there is too much to do and it is not humanly possible to accomplish it all	**Elm,** to reduce overwhelmed feeling and restore confidence
Feel disinterested and apathetic; gliding through life	**Wild Rose,** to restore enthusiasm and interest

The Healing Touch of Craniosacral Therapy

Developed in the 1970s by osteopathic physician and surgeon John E. Upledger, craniosacral therapy is designed to release restrictions in the membranes that surround and protect the brain and spinal cord so the central nervous system can perform at optimum efficiency. The craniosacral system consists of the membranes and cerebrospinal fluid that surround and protect the brain and spinal cord; it extends from the bones of the skull, face, and mouth (cranium) down to the tailbone area (sacrum).

Craniosacral therapy is performed while you lie on a massage or treatment table, and lasts 15 minutes to one hour. Using a light touch, the practitioner tests for restrictions in the craniosacral system by monitoring the rhythm of the cerebrospinal fluid as it flows through the system. By using techniques to release restrictions, the practitioner helps your body heal itself.

All is revealed in craniosacral therapy. Physical, mental, *and* emotional stresses can be reflected in the body and will show up in the tissue for practitioners to evaluate. Because of this, craniosacral therapy can also help restore emotional balance. To find a craniosacral practitioner near you and for more information, visit the Upledger Institute at www. upledger.com.

natural news

Research shows that acupuncture is a promising treatment for depression in women, who are more prone to depression. A study at the University of Arizona with 38 women with mild to moderate depression showed that, after 12 sessions, 70 percent of women experienced at least a 50 percent reduction in symptoms. These results are comparable to the success rate of psychotherapy and medication.

Emotional Freedom Techniques

Okay, we admit that it sounds a little out there, but it just might work for you. Basically, Emotional Freedom Techniques (EFT) is a psychotherapeutic treatment based on a theory that you feel depressed because you have unresolved emotional issues that are disturbing the body's energy field. To get rid of these disturbances, a practitioner taps on energy meridian points (think of it as a kind of acupressure) to release negative emotions and bring the body back into balance. It's a kind of healing touch. If you think EFT could be helpful for you, visit www. emofree.com for more information.

Seasonal Affective Disorder

Sometimes winter seems to drag on forever. For those with seasonal affective disorder (SAD), this can be a real problem. That's because when the days get shorter, it means less light, and less light can lead to depression, oversleeping, and fatigue, even though you aren't doing much. Not to fear, natural remedies are here!

Moving Toward the Light

Since lack of exposure to sunlight seems to be a key cause of SAD, light therapy can make a huge difference in your mood. Using both a full-spectrum light box and a dawn simulator can help by giving you a dose of sunshine. Using, say, a light box while you read, means sunlight exposure for your pineal gland. This stimulates serotonin and melatonin production and vitamin D. A dawn simulator (a small computer that allows you to turn any table lamp into a simulated dawn or dusk used with opaque blinds) is timed and progressive, so a light slowly gets brighter over a programmed period of time. Think of it as a natural alarm clock! Visit www.lighttherapyproducts.com to find these products.

Using Nutrients to Treat SAD

First, take a look at what you are eating. Chances are, because you're feeling blah, you are taking in lots of sugar, simple carbs, and caffeine to get you going. This may give you a temporary burst of energy, but eventually you will end up more tired than you were before. Instead, choose foods that keep your blood sugar stable (this is important if you suffer from depression), like proteins, complex carbohydrates, whole grains (which also contain vitamins B_6 and B_{12}, which are important for brain health), vegetables (green leafies have folic acid), and fruit. Try not to let yourself get too hungry, either. This means eating every two to three hours, eating three regular meals, and then snacking in between on healthy foods like low-fat mozzarella sticks, cashew nuts, or sunflower seeds. Combining protein and a complex carbohydrate is very effective at stabilizing blood sugar, so a whole-wheat cracker with cheese or peanut butter is a good choice, provided that you don't have any allergies.

Focus on Tryptophan

Be sure to include foods and snacks with tryptophans in them, since folks with SAD tend to be tryptophan deficient. Why is tryptophan important? We need it to make serotonin, that feel-good brain chemical. Tryptophan foods to choose include turkey, chicken, tuna, soybeans, shrimp, and salmon.

Get Your Vitamin D

When you sit in the sun, your body goes to work manufacturing vitamin D. But in the winter months, when you aren't getting enough sun time, you may not be getting enough vitamin D. No worries—taking a supplement can help boost the activity of neurotransmitters in your noodle. A good choice is Nordic Naturals Arctic-D Cod Liver Oil Omega-3 with Vitamin D. This way, you get your vitamin D and your omega-3! For more information, visit www.nordicnaturals.com.

dial your doc

Dietary changes and dietary supplements are not a substitute for proper evaluation and mental health care. If depression is not adequately treated, it can become severe and, in some cases, may be associated with suicide. Consult a mental health professional if you or someone you care about may be experiencing depression.

Natural R$_x$

5-Hydroxytryptophan (5-HTP): 50–100 mg three times daily with meals. Can help ease SAD and depression; take in spray or pill form; do not take with Prozac (fluxotine) or mix with antidepressants.

Folic acid: 800 mcg.

Gamma-aminobutyric acid: GABA. As directed. Good for depression, especially if it's connected with anxiety.

Ginkgo biloba: 240 mg daily. May give you the boost you need—can improve blood flow to the brain and can help preserve omega-3 fatty acid levels.

Melatonin: 1–3 mg. Small doses of this hormone may help if you have trouble sleeping due to SAD—if you feel too groggy, reduce your dose.

Omega-3 fatty acids: 1,000–3,000 mg. Important for optimum brain function.

SAM-e: 800 mg daily.

Selenium: 200 mcg. The antioxidant in the diet that protects the brain and influences energy levels; studies show that lower levels can influence your mood.

St. John's wort: 900 mg daily. Can also help alleviate the symptoms of SAD; do not take with antidepressants.

Valerian tincture: ½ tsp., 40 drops, or 2.5 mL. Capsules and tablets: 250–400 mg.

Vitamin B6: 50–100 mg.

Vitamin B12: 1,000 mcg. Low levels have been found in people with depression.

Vitamin D: 1,000 IU.

Zinc: 15–50 mg. Research shows that 25 mg on top of antidepressants significantly improves depression.

Diabetes

If you have diabetes, your body has trouble with insulin, the big "I." Insulin is a hormone released by the pancreas in response to increased levels of blood glucose, or blood sugar—the main sugar found in blood and the body's main source of energy. Insulin's number-one job is to take glucose from the blood into the cells.

Diabetes comes in two types, type 1 and type 2. If you have type 1 diabetes, your pancreas no longer makes insulin, so you need to take insulin to get the glucose you need. If you have type 2 diabetes, the most common form of diabetes (more than 15 million folks in the United States have it), either you don't produce enough insulin or your cells are what we call *insulin resistant*, which prevents the insulin from getting to them. Often type 2 diabetes can be controlled with healthy eating and exercise.

def•i•ni•tion

Insulin resistant means that the insulin your pancreas produces has trouble connecting with fat and muscle cells to let glucose inside and produce energy. The more overweight you are, the more fat hinders the way insulin works in the body. The good news is any weight loss, even 10 or 20 pounds—can reduce your risk of diabetes.

How Diet Plays a Part

Diet is essential for diabetes when it comes to both controlling blood sugar and helping you maintain a healthy weight. One of the simplest places to start is with breakfast. According to the May 2008 issue of the *Harvard Heart Letter*, eating breakfast reduces your risk for diabetes, heart attack, stroke, and heart failure—especially if it includes a whole-grain cereal like steel-cut oatmeal; or a whole-grain English muffin with, say, peanut butter; or a smoothie with added oat bran, ground flax seeds, or wheat germ.

Fill Up Your Tank

Have you ever noticed that when you eat breakfast, you are less hungry throughout the day? This can keep us from overeating and gaining weight. Studies also show that when we eat breakfast, it keeps our blood sugar and insulin more stable. When we get off to a good start by having breakfast, it also helps reduce levels of LDL, or so-called "bad" cholesterol and triglycerides.

Refuel on These Foods

To help stabilize your glucose levels and insulin production, throughout the day, never let yourself get too hungry. You may want to have three main meals and three mini-meals or snacks to keep your energy up and blood sugar stable. When you choose foods, opt for low-fat dairy and protein, beans, and more whole grains (brown rice, multigrain bread). Include in your routine a half-cup to a cup a day of fruits and vegetables that are high in bioflavonoids (nutrients with antioxidant properties) like blueberries, grapefruit, red grapes, cherries, strawberries, oranges, cranberries, blue plums, black currants, onions, and raspberries, too. This will also help protect your vision, something that is especially important for diabetics. Eating two to three cloves of raw garlic and ½ cup of onions daily can also help regulate blood sugar.

Friendly Fiber

We've already seen how whole grains with fiber can get us off to a good start with breakfast, but it's just as important to add fiber throughout the day, says Beverly Yates, N.D., founder of the Naturopathic Family Health Clinic in Mill Valley, California, and author of *Heart Health for Black Women*. "When you have meals with fiber and snacks with fiber, it helps the regulation of glucose and keeps it even in the blood stream." This means you'll avoid symptoms like brain fog, sexual dysfunction, and peripheral neuropathy, where you can't feel your fingers or toes. Fiber and exercise together not only help keep blood sugar stable, but also make the insulin you do have work better.

Stabilize Blood Sugar with Yogurt

If you have type 2 diabetes, it can be smart to add low-sugar, fermented, soy-based blueberry yogurt to your diet on a regular basis. According to University of Massachusetts Amherst researchers, soy yogurt and fruit both contain phytochemicals that help moderate blood glucose levels by slowing the way sugar is taken into our cells. Together, soy yogurt and fruit block the enzymes known as alpha-amylase and alpha-glucosidase, which trigger absorption of glucose by the small intestine. Type 2 diabetes medicines work in the same way. Because of this, you avoid sugar spikes. The phytochemicals in soy and fruit are also potent antioxidants, which are important because diabetics need protection from free radical damage even more than most folks.

Researchers at Massachusetts Amherst also recently found that red wine and black tea are helpful in keeping blood sugar stable if you have type 2 diabetes. Both red wine and tea contain antioxidant compounds known as polyphenolics that inhibit alpha-glucosidase, which slows the passage of carbohydrates into the bloodstream. Like soy and blueberries, wine and black tea contain potent antioxidants, an added benefit.

natural news

The Nurses' Health Studies (Part I was established in 1976, Part II in 1989) were developed by organizations such as Harvard Medical School and the Brigham and Women's Hospital to track more than 120,000 female nurses for risk factors for diseases. One of their findings? The risk of developing diabetes triples if your diet is full of products that produce inflammation in the body, like regular and diet soda, refined grains (white rice and bread), and processed (deli) meats.

Stabilize Blood Sugar with Exercise

Exercise makes your body use fat and glucose more efficiently. By staying lean and exercising every day, you'll improve insulin sensitivity and your body will be better able to regulate blood sugar levels. When you exercise regularly, you're also likely to be in a better mood, have a better outlook on life, and keep your commitment to your health day after day. "If you have diabetes, exercise is your friend," says Dr. Yates. "It makes the glucose-insulin mechanisms more efficient and helps keep the blood sugar levels even. Try to exercise every day of the week, if you can." Ideally, it's best to exercise more intensely for one hour five times a week and then do something gentler, like walking, three times a week.

Try Tai Chi

You may want to try tai chi, a new study in the *British Journal of Sports Medicine* suggests. Those who engaged in this Chinese martial art practice that combines breathing and movement benefited from better blood glucose levels and blood glucose metabolism. Another study showed that practicing tai chi and qigong together for 12 weeks produced improvements in blood glucose levels and blood pressure. These practices like yoga also have the added benefit of stress reduction and of mind-body effects like strengthening of the immune system. The program also helped them have more energy and sleep better, too.

Flex Your Muscles

Weight training can also help metabolism by ensuring that you burn fat rather than store it. So if your body is not particularly efficient at managing glucose and tends to be more efficient at making fat, weight training discourages that phenomenon. (This is why some diabetics tend to be thin, while others tend to put on weight.) It's best for energy management and glucose regulation to exercise at the same time of the day every day. You may want to do it first thing in the morning or when you finish work.

Type 1 Diabetes: A Note About Early-Morning Exercise

One caveat if you have type 1 diabetes is that you may experience what's known as rebound phenomenon upon waking in the morning. This means your blood sugar may not be stable enough for exercise. In this case, says Dr. Yates, eat a small meal first. "Afterward, do a finger stick with a glucometer to make sure you've got enough energy. If you do, go ahead and exercise." If you have type 2 diabetes, go ahead and exercise first.

natural news

Trans fats, which are made by adding hydrogen to vegetable oil to increase shelf life (a process known as hydrogenation), interfere with insulin function and also raise LDL, or so-called bad cholesterol. You'll find trans fats in veggie shortenings, margarine, and many hard-to-resist foods, like cookies, cakes, crackers, and other snack foods. "Trans fats just make everything sticky," says Dr. Yates. "If you've got an issue with insulin function, the last thing you need to do is gum up the cell wall with trans fats and set yourself up for heart disease." Cutting down on processed foods and limiting your fat intake is a good practice for preventing diabetes and heart disease.

Supplemental Help

Herbal and nutritional supplements can strengthen the response to insulin and bring down blood glucose levels. Studies have found that antioxidants such as vitamins C and E can reduce insulin resistance, and milk thistle extract has a similar effect. Antioxidants from herbs such as bilberry and other nutrients are also important because high blood sugar levels in people with diabetes increase the oxidative damage to cells, leading to diabetic complications such as neuropathy (numbness of the hands, legs, and feet) and retinopathy (damage to the eyes).

Milk thistle: Milk thistle seeds are high in antioxidants and known for their ability to promote detoxification and prevent damage to the liver from toxins and viruses. But did you know they can also help control blood sugar? A study published in the medical journal *Phytotherapy Research* showed that when people with type 2 diabetes were given 200 mg three times a day of silymarin, a milk thistle extract, average fasting blood glucose level (measures your blood sugar [glucose] level after you have not eaten for at least eight hours) fell 15 percent. Since this herb is low cost and safe, it may be a good addition to your daily regimen.

natural news

When you have type 2 diabetes, you double your risk for high blood pressure. The good news is, research shows that taking zinc sulfate, magnesium oxide, and vitamins C and E can help reduce that number.

Gymnema sylvestre: A traditional treatment for diabetes in India, the herb Gymnema sylvestre is good herbal therapy when it comes to blood sugar control. That's because this woody, vinelike herb with yellow flowers helps stimulate insulin secretion. This means your body can use insulin more effectively.

Fenugreek: Studies have also shown that the herb fenugreek (the name is Latin for "Greek hay") can also help make cells more receptive to insulin and, in turn, lower blood sugar levels, thanks to phytochemical compounds in the leaves. The plant is also a good source of fiber. Fenugreek is used extensively in ayurvedic cooking. If you are interested in using Gymnema sylvestre or fenugreek to treat your diabetes, it's best to talk to a nutritionally oriented health practitioner for guidance.

natural news

Gotta have that cup of coffee? It may be a good thing, according to the recent Nurses Health Study II. Drinking a moderate amount of either caffeinated or decaf coffee may lower type 2 diabetes risk for middle-aged and younger women (ages 26 to 46). Researchers still aren't sure which compound in coffee is responsible for the benefit.

Chromium and Vanadium: Chromium picolinate and Vanadium are two minerals that you may want to consider using. "They help bind insulin to the wall of the cell membrane," says Dr. Yates. "This is important because it enables insulin to be more effective at grabbing glucose out of the bloodstream." Chromium can also help you resist that cookie, as it can ease sugar cravings.

Bitter melon (Momordica charantia): Also known as balsam pear, this unripe fruit has been used extensively in folk medicine as a remedy for diabetes. "It helps make the insulin receptors more sensitive," says Dr. Yates. "It also helps lessen insulin resistance." It's available primarily at Asian grocery stores, as well as in a supplement.

dial your doc

If you'd like to use chromium picolinate supplements, check with your health practitioner first. High doses can be dangerous.

Aloe vera: Got an aloe vera plant on your window sill? Let it be your inspiration. Some cultures in the world use aloe vera juice from the dried inner leaves of this plant to lower fasting blood glucose levels. Studies show that aloe vera gel may be useful to help wound healing in diabetics.

Alpha lipoic acid: This antioxidant is your ace in the hole for preventing nerve dysfunction and maintaining a healthy nervous system, says Dr. Yates. Antioxidants are especially important when it comes to diabetes because, as we said, this condition creates a great amount of free-radical damage. Research published in the medical journal *Diabetes Care* in 2006 showed the effectiveness of using 600 mg once daily of alpha lipoic acid over five weeks to treat diabetic neuropathy (burning pain, tingling, and numbness).

dial your doc

If you are a type 1 diabetic, it's especially important to exercise caution when you begin supplementation. So start with low doses and regulate your blood sugar. "It's easy to get on autopilot and stop using your glucometer," says Dr. Yates. "But if you're going to add supplements, nutraceuticals, and herbs, you have to be scientific so you don't overdo it. Some of these things have a profound effect on the body, and you don't want to bottom out and have a crash." If you have any questions or concerns, it's best to work with a nutritionally oriented doctor, a naturopathic physician, or a certified nutritionist.

Natural R~x~

Aloe vera gel: 1 TB. Use topically for wound care.

Alpha lipoic acid: 600 mg.

American ginseng: 3 g two hours before a meal. Research shows it improves fasting blood glucose levels.

Bilberry: 100 mg three times daily.

Bitter melon, balsam pear (Momordica charantia): 50–100 mg; build from there to curb your craving for sweets. Be vigilant about monitoring your blood sugar while taking this supplement.

Capsaicin cream: Active component of cayenne pepper. Studies show topical application may relieve pain of diabetic neuropathy.

Chromium: Start with 200 mcg and work up, depending on how you feel.

Fenugreek (trigonella foenum graecum): Start with 200–300 mg. Part of ayurverdic treatment, used extensively in cooking; helps make cells more receptive to insulin; research shows it may help glycemic control in type 2 diabetes.

Ginkgo biloba: 40–80 mg three times daily. Effective in treating diabetic retinopathy and neuropathy.

Gymnema sylvester: 100 mg twice daily. Makes cells more insulin sensitive. Be vigilant about monitoring your blood sugar while you are taking this supplement.

Holy basil (basil leaf): As recommended by your practitioner. Research shows it may improve fasting blood glucose levels.

Magnesium: 300–700 mg daily.

Milk thistle: 200 mg three times daily.

Multivitamin and mineral: As directed.

Panax ginseng: 200 mg daily. Research shows that it can improve fasting blood glucose levels.

Vanadium: 25 mcg to start; can build up to 100 mcg daily.

Vitamin C: 500-2,000 mg daily in divided doses.

Vitamin E: 400–800 IU daily.

Zinc: 15–50 mg daily.

Diarrhea

You hope it doesn't happen when you're at a concert, on a train or plane, or at the movies, because when you really need to go, you don't want to wait in line. If you're human (and since you're reading this book, we assume you are!), you've had a bout or two of diarrhea. Usually diarrhea is mild and lasts a few days. Diarrhea can be caused by bacteria, an infection, or an overgrowth of yeast or parasites. Or it can be the result of antibiotics, laxatives, inflammatory bowel disease, improper absorption of food, food poisoning, food allergies, or stress.

Depletion Dangers

The main dangers diarrhea poses to the body are dehydration, mineral or electrolyte imbalance, nutrition deficiencies (because of improper absorption), and weight loss. If diarrhea is severe and prolonged, where loss of important electrolytes such as sodium, potassium, and magnesium becomes problematic, it's often recommended to replace them with sports drinks like Gatorade for adults and Pedia Lyte for kids. For most mild cases of diarrhea, broths such as chicken stock and miso (soy), along with water and diluted vegetable juice (avoid sugar, as it will loosen the stool further), will work just fine.

Bringing the Body Back into Balance

If you swing between diarrhea and constipation, you probably have a food sensitivity issue. The most common food sensitivities are wheat, dairy, corn, eggs, soy, peanuts, sugar, and caffeine. Using an elimination diet can help: you stop eating what you suspect are offending foods for two weeks and evaluate whether your condition improves.

But many people find it's tough to give up wheat. That's because a lot of the bacteria you develop is the result of a yeast overgrowth in the digestive tract, says Brenda Watson, N.D., C.N.C. and author of *The Fiber35 Diet: Nature's Weight Loss Secret.* "Yeast is an organism that likes simple carbohydrates, sugar, or bread. So you set up a yearning for them to be fed. When you stop eating the bread, it's like they are saying, 'Feed me!'" Initially, when you stop eating bread and sugar, you'll experience a yeast die-off. But this lasts for only three or four days, and then you'll begin to feel better.

Foods that may help relieve diarrhea include bananas, rice, applesauce, tea, and toast, what is referred to as the BRATT diet, an acronym for those foods. Antibacterial herbs bayberry, chamomile, gentian, goldenseal, Oregon grape, and wormwood in any combination as a tea or tincture can also help. Chamomile tea can sometimes relieve cramps and gas, and colostrum can be very helpful in severe cases of diarrhea.

natural news

Is something bugging you? It's not uncommon, says Dr. Watson, for people to have diarrhea with flulike symptoms caused by parasites. "The diarrhea is the body's attempt to send the parasites packing, but when that doesn't work, the body settles into a kind of symbiosis with the invader. If you have ongoing, chronic diarrhea that comes and goes, you should probably be tested. The best way to be sure is to have a stool analysis from either the Doctor's Data Lab in Chicago or The Institute of Parasitic Diseases in Tempe, Arizona.

Remedies for Relief

To help stop a bout of diarrhea, Dr. Watson has a home remedy that can bring you some relief. Simply boil brown rice (double the amount of water—if it's 2 cups, make it 4), add a little bit of sea salt, and then drink the liquid. "Brown rice has B vitamins, so it's a very good nutrient. It's very good for you when you have diarrhea." Bouillon broths can also be soothing. Avoid juices or drinks with sugar because this will loosen the stool. Adults and children alike can also take DiarEASE. Find it at www.renewlife.com/Natural/.

Activated charcoal capsules can also be a big help. Think of them like a big sponge. When you have diarrhea, your bowel is irritated and has a lot of negative bacteria. Charcoal acts like a sponge that soaks up the negative bacteria and makes your stool harder. You can find charcoal capsules at your local health food store.

dial your doc

Since diarrhea is a symptom, you should see a health care practitioner to determine the cause if it lasts longer than two days.

If your diarrhea is a result of food poisoning, it's a good idea to add a probiotic as well, so the good bacteria will fight off the negative bacteria. Look for a probiotic that is half bifidus, because that's the bacteria that's most prevalent in the colon. Aim for 50 billion units. Check the label before you buy; if it's over one year old, find a newer brand.

Natural R_x

Acidophillus bifidus multilayered pearls: 50 billion

Antibacterial herbs in tincture: bayberry, chamomile, gentian, goldenseal, Oregon grape, and wormwood: ½ tsp., 40 drops, or 2.5 mL.

Chamomile tea: 1 TB. per cup of water, 4 cups a day.

Charcoal in capsule form: Warning! Don't use charcoal briquettes! 520–975 mg after each meal and up to 5 g per day.

Colostrum: As directed.

DiarEASE: As directed.

Ear Infections

Kids and ear infections seem to go hand in hand, kind of like peanut butter and jelly. The infection or inflammation of the middle ear is officially known as otitis media. The inflammation often begins when viral or bacterial infections that cause sore throats, colds, or other respiratory or breathing problems spread to the middle ear. Antibiotics are often the treatment of choice by doctors, but if the infection is caused by a virus or allergy, antibiotics will be of little use. For this reason, it can make sense to consider your "natural" options as well. These remedies can help you treat your child's discomfort and speed healing.

Allergy Connection

To get to the root of chronic ear infections, think allergies, says Deborah Wiancek, N.D., a naturopathic doctor whose practice, the Riverwalk Natural Health Clinic, is in Colorado's Vail Valley. "The number-one cause for kids is dairy products, which leads to mucus, which leads to constant runny noses," says Dr. Wiancek. "When kids lie down, the mucus drains into the ears and stays there, and they are more likely to get ear infections." So one of the first steps she takes is having patients eliminate dairy to eliminate the mucus buildup.

Herbal Help

For pain, Dr. Wiancek recommends garlic oil and mullein drops, five drops in each ear twice a day. (You need to do both ears because infections can travel from one ear to the other.) "The garlic is a natural antibiotic and it kills bacteria, and the mullein is an anti-inflammatory that will help stop the pain and help the healing process," she says. "It's really soothing. It's definitely better to use them together." You can get these premixed at health food stores. You may also want to try Otikon Otic Solution. A study in the medical journal *Archives of Pediatrics & Adolescent Medicine* in 2001 showed that children with ear infections who received Otikon Otic Solution, which is an olive oil solution with herbal extracts of calendula, mullein, garlic, and St. John's wort, experienced as much pain relief as from medicated ear drops.

natural news

A study in the medical journal *Pediatrics* (2003) showed that Naturopathic Herbal Extract Ear Drops (NHED), which contain allium sativum, verbascum thapsus, calendula flores, hypericum perfoliatum, lavender, and vitamin E in olive oil, may be beneficial in treating ear infections (using five drops three times daily).

The Healing Power of Homeopathy

Homeopathy, the principle of "like treating like" can work well for ear infections. The practice of homeopathy aims to stimulate the body's own healing responses by giving extremely small (and quite safe) doses of substances that produce symptoms of illness when given in larger doses. The homeopathic remedy Aconite is recommended for throbbing ear pain that develops quickly after exposure to cold air. Chamomile works well with ear infections associated with teething.

Hot and Cold Remedy

Hydrotherapy can soothe earache pain, too, says Dr. Wiancek. Here's how to do it:

1. Put a warm towel, compress, or heating pad on the ear for five minutes.

2. Then put a cold compress on the ear for one minute.

3. Do this three to five times in a row, and always end with the cold. This drains and soothes the ear.

Important Nutrients

Beta carotene, a form of vitamin A, fortifies the immune system and can help prevent ear infections. (Check with your child's health care practitioner for the appropriate dose.) Flaxseed oil can also be helpful to boost immunity: a teaspoon for kids and a tablespoon for adults can do the trick. If kids are prone to ear infections, they can keep taking these two nutrients, beta carotene and flaxseed oil, for a month.

dial your doc

Be aware that natural remedies are not a substitute for proper medical care. According to the National Institutes of Health, if your child has these symptoms of a possible ear infection, call your doctor: unusual irritability, difficulty sleeping, tugging or pulling at one or both ears, fever, fluid draining from the ear, loss of balance, unresponsiveness to quiet sounds, or other signs of hearing difficulty, such as sitting too close to the television or being inattentive.

Natural R~x~

Beta carotene: Children, consult doctor for dose; adults, 50,000 IU.

Flaxseed oil: Children, 1 tsp.; adults, 1 TB.

Homeopathic Aconite: As directed.

Homeopathic Chamomile: As directed.

Multivitamin and mineral: As directed.

Naturopathic Herbal Extract Ear Drops (NHED): As directed.

Otikon Otic Solution: As directed.

Vitamin C: Children, 500 mg; adults, 3,000 mg in divided doses; good for the immune system; antiviral.

Zinc: Children, 15 mg; adults, 15–50 mg; antiviral.

Eczema

If you've got dry, hot, itchy skin, you could be one of more than 15 million folks in the United States who have eczema. Although eczema is chronic, sometimes you have no symptoms at all. Other times the skin has what are known as "flare-ups," or times when the skin feels extremely itchy and uncomfortable. In more severe cases, the skin can become broken, raw, and bleeding. Forms of eczema include *allergic contact eczema*, *contact eczema*, and *seborrheic eczema*. People with eczema often have a personal or family history of allergic conditions like asthma or hay fever, but you can't "catch" it from someone else. There is currently no cure for eczema, but natural remedies can help ease symptoms.

def•i•ni•tion

Allergic contact eczema: This happens when your immune system reacts to something you've touched, like poison ivy, and becomes inflamed.

Contact eczema: Your skin becomes irritated due to frequent contact with a normally harmless substance, like laundry detergent.

Seborrheic eczema: The inflamed skin is yellow, oily, and scaly. Dandruff is an example of seborrheic eczema.

Check Your Home and Diet

To treat the cause of eczema, you have to know what is creating it, says Barbara Close, the author of *Organic Beauty Basics* and the founder of Naturopathica in East Hampton, New York. So become a detective in your own home. Check out your surroundings. Are you using a new laundry detergent? Have you recently switched cleaning products? Or maybe you are wearing new clothes. If the detergent, cleaning products, or fabric don't agree with you, all of these "irritants" can potentially cause an eczema flare-up.

Next, it's important to look internally to eliminate triggers. Close suggests a two-week cleansing diet, eliminating offending foods and beverages like caffeine, dairy products, wheat, processed foods, sugar, and alcohol. Other top allergen triggers? Peanuts, soy, eggs, and fish. Foods high in saturated fats like red meat and fried foods can also trigger inflammation, which can aggravate eczema. To cool off your skin, it's wise to switch to a whole-foods diet with whole grains, lean protein, and lots of fruits and veggies.

You'll also want to include coldwater fish (avoid it if you're allergic) that are high in omega-3 essential fatty acids, like salmon or mackerel, because these will also lower the inflammation response in the skin. According to a 2008 study in the medical journal *Current Opinion in Clinical Nutrition and Metabolic Care*, when pregnant women supplemented with fish oil, it helped to decrease their children's allergy sensitivities. Be sure to supplement with a fish oil that has been screened for contaminants, especially if you are pregnant. Nordic Naturals (www.nordicnaturals.com) has stringent safety testing.

Keeping a food diary can help you identify which foods cause eczema flare-ups. People who suffer from migraine headaches often do the same thing to identify foods that trigger headaches.

dial your doc

Several different types of eczema exist, with very different causes and treatments. As a first step, it's important to get a correct diagnosis. See your health care practitioner, who should refer you to a dermatologist for further diagnosis and treatment.

Skin-Cooling Herbs

In addition to cleaning up your diet, it's important to reduce the heat in the body, says Close. She recommends calendula as a hydrating, cooling herb that can calm eczema. "It's one of the best herbs you can use." You can find a calendula hydrating cream at www.naturopathica.com.

Close also recommends German chamomile essential oil diluted into a serum for inflamed or aggravated skin conditions to reduce inflammation and speed wound healing.

1. Fill a ½-ounce glass bottle halfway with a vegetable oil such as hazelnut oil.

2. Add 5 drops of German Chamomile essential oil, cover, and shake well.

3. Top off with hazelnut oil, cover, and agitate a second time.

4. Apply three to four drops to a moist cotton pad and wipe over damp skin.

You can find excellent essential oils at Floracopeia (www.floracopeia. com) and at many health food stores. Close also recommends evening primrose or black current oil to help soothe itching.

Soothing "Baths"

Want to soothe dry and inflamed skin? Think of breakfast cereal—specifically, oatmeal. An oatmeal bath soothes "hot" skin because it contains a compound called oat beta-glucan, which forms a gel that helps to hold moisture in the skin. Here's how Close suggests you take an oatmeal bath:

1. Put ½ cup of rolled oats inside a washcloth.

2. Tie it off with a rubber band

3. Fill the sink with warm water.

natural news

Epsom salts, sea salts, and sulfur bath salts can all help relieve the symptoms of eczema. Just add them to your tub and enjoy!

4. Place the washcloth with the oats in the water, and squeeze the ball to create oat milk.

5. Splash the milk over your face and hands. You can also use it as a poultice and apply it directly wherever you need it.

Maintain Moisture

One mistake people with eczema often make is to overwash their skin, says Valori Treloar, M.D., CNS, the co-author of *The Clear Skin Diet.* "Soap and hot water strip the protective oils off the surface of your skin, which serve as a barrier to the evaporation of moisture." Dr. Treloar advocates minimal soap use. "Soap is harsh and irritating. You need it in the armpits, in the groin, and on the feet, but unless you've played touch football in the mud, then you don't need soap all over. Use nonsoap cleansers, like milky cleansers, instead. If you get out of the shower and you feel dry, you are overusing soap or you're not getting your moisturizer on soon enough."

For a natural moisturizer the next time you step out of the shower (especially in the winter, when humidity is minimal), consider applying food-quality organic extra-virgin olive oil or coconut oil after you towel off, while your skin is still moist. "The advantage to these oils is, you are putting a film on top of the water," says Dr. Treloar, whose practice, Integrative Dermatology, is in Newton, Massachusetts. "They also have bioflavonoid antioxidant-type molecules in them that are wonderful for your skin." Even these natural products can cause an allergic reaction in some people. If you experience stinging, burning or itching after application, you may be allergic and should wash it off promptly. Pay attention to the humidity level in your environment, too, says Dr. Treloar. The optimal level is 35 to 40 percent, and you can buy a hygrometer (a device for measuring humidity) to keep track. To increase moisture in your home in the winter, run a vaporizer or a fountain. In the summer, dehumidifying is important. Keeping the humidity around 40 to 50 percent will keep your skin more comfortable.

natural news

People who have eczema may be affected by allergens in the droppings of house dust mites. These mites like warm, moist environments and live in bedding, mattresses, curtains, and carpets. Reducing the number of house dust mites in the home may improve the condition of your skin. Dr. Treloar suggests these guidelines to help clear out your environment:

- ◆ Go for Asian or Scandinavian decor (no rugs, no overstuffed furniture, no heavy drapes).
- ◆ Clean bedding regularly.
- ◆ Cover mattresses and pillows.
- ◆ Clean kids' stuffed animals on a regular basis.
- ◆ Vacuum regularly.
- ◆ Make it a practice to damp dust.

Ah, Aromatherapy!

Holistic aromatherapist Jade Shutes, B.A., Diploma AT, recommends this aromatherapy remedy for eczema:

Skin-Soothing Salve

1. Place ¼ cup calendula and ¼ cup sunflower oil (or use a combination of vegetable or herbal oils) with ½ ounce beeswax.

2. Melt down in a double boiler at medium temperature. Stir often to ensure the merging of oils with the beeswax.

3. Remove from the stove and add to small glass jars (usually 1 to 2 ounces).

4. In another salve jar, add the following:

   10 drops lavender
   4 drops German chamomile
   4 drops helichrysum

5. Add the oil mixture to each salve jar. Each jar should have 30 to 40 drops of combined essential oils.

6. Put the lid on the jars and shake; then let stand until hardened. Once hardened, the salve is ready for use.

Apply the salve to the eczema two to three times a day or as needed to reduce inflammation and itchiness.

Note: Test the consistency of a salve before blending it with other essential oils by placing a spoonful of the salve in the refrigerator. Allow the salve to harden. If the salve comes out too hard or thick, you can melt the mixture down again and add more oil. If the salve is too fluid or thin, you can melt it down and mix in some more beeswax. Experiment with different herbal oils or infusions, and notice how and when the consistency differs. By working with herbal oils, you can increase the potential therapeutic benefits of the salve.

natural news

Eczema can also be stress related, so it's important to learn ways to relieve tension and relax. One of the most useful relaxation tools is called biofeedback, a practice that uses your mind to improve your health by controlling involuntary body responses such as brain activity, blood pressure, muscle tension, and heart rate. A new do-it-yourself bio-feedback program, called Healing Rhythms, created by Deepak Chopra and Andrew Weil, M.D., can be helpful for stress reduction and relaxation. Learn more about it at www.wilddivine.com.

Natural R$_x$

Black currant oil: 500 mg twice daily.

Burdock root (Arctium lappa): Apply topically as directed. Anti-inflammatory.

Calendula: Apply topically as directed.

Evening primrose oil: 1 TB. daily.

German chamomile (Matricaria recutita): Apply topically as directed. Essential oil.

Goldenrod (Solidago virgaurea): 1,000 mg. Apply topically. Anti-inflammatory; wound-healing properties.

Omega-3 essential fatty acids: www.nordicnaturals.com. 1,000 mg.

Red clover (Trifolium pratense): Apply topically; anti-inflammatory properties.

Rhus toxicodendron homeopathic remedy: As directed.

Endometriosis

Endometriosis is a common health problem for women, but it can cause uncommon problems, like infertility, severe pain, and fatigue. It's a condition in which tissue similar to that in the uterus is found elsewhere, especially in the abdominal cavity, leading to abdominal pain, pelvic pain, and very heavy periods. Monthly hormonal surges also produce extra tissue growth in the ovaries and fallopian tubes, which results in inflammation and scarring. Over time, this scarring blocks the ovaries and fallopian tubes and leads to infertility. Thirty to 40 percent of women with endometriosis are estimated to be infertile.

We don't know for sure what causes endometriosis. Heredity may play a part (research shows that having a first-degree relative with endometriosis can up your risk) and so may a dysfunctional immune system. Some believe it may be due to metaplasia, which means the ability of one type of normal tissue to change to another and replace it—in this case, outside the uterus. Naturopathic experts believe that exposure to environmental estrogens, such as byproducts of synthetic chemicals, can cause an imbalance in estrogen that can lead to endometriosis. Environmental estrogens are often referred to as *endocrine* disruptors because of their ability to affect endocrine function when humans and animals are exposed to them.

def•i•ni•tion

The **endocrine** system includes the thyroid, the pituitary gland, and the reproductive organs. The endocrine glands secrete, produce, and store hormones to regulate metabolism, growth, mood, and functions of various tissues.

Endometriosis is made worse by estrogen, so conventional treatment involves gonadotropin-releasing hormone agents (GnRH), which are hormones that actually suppress the ovaries' estrogen production and stop ovulation. GnRH agonists, a group of drugs that have been used to treat endometriosis for over 20 years, come in monthly injections, daily injection, and nasal sprays. It usually takes about four to eight weeks for women to notice an improvement in symptoms. Unfortunately, side effects of this treatment can include hot flashes, vaginal dryness, and irregular vaginal bleeding. Severe cases of endo-metriosis may need surgery, but natural remedies can bring relief.

How Diet Can Make a Difference

From a naturopathic perspective, endometriosis is caused by too much estrogen in the body—estrogen tells cells to proliferate. Changing what you eat by reducing red meat and dairy products that are filled with hormones can help, says Deborah Wiancek, N.D., a naturopathic doctor whose practice, the Riverwalk Natural Health Clinic, is in Colorado's Vail Valley. "Red meats and dairy products are two main causes, so you want to reduce these in your diet or go organic so it has no hormones. Use organic dairy, too."

Strike Oil

Adding plants like those found in flaxseed oil, which contain estrogens that are much less potent than synthetic estrogens such as those given in Hormone Replacement Therapy (HRT), is also very good for reduc-ing estrogen in the body. Flaxseed oil helps reduce cramps because it's anti-inflammatory. You need to take it every day because it may take a month to see a difference. Borage oil, evening primrose oil, and black currant oil can also help reduce inflammation in the body.

Tap the Power of Phytoestrogens

Agatha M. Thrash, M.D., the co-founder of the Uchee Pines Lifestyle Center in Seale, Alabama, says a diet high in plants with estrogens or phytoestrogens has helped many of her clients with endometriosis. That's because plant estrogens bind to the estrogen receptor sites in the body, blocking excess estrogen produced by the body. Plant estrogens are also easier for the body to eliminate. So it's smart to include apples, cherries, olives, plums, wheat germ, whole grains, carrots, peanuts, dried

natural news

If you have endome-triosis, it's important to avoid sugar as much as pos-sible because it can increase inflammation around the uterus and make cramping worse. For this reason, you'll also want to eliminate caf-feine and alcohol.

beans and peas, yams, bell peppers, eggplant, potatoes, tomatoes, parsley, sage, clover, alfalfa leaf tea, licorice root tea, red raspberry leaf tea, food yeast, garlic, anise seed, coconut, and nuts.

The Function of Fiber

Including fiber in your diet is essential because it helps to move excess estrogen out of the body, which, in turn, eases the symptoms of endometriosis. To this end, you'll want to put these high-in-fiber veggies on your shopping list: broccoli, cabbage, and Brussels sprouts. Other good sources? Oat bran, nuts, seeds, flaxseed, psyllium seed husks, pears, apples, dried beans, and legumes.

Soy Wonderful

Soy can regulate hormones and help with cramping, too. Add it in your diet as food sources, like tofu, soy milk, soy nuts, and soy nut butter as snacks.

natural news

Since women with endometriosis have too much estrogen and not enough progesterone, striking a balance with natural progesterone creams may help, says Holly Lucille, N.D., author of *Creating and Maintaining Balance: A Woman's Guide to Safe, Natural Hormone Health.* "Use it for just three months at a time while you work on your diet, exercise, and adding nutrients." One brand of progesterone cream, called Progest, is natural and paraben free. For more information, visit www.emerita.com.

Herbal Health

Herbs can ease the symptoms of endometriosis, like cramping, and prevent scar tissue buildup. Dr. Wiancek recommends a combination tincture of red clover, wild yam, cranberry bark, red raspberry, and motherwort. You can find them at your local health food store as a Menstrual Cramp Formula to ease endometriosis. Antioxidants like vitamin E and grape seed extract can help prevent scar tissue buildup, too.

Dr. Thrash recommends this tea for endometriosis. Make it fresh daily:

1. Boil 3 cups of water.

2. Add 1 teaspoon black cohosh, ¼ teaspoon licorice powder, and 1 teaspoon ginseng. Gently boil for 30 minutes.

2. Add 3 teaspoons catnip tea, 3 teaspoons red raspberry leaf, 1 teaspoon alfalfa leaf, and 1 teaspoon hops.

3. Steep for 30 minutes, then strain.

4. Drink 3 cups daily.

Enhance Liver Function

Lipotropics, compounds that help break down and metabolize fat in the body, can enhance liver function and promote detoxification. "Lipotropics help endometriosis by getting extra estrogen and toxins out of the body, which, in turn, relieves symptoms," says Dr. Lucille. Lipotropics include choline, a B vitamin, and methionine, which promotes the flow of fat and bile. Use dandelion root, too, one of the most detoxifying herbs; it works in the liver and the gall bladder to remove waste products from the body. Dr. Lucille advocates making your beverage your medicine. Why not have a nice cup of dandelion tea?

Add a Multivitamin and Mineral Supplement

It's also a good idea to take a good multivitamin that contains vitamins C and E, beta carotene, and selenium to cover all your nutritional needs when you have endometriosis. Dr. Lucille likes Enzymatic Therapy's Doctor's Choice for Women multivitamin and mineral. It also contains angus castus, or chaste tree, which is helpful for hormonal balance because it increases the levels of progesterone while reducing the levels of estrogen. Shifting this balance can help relieve the symptoms of endometriosis. Visit www.enzy.com for more information.

natural news _____

A study published in the *Journal of Reproductive Medicine* shows that a natural antioxidant and anti-inflammatory plant extract from the bark of the maritime pine tree in France significantly relieved symptoms of endometriosis by 33 percent. (Previous studies have shown a reduction in menstrual cramps and pain in 73 percent of women following administration of 30 mg of Pycnogenol a day for one month.) The extract not only reduced pain and spasm, but it also improved the overall function of the reproductive system and the body in general. In addition, five women became pregnant, which is remarkable because endometriosis is one of the main causes of infertility. For more information, visit www.pycnogenol. com.

Bust a Yoga Move

The Child's Pose in yoga can help ease the cramps of endometriosis. Here are instructions on how to do it from Stephen Hartman, the director of professional training and association at the Kripalu Center for Yoga & Health in Stockbridge, Massachusetts:

1. Sit in Vajrasana (on your knees). Press down through the sitz bones and up through the crown.

2. Exhale, contracting the abdominal muscles. Hinge forward at the hips, extending the torso over the thighs. Bring the forehead toward the floor and extend the arms along the sides, palms up or down.

3. Breathe deeply and relax.

4. To release, exhale, engaging core stabilization. Inhale, raising the torso back to vertical.

The Child Pose offers these benefits for those with endometriosis:

◆ Increases flexibility in the hips and legs

◆ Massages, oxygenates, and decongests abdominal organs, improving peristaltic action

◆ Provides a counterstretch for backward-bending postures

◆ Helps relieve constipation and hemorrhoids

- ◆ Deeply tranquilizes the nervous system, calming the mind and emotions

- ◆ Puts the head below the heart, increasing blood flow to the brain and reducing the possibility of strokes and aneurisms

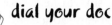

dial your doc

Your obstetrician/gynecologist (OB/GYN) has special training to diagnose and treat endometriosis. Your doctor likely will talk to you about your symptoms and health history, do a pelvic exam, and run tests, including an ultrasound, magnetic resonance imaging (MRI), and a laparoscopy and biopsy of the uterus to diagnose you.

Natural Rx

Black currant oil: 1 TB. daily.

Borage oil: 1 TB. daily.

Chaste tree (Agnus castus): As directed. Different brand formulations are available, including Agnoly and Femicur.

Choline lipotropic: 500–1,000 mg daily.

Dandelion root tincture: ½ tsp., 40 drops, or 2.5 mL three times daily. Tea: 1 TB. per cup of water, 3 cups daily.

Evening primrose oil: 1 TB. daily.

Flaxseed oil: 1 TB. daily.

Grape seed extract: 300 mg.

Menstrual Cramp Formula: As directed.

Methionine lipotropic: 500–2,000 mg daily. Should not be used by individuals with coronary heart disease and cancer.

Multivitamin and mineral: As directed. Enzymatic Therapy's Doctor's Choice for Women. www.enzy.com.

Omega-3 essential fatty oils: 1,000 mg daily.

Progest topical cream: As directed. www.emerita.com.

Vitamin E: 400–800 IU.

First Aid

Being prepared is the Boy Scout's motto, and it's a smart one. By keeping the right natural first-aid supplies on hand, you can reduce the discomfort of minor emergencies like burns, bruises, blisters, wounds, scrapes, insect stings, and more. Often one remedy has more than one use. Of these, lavender oil and Rescue Remedy are two of the best. (More about this dynamic duo in a minute!) Speaking of being prepared, it's a good idea to have a first-aid kit handy, so you'll want to keep one in the car, at home, and in the office. Of course, if a severe accident happens, see your health care professional immediately.

Burns

A burn is one of the most uncomfortable ailments you can have, which can lead to wrong-headed decisions in treating it. "A lot of people make the mistake of putting something on the burn right away, and it actually traps the heat in," says Brigitte Mars, A.H.G., author of *The Desktop Guide to Herbal Medicine*. "Instead, soak the inflected area in cold water. Don't use running water because it can further irritate the skin if the water pressure is high." Soak it until the pain of the burn is relieved.

Afterward, reach for your aloe vera plant and slice it open lengthwise. (You may have one on your windowsill—if not, you may want to get one!) Slather the gel over the burn. If you will be using a gel from the store, find one that is 100 percent aloe vera. Mars suggests using a salve that contains the healing herb calendula, vitamins A and E, beeswax, and St. John's wort, which can heal the skin because it has both antiviral and antibacterial properties. It's up to you, but you may feel more comfortable covering the burn with a light bandage to give it some protection. Finally, drink a lot of water, to help lower your inner thermometer.

Ah, Aromatherapy! For Burn Relief

Aromatherapy actually got its name after its founder, Rene Gattefosse, experienced burns due to a laboratory accident and applied lavender essential oil to treat them. You can do the same thing to help heal your own burns. First cool the burn with cold water and then apply lavender oil to it, says holistic aromatherapist Jade Shutes, B.A., Diploma AT. Continue to place drops of lavender on the burn throughout the day. Shutes also recommends applying the following therapeutic aloe vera gel base (there's the power of aloe vera again!) after the initial application of undiluted lavender:

1. In a 1-ounce salve jar, place 1 ounce aloe vera jelly with 10 drops lavender and 5 drops helichrysum.

2. Stir with the end of a spoon.

3. Apply salve to the burn site frequently throughout the day.

Ancient Chinese Secret

Some "Chinese Patent Medicines" work well for burns, according to Deborah Wiancek, N.D., a naturopathic physician whose practice, the Riverwalk Natural Health Clinic, is in Colorado's Vail Valley. "I use Jing Wan Tong salve. It's excellent for really bad burns. If you put it on as soon as possible, you won't have a scar." You can find Chinese Patent Herbal Formulas at Chinese pharmacies.

dial your doc

If the burn is severe—say, it covers more than 5 percent of the body or is still red and inflamed after a day or so—it's time to head to the emergency room or see your health care practitioner.

def•i•ni•tion

In **Chinese patent medicines**, each medicine is a specific combination of herbs. The word *patent* refers to the standardization of the formula. All Chinese patent medicines of the same name can be expected to have the same proportions of ingredients.

Cuts and Scrapes

When you get a cut or scrape, it's no fun. Taking steps to clean and help heal the wound will make it go away faster. Bleeding will help to cleanse a wound naturally, says Mars, but follow up with hydrogen peroxide at least initially to make sure all the dirt is removed. After that, switch to an antiseptic soap made out of lavender or tea tree oil so you don't destroy new cells that are trying to heal the wound. Disinfect with lavender oil afterward.

Finally, Mars suggests applying a good herbal salve with infection-fighting and healing properties like those that contain plantain, comfrey, or calendula, or antiseptic herbs such as echinacea, chaparral, golden seal, calendula, vitamin E, or lavender. Good brands include Burt's Bees and Herbal Ed's Salve by Herb Pharm. Cover the cut or scrape with a gauze bandage and tape so the wound can "breathe."

Homeopathic remedies for wounds include Hypericum (St. John's wort). "It's good for wounds where there are a lot of nerve endings, like the fingertips," says Mars. Use the homeopathic remedy Ledum for deep puncture wounds.

dial your doc

When you have a cut that is bleeding, it's important to apply pressure to the wound and to rest and elevate the area. You can also try applying Cayenne powder, says Nancy Eagles, a Chartered Herbalist whose website is www.inannaherbs.com. Of course, if the wound is bleeding uncontrollably and doesn't stop, see your doctor.

Bruises

When you get a bruise, nothing is better than arnica montana, a flower in the daisy family. "When you get bonked, however that happens, fibrin, a blood protein, forms at the site of the injury and that tends to cause bruising," says Mars. "When arnica is taken homeopathically or applied topically, it helps move fibrin, and swelling and inflammation are greatly minimized." You can even take arnica pellets after you have surgery or visit the dentist, to reduce bruising. Boiron, www.boiron. com, is a good brand for homeopathic arnica. Good brands of arnica oil include Weleda (the smell is fantastic!) and Peaceful Mountain. Arnica is not an herb to use as a tea or a tincture unless you see a professional herbalist. Don't apply arnica topically to broken skin.

Blisters

If you're breaking in a new pair of shoes or are just on your feet for too long, you can get a nasty blister. Your first step is to cleanse the area well with an antiseptic soap like lavender, echinacea, tea tree essential oil, or Dr. Bronner's peppermint soap. Next, Mars suggests disinfecting the wound with lavender essential oil, which is also anti-inflammatory. "Lavender reduces the risk of infection, reduces pain, and stimulates skin regeneration," says Mars. "During World War I, it was even used topically to treat gangrene."

Whether your blister is broken or unbroken, apply lavender oil three times a day, says Mars. Cover the blister with light gauze so air can circulate around the wound.

Toothache

One of the biggest nightmares is to have toothache strike in the middle of the night or while you are camping or on a trip. Although there is no substitute for seeing a dentist as soon as possible, these natural remedies from Eagles may help provide some comfort:

◆ Suck on a dried clove near the painful tooth.

◆ Put ½ teaspoon of Valerian herb tincture in a half glass of water and take it every half-hour.

Insect Bites and Bee Stings

If it's the first time you or your child has been stung by a bee and you are having trouble breathing or find your throat swelling up, seek help immediately! This is not the time to self-treat. People who know they are allergic to bees carry an Epi pen (an autoinjector of epinephrine, or adrenaline) for emergencies and seek immediate medical attention.

If you're not allergic, your first step is to remove the stinger. That's because the longer the stinger stays in your skin, the more venom is released, says Mars. You can remove the stinger with a credit card or tweezers. Next, wash the area and apply lavender or tea tree essential oil. Antifungal and antiviral, tea tree oil is a multipurpose antiseptic remedy you can apply to stings, mosquito bites, burns, cuts, rashes, and even sprains. You can even dab it onto pulse points on your neck (by your carotid artery) and wrists (radial artery) as an insect repellent. Once you are stung, it can help reduce itching and irritation, says Eagles. Just don't ingest it internally.

Mars also recommends a paste of apple cider vinegar and baking soda. In a pinch, you can apply mud because it has a very drawing effect. Leave it on as long as you like, and reapply as often as necessary. Another handy remedy for treating stings and bites, says Mars, is papaya (papain). (It's also used as a digestive aid.) Mars also likes Sting Stop, a homeopathic topical application that is good for a wide range of stings, from bees to wasps to mosquitoes. Or try Burt's Bees Bug Bite Relief. You can find both at health food stores and natural pharmacies.

For eensy-weensy spider bites, you can apply charcoal as a poultice by mixing the contents of a charcoal capsule with just enough water to moisten it and make a paste, says Mars. "Charcoal capsules are made of pure carbon from burnt wood and bones so they can absorb toxins." One charcoal capsule can absorb 40 times its weight, preventing poisons from entering the bloodstream. Leave it on as long as you like and reapply as often as necessary. Do not use charcoal briquettes, which contain petrochemicals!

Rescue Remedy

Finally, one of the best things to include in your natural first-aid kit is Bach's Rescue Remedy, a combination of flower essences, because it can help to calm you down when emergencies occur. Rescue Remedy contains Star of Bethlehem to ease trauma and shock, rock rose to relieve panic or terror, cherry plum to teach trust in one's own wisdom, impatiens for relieving stress, and clematis to bring clarity and alertness to the present moment.

You can take four drops of Rescue Remedy under the tongue or add the drops to a glass of water and sip it. You can also take it as a spray or as a pastille, which is a medicinal pill, or apply five drops of Rescue Remedy to a cloth and use it as a compress. You can find Rescue Remedy in any natural health food store or at www.rescueremedy.com.

Natural Rx

Along with the following items, keep Band-Aids, butterfly bandages, gauze pads, rolls of adhesive tape, and a small pair of scissors in your natural first-aid kit. Tweezers are good, too, for removing splinters, thorns, and other foreign objects.

Apple cider vinegar/baking soda: Apply topically.

Arnica homeopathic remedy: As directed.

Arnica montana essential oil: Apply topically.

Burt's Bees Res-Q Ointment: Apply topically. www.burtsbees.com.

Ching-wang-hong salve: Apply topically.

Cloves: As directed.

Dr. Bronner's peppermint soap: Wash topically. www.drbronner.com.

Echinacea *essential* oil: Apply topically.

Herbal Ed's Salve: Apply topically. www.herbaled.org; www.enatural-life.com.

Lavender essential oil: Apply topically.

Ledum homeopathic remedy: As directed.

Papaya powder: Apply topically.

Rescue Remedy: As directed.

St. John's wort homeopathic remedy: As directed.

Tea tree oil: Apply topically.

Valerian: As directed.

Flu

The flu is no fun, and 5 to 20 percent of us come down with it every flu season, which usually begins in January and can last as late as May. When you get the flu, it can feel like getting hit by a truck. The flu is an illness caused by the influenza virus that affects the respiratory tract. Unlike colds, flu symptoms of headache, chills, muscle aches, fatigue, high fever, cough, and runny nose begin suddenly. If you do get the flu, antibiotics are of little use, since they target bacteria. You also don't want to take them for the flu because antibiotics often lower susceptibility and your immune response, because they kill the healthy bacteria.

We all know that the flu is pretty darn contagious. That's why you can get the flu if someone who has the flu coughs or sneezes around you. If you touch a surface, like a grocery cart, telephone, or doorknob, that has been contaminated by someone who has the flu, you can get it that way, too. Exposure to cold, damp, wind, and rapid temperature change can also make us more susceptible.

Once you get "infected," you'll usually feel the symptoms pretty quickly, usually within one to four days. But be aware that you can spread the flu to others before your symptoms start and for another three to four days after your symptoms appear.

A good diet, exercise, enough sleep, and less stress all help the immune system stay strong and lessen your risk of catching the flu. But if you do catch it, natural remedies can help shorten the duration and ease your symptoms. Let's start with which foods to use and which to nix.

Foods to Embrace and Avoid

When you get the flu, you just can't beat one of the oldest and best natural cures around: chicken soup. "Every culture around the world has some version of chicken soup," says Beverly Yates, N.D., founder of the Naturopathic Family Health Clinic in Mill Valley, California. "Chicken broth seems to have medicinal benefits in part because of garlic, which is a powerful immune booster, and ginger, which is a warming herb." Chicken soup is also effective at easing congestion.

In fact, garlic contains several helpful compounds, including allicin, which acts as an herbal antibiotic and antibacterial. Garlic also dilates bronchioles (airways), improving congestion, while ginger improves circulation.

When you have the flu, you'll also want to "drink up"—that is, increase your intake of fluids to prevent dehydration. Include herbal teas in the mix too. Brigitte Mars, author of the *Desktop Guide to Herbal Medicine*, suggests reaching for lemon in hot water to ease your symptoms.

On the not-to-do list, avoid dairy, sugar, alcohol, and coffee, which promote more inflammation in the body. Avoiding dairy and sugar (including that in fruit juices) is also smart because it helps curb mucus production.

natural news

Like medicines, herbs have different properties. Knowing what each herb does can help you choose. For example, if you want to fight a virus and bacteria, you reach for an antiseptic herb, like echinacea. Although fever can help to fight infections, it can also be uncomfortable, so a febrifuges herb like elderberry, ginger, peppermint leaf, or boneset can help. So can diaphoretic herbs like lemon balm and yarrow because they increase perspiration. If you need help with a cough, instead of a cough syrup, you can reach for an antitussive herb, like elderberry (a versatile herb), nettle, and mullein.

Build Immunity

When you have the flu, your immunity is clearly not all it could or should be. Herbs like these can put your immune system on alert so you can feel better faster. Why not put a few of these in your natural medicine cabinet?

Echinacea

One of the go-to herbs to shorten the duration and severity of the flu is echinacea, which is like the carrot at the end of the stick when it comes to the immune system; it urges it into action to fend off bacteria and viruses. It does this by increasing white blood cell activity, or what is known as phagocytosis. Echinacea also works in the body to boost levels of a natural compound called properdin, which helps our cells resist infection. A study in the medical journal *Alternative Medicine Review* showed that treatment with two different species of Echinacea, E. purpurea and E. angustifolia, raised levels of properdin by 21 percent. Commission E, which is Germany's equivalent to our FDA, endorses echinacea to help ease symptoms and shorten the length of the flu.

natural news

Esberitox is super—a super-concentrated form of echinacea, that is. "Esberitox really helps chase the flu bug away," says Dr. Yates. "It can make a big difference." Esberitox comes in a convenient chewable tablet that contains Echinacea purpurea, Pallida (purple coneflower), Thuja (white cedar), and Baptisia (wild indigo). Although Echinacea doesn't cause auto-immune diseases, it can aggravate an existing condition. Don't take Esberitox if you are echinacea.

Echinacea and Goldenseal: Together Is Better

Echinacea and goldenseal, an herb with both antibacterial and antiviral compounds, are often used together to stimulate the immune system to activate white blood cells, to do more damage to invaders. This is thanks to the alkaloids in this buttercup-like flower known as berberine and hydrastine. Many studies show that echinacea and goldenseal shorten the duration of cold and flu. The Iroquois and Cherokee thought goldenseal was good medicine and used it to treat a variety of infections and other complaints. Interestingly, goldenseal got its name because the markings on its stem resemble wax seals that were used in times of yore to certify documents.

Elderberry

As we've seen, elderberry is a truly versatile herb. Also known as Sambucus nigra, this antiviral herb packed with flavonoids, including quercetin (more about this fabulous nutrient in a moment), has been used for hundreds of years in Europe to treat the flu (and colds, too.)

That's because it can shorten the time you spend in bed with the flu and make your symptoms more bearable, too. Its special compounds make you sweat, but in a good way, getting rid of nasty toxins and also decreasing inflammation, helping you to breathe easier and cough less.

In fact, in 2004, when patients with flu symptoms took a specific type of elderberry syrup, they recovered faster, according to a study in *The Journal of International Medical Research.* Here's how it worked. Researchers gave Sambucol, a patented elderberry compound, to volunteers four times a day for five days. After just one day, 20 percent of people felt relief from flu symptoms; 73 percent were feeling perkier by day two; and by day three, 90 percent felt like themselves again. By contrast, it took almost a week for the control group, who didn't take the Sambucol, to feel better. Pretty amazing, huh? You can find Sambucol patented extract at www.vitacost.com, CVS, or RiteAid.

Astragalus

For over 2,000 years, astragalus, an herb native to China, has been used to strengthen chi (the vital energy thought to flow through all beings) and the body's resistance to invading pathogens such as bacteria and viruses. In more practical terms, it wakes up the immune system and increases levels of white blood cells called macrophages, so it's more prepared to fight off viral and bacterial infections that cause the flu. This can help you feel better faster.

natural news

Flu can mean nausea. When this happens, make a nice cup of ginger tea. Not only will this "warming herb" soothe your overall symptoms, but it can ease that icky feeling, too. You can also take ginger in a candied form. Want to go really natural? You can get ginger mints from Newman's Own Organics, at your health food store, or visit www.newmansownorganics.com for more information.

Quercetin: Powerful Antioxidant Medicine

You'll find this superstar antioxidant plant compound in various fruits and veggies, including green tea, apples, and red onions. We say "superstar" because it is the first plant compound proven in a "gold standard" type of study: double-blind, randomized, placebo-controlled to actually help prevent us from getting sick from a virus. This, folks, is a big deal.

First, researchers at Appalachian State University asked 20 cyclists to bike vigorously three hours a day for three days, after taking a 1,000 mg dose of quercetin. (You and I probably eat 25 to 50 mg of quercetin in our food each day. Vegetarians get up to 250 mg!) They did this for three weeks. Then researchers asked cyclists to continue to take quercetin for two weeks after the study. The other 20 cyclists took what they thought was quercetin but was actually a placebo or a kind of sugar pill. The results? While nearly half of the cyclists who received the placebo got sick after their extreme sporting, only 5 percent in the quercetin group did. The antiviral effects were proven so strong that there is now talk of producing a "cocktail" of supplements that includes quercetin to help people cope with the flu virus.

natural news

Need to soothe sore throat pain? Brigitte Mars recommends a nice cup of licorice and marshmallow root tea, along with Osha root tincture, which also relieves congestion.

Medicinal Mushrooms

Medicinal mushrooms have been used traditionally for thousands of years to promote healthy immune system function. Many studies now validate the remarkable healing potential and therapeutic value of reishi, shiitake, and maitake mushrooms and their extracts, and the fact that they enhance immune system function. In addition, they may have antiviral and antibacterial properties. To boost your immunity to the flu, you can use them in a stir-fry or take them as a supplement. A good brand is Garden of Life.

Homeopathy Remedies

As soon as you feel run down and get that I'm-coming-down-with-the-flu feeling, it's time to reach for a favorite homeopathic medicine:

Oscillococcinum (Oscillo). That's because taking this compound early may help shorten your bout with the flu. Millions of people around the world swear by it. You may find it helps you, too. You can find Oscillo at your health food store.

Once you have the flu, you may want to choose Allium Cepa, which comes from the red onion, of all things. This makes sense when you think that it's used to ease symptoms like watery eyes. That's because homeopathic medicines use tiny amounts in a "like treats like" methodology. It also is helpful for a runny nose and a sore throat.

Ancient Chinese Secret

Patented Chinese formulas can also be taken at the first hint of the flu or a cold. For centuries, the Chinese have taken the formulation known as Yin Chiao, which contains ingredients like honeysuckle, peppermint, and Chinese licorice root. These ingredients and others work to benefit the chi, remove toxins and clear your head. You can find Yin Chiao or Cold Stop at www.yinchiao.com.

Ah, Aromatherapy!

Once you use an aromatherapy diffuser, you'll never want to be without it. That's because you can fill it with different essential oils or blends of essential oils and find relief from a wide variety of conditions. One of the best for the flu is Anti-Viral Plus aromatherapy blend from Leyden House (www.leydenhouse.com). Saturating the air with this combination of eucalyptus, lavender, tea tree, clove bud, geranium, and more will help to relieve a stuffy head, cough, fever, and congestion in the lungs. Running a diffuser in your household may also keep others from coming down with the flu by helping to eliminate airborne viruses. And we know how they love to travel!

Holistic aromatherapist Jade Shutes, B.A., Diploma AT, founder of the East West School for Herbal and Aromatic Studies in Willow Spring, North Carolina, recommends this remedy for the flu:

Immune scrub:

> 1 cup fine sea salt
>
> 2 TB. of sunflower vegetable oil
>
> 8 drops eucalyptus globulus (for adults only)
>
> 6 drops grapefruit (Citrus paradisi)

While in a warm/hot shower, scrub the arms, legs, feet, and hands with the salt scrub.

Try Hydrotherapy

Feeling funky? Fill that tub. To promote sweating and the release of toxins, says Mars, just add a cup of Epsom salts and seven drops of essential oil of eucalyptus or ginger to the water. To make it even more effective, sip a cup of diaphoretic herbs, such as elder flower or ginger, while you're in the tub.

Rest Remedy

Rest is critical when you get the flu. "The second you start feeling yucky, it's so important to rest for two to three days," says Dr. Yates. "If you can just slow down and say no to anything new, it really helps."

If you find it difficult to slow down and rest, you may want to try the Bach Flower Remedy called Impatiens. It will help if you are feeling impatient and tired of being sick. Take this remedy three times a day for three days.

Natural R$_x$

Allium cepa homeopathic remedy: 3 or 4 30C pellets every two to three hours until symptoms improve.

Astragalus: 500 mg four times daily at onset of flu; afterward, 500 mg twice daily for a week.

Boneset (Eupatorium perfoliatum): As directed, capsules.

Echinacea tincture: ½ tsp., 40 drops, or 2.5 mL three times daily. Tea: 1 TB. per cup of water, 3 cups daily. Capsules and tablets: 200 mg twice daily. Has been shown to lose its immune-boosting effects when taken for more than two weeks at a time.

Elderberry tea: 1 TB. per cup of water, 3 cups daily. Extract: 500 mg twice daily.

Esberitox: Adults and children 12 and older: 3 tablets, 3 times daily; ages 8–12: 2 tablets, 3 times daily; age 7 and younger: 1 tablet, 3 times daily. Tablets can be chewed.

Gan Mao Dan: Chinese herbal formula for flu. As directed. Reduces fever; relieves chest congestion; stops cough.

Garlic: 400 mg, containing 5,000 mcg of allicin, two to three capsules daily.

Gelsemium: Take 3 or 4 30C pellets under the tongue every two to three hours at the first sign of symptoms until they improve.

Ginger tea: 1 TB. per cup of water, 3 cups daily.

Goldenseal: ½ tsp., 40 drops, or 2.5 mL three times daily for a maximum of two weeks. Capsules or tablets: 100 mg three times daily for a maximum of two weeks.

Honeysuckle flowers (Lonicera japonica): As directed, capsules.

Impatiens Bach Flower Remedy: Add 2 drops to a glass of water or juice and sip at intervals. www.bachremedystore.com.

Isatis root (Isatis tinctoria): As directed, capsules. Traditional Chinese medicine for flu.

Licorice root (Glycyrrhiza glabra) tincture: ½ tsp., 40 drops, or 2.5 mL three times daily. Tea decoction: 1 TB. per cup of water, 3 cups daily.

Marshmallow root (Althaea officinalis) capsules: 100–200 mg twice daily.

Myrrh resin (Commiphora myrrha) tincture: ½ tsp., 20 drops, or 1.3 mL three times daily. Tea: 1–2 TB. per cup of water three times daily. Increases white blood cell motility and facilitates mucus drainage.

Oscillococcinum, by Boiron (Anas barbariae): Adults and children 2 years of age and older: one dose at the onset of symptoms, repeat for two more doses at six-hour intervals; allow pellets to dissolve in the mouth at least 15 minutes before or after meals. Stop using this product and consult a doctor if symptoms persist for more than three days or worsen.

Osha root (Ligusticum porterii): As directed.

Peppermint leaf (Mentha piperita): As directed.

Propolis: As directed, lozenges. Produced by bees from tree resin.

Usnea lichen (Usnea barbata): As directed. Acts as a wide-spectrum herbal antibiotic.

Vitamin A and/or beta carotene: 5,000 IU. Strengthens the mucus membranes, making them more resistant to infection.

Vitamin C: 3,000–4,000 mg to start, reducing over three to four days to 500 mg until you recover.

Yarrow leaf and flower (Achillea millefolium) tincture: ¼ tsp., 20 drops, or ⅓ mL three times daily. Tea: 1 TB. per cup of water, 2–3 cups daily.

Yin Qiao Chinese botanical formula: As directed.

Zinc: 15–50 mg daily; lozenges, capsules, and tablets. Helps stimulate the immune system.

Food Poisoning

"When in doubt, throw it out" is the tried-and-true saying when it comes to food that you may suspect has passed its prime. Still, when you travel, eat out, or even eat at home, mistakes can happen and food poisoning can result. Here's the 411 on what to be aware of and how natural remedies can help.

Eek! E. Coli

When it comes to food poisoning, we've all heard about the big E— E. coli (Escherichia coli), that is. Although many strains of E. coli are quite harmless, when beef or veggies become contaminated with strains that don't agree with us, we can get sick, with symptoms that can include everything from severe cramps and diarrhea to urinary tract infections and respiratory problems.

Food poisoning is especially dangerous when kids eat undercooked burgers: when meat gets ground up and made into burgers, any contamination that is on the beef, chicken, or turkey gets spread throughout the patty, so the whole thing is infected. The fact that children's immune systems are not fully formed, and that they love burgers, puts them at higher risk of getting food poisoning from E. coli.

Salmonella

A group of bacteria called salmonella, which is closely related to E. coli, can also cause food poisoning. Salmonella bacteria comes from … wait for it … poop. Yuck, right? If you get infected with it, expect diarrhea, fever, and tummy cramps 12 to 72 hours later. This is why it's very important to be very careful whenever you are handling chicken, beef, fish, or pork. Get into the habit of washing your hands thoroughly (one way to be sure you do it long enough is to sing "Happy Birthday") while you are preparing the food, and before you eat, too. Be alert to cross-contamination, too. For example, if you want to use a marinade on some chicken cutlets, never use the same plate for the cooked pieces of chicken. Ditto goes for, say, using the same carving knife you cut up the chicken to eat with.

Beware These Bacteria, Too!

High-risk individuals like pregnant women and those with impaired immune systems should avoid raw or partly cooked fish. Shellfish, especially mollusks (oysters, clams, mussels, and scallops), may carry the bacterium Vibrio vulnificus, which multiplies even during refrigeration. To reduce the risk, ask to see the certified shipper's tag and be sure to cook seafood properly (see "Safe Cooking Practices" to do so.) Symptoms of food poisoning from seafood include fever, muscle aches, nausea, and diarrhea.

Listeria monocytogenes, a bacteria found in soft and raw cheeses, hot dogs, and deli meats, can cause food poisoning, too. This can be especially dangerous for pregnant women, who already have naturally suppressed immune systems so their body will not reject the baby-to-be. If you are elderly or have a weakened immune system, you also need to be extra careful when it comes to listeria. Symptoms of food poisoning from this bacteria can occur even weeks later and include fever, muscle aches, nausea, and diarrhea.

dial your doc

If you have diarrhea and have trouble keeping liquids down for more than a day, see a doctor. This is especially true for young children. Because they are smaller, they get dehydrated more easily.

With all types of food poisoning, you want to be careful about becoming too dehydrated. It's important to be sure you are drinking enough water. Visit www.foodsafety.gov for more information.

Safe Cooking Practices

For beef, make sure hamburger is well done and isn't pink in the middle. Use a meat thermometer to make sure it's cooked to 160°F. If you like your beef rare, make a steak instead: with whole cuts of meat, searing them kills the harmful bacteria.

As with beef, it's important to cook poultry thoroughly. The USDA recommends cooking it to 170°F. Use a food thermometer to be sure. If you are roasting a chicken or a turkey, put the thermometer into the thickest part of the breast, since it's the coldest, slowest-cooking part. When cooking turkey, follow the manufacturers' directions.

In seafood, if fish is sushi grade, it's generally safe, since reputable restaurants have highly trained chefs who know how to buy fish that meets safety and sanitation standards, and how to handle it safely. When you prepare raw fish at home, start with high-quality, very fresh seafood and use it within two days of purchase. Cook fish to an internal temperature of 145°F to destroy parasites. A good rule of thumb is to cook it until it's translucent and flakes with a fork. Scallops and clams take three to five minutes, depending on size.

Most dairy foods, like milk, cottage cheese, yogurt, and hard cheeses, are made from pasteurized milk, so they're safe. Just be sure to check the dates on the packaging, to consume them when they are freshest.

Use a thermometer to make sure your refrigerator is set at 40°F or less. Set the freezer at 0°F or less. During the summer, it's particularly critical; with warmer temperatures, bacteria can grow even more rapidly.

Eating Out—and In—Safely

The U.S. Food and Drug Administration Center for Food Safety and Applied Nutrition suggests some guidelines to help you eat out safely.

Check out the restaurant before you sit down. If it's not as clean as you would like, eat somewhere else.

Order your food cooked thoroughly, especially meat, poultry, fish, and eggs. When you're served a hot meal, make sure it's served to you "hot" and completely cooked; if not, don't be afraid to send it back. Avoid eating raw or undercooked eggs; they can be a hidden hazard in foods like Caesar salad. If you are unsure about the ingredients in a dish, ask before ordering.

If you won't get back home within two hours of being served, leave the leftovers at the restaurant. Bacteria can grow quickly on food that is left out.

When preparing food at home, get in the habit of washing your hands often as you prepare food and before you eat. Keep your kitchen, including appliances, countertops, and utensils, spick-and-span.

Wash fruits and vegetables before preparing and eating them. Also wash the tops of cans and jars (make sure safety buttons are depressed) before opening them, and wash can openers after each use.

Avoid countertop thawing, and leave foods at room temperature no longer than two hours.

Pay attention to the "sell by" date, and, finally, when in doubt, throw it out!

Don't Leave Home Without These Remedies

If, despite your best efforts, you still get food poisoning, natural remedies can help at home and on the road. Brigitte Mars, A.H.G., author of *The Desktop Guide to Herbal Medicine*, recommends ume, which is a concentrate made from the umeboshi plum, for digestive troubles. Not only does it help relieve diarrhea, but it also helps prevent parasites—and eases a hangover, if you've had one too many margaritas. You can even take ume concentrate as a preventative. You can also take it if you eat something questionable, like potato salad that sat in the hot sun too long, or if something tastes a little "funny."

You may also want to try a cup of peppermint tea, says Mars, or you can add two drops of essential oil of peppermint to a cup of purified water to ease tummy troubles.

Put the Brakes on Diarrhea

Getting ready to leave on a trip? You may want to stock up on probiotics, or what are known as "friendly bacteria" like acidophilus, a week before you go, to give your bowel flora a boost. Bowel flora include certain kinds of bacteria in the gut that we need to help us maintain good health, by protecting us from harmful bacteria and viruses. When you add probiotics, you give your bowel flora a healthier starting point in case you encounter foods that are a little "off." Once you're traveling, you may want to add some enzymes, such as betaine hydrochloride, to help you more easily digest foods you may not be accustomed to eating.

If you can't stop "going," Mars also recommends charcoal capsules. No, these have nothing to do with the briquets you put on your barbeque. You can find them at your local health food store. If you are traveling to the tropics, where parasites and bacteria party all year long, you may want to invest in an activated charcoal water filter or purification system, says Mars, who suggests you get one that will remove giardia, a germ that causes diarrhea. Use your purified water for everything from washing veggies to brushing your teeth.

natural news

Feeling dehydrated after an attack of food poisoning? Mix 8 ounces of water with ¼ teaspoon baking soda and ¼ teaspoon salt. You can also find ready-to-mix electrolyte powder in your local health food store.

Natural Rx

Acidophilus pearls supplement: One pearl daily as a preventive; if you get sick, take one pearl three times daily.

Betaine hydrochloride: As directed.

Charcoal capsules: As directed.

Electrolyte powder: As directed.

Garlic standardized extract: 400 mg, containing 5,000 mcg of allicin, two to three capsules daily.

Peppermint essential oil: 2 drops to a cup of water. Find it at www.leydenhouse.com.

Peppermint tea: 1 TB. per cup of water. Drink as needed.

Ume concentrate, umeboshi plum: Paste: stir 1 tsp. into a cup of warm water. Pills: 9 daily.

Healthy Aging

What if we never had to get old? It's a tantalizing thought, and one that keeps plenty of researchers looking feverishly for ways to stop the march of time. One theory on why we age is oxidative damage to tissues in the body. Free radicals, those party poopers, can alter the membrane of a cell and affect DNA production or protein synthesis. They can also damage the skin and collagen, speeding wrinkling, and contribute to the hardening of your blood vessels, increasing your risk of a heart attack or stroke. Sunlight, smoking, radiation, and other environmental factors can also produce free radicals, and as we age, the body's ability to neutralize them is reduced.

You can tell how old you are in oxidative terms by how you feel. If you're out of energy, your joints hurt, and you feel stiff, then you're probably a lot older than that number on your birth certificate, unless you're in your 80s. But it doesn't have to be that way. Antioxidants work to quench that active energy from free radicals so you don't have as much oxidation or aging. Combine careful eating with large amounts of antioxidants, and you'll raise your odds of living a long and healthy life.

Slow Aging with Antioxidants

Antioxidants are the closest thing we have to the Fountain of Youth, the key to living long and well. Essentially, antioxidants are our first line of defense. Think of them as toy soldiers on a battlefield. Their "job" is to prevent unstable molecules called free radicals, byproducts of our energy metabolism, from damaging our cells and DNA. If we don't have enough soldiers on the battlefield, we can be prone to diseases of aging like cancer, heart disease, and diabetes. When we eat foods that are high in antioxidants like fruits and vegetables, we have a better defense against the diseases that can come with getting older.

Antioxidant nutrients, such as vitamin A with beta carotene, vitamins E and C, and coenzyme Q10, protect against the development of heart disease, cancer, and other chronic degenerative diseases; help minimize oxidative damage; and are key to slowing the aging process and keeping you young and vital.

Vitamin C is a water-soluble antioxidant, which means it's easily absorbed by the body, although it can't be stored. This means you need to eat fruits and vegetables with vitamin C every day to benefit from this antioxidant. Top food sources include mangoes, sweet potatoes, black currants, broccoli, Brussels sprouts, cauliflower, lemons, oranges, spinach, and peas.

Originally, it was thought that vitamin C's power as an antioxidant was to scavenge free radicals before they can cause harm by, say, damaging DNA and causing mutation that can cause cancer. Now, though, a new study by Johns Hopkins researchers in the medical journal *Cancer Cell* showed that the role of antioxidants in vitamin C and in N-acetylcysteine (NAC) is actually to hinder a cancer cell's ability to thrive in oxygen-starved conditions. Vitamin C's antioxidants quench free radicals before they can provide HIF-1 (hypoxia-induced factor), a protein that is dependent on free radicals and helps oxygen-needy cancer cells grow.

According to Michael Janson, M.D., author of *Dr. Janson's New Vitamin Revolution*, "Vitamin C is one of the most important antioxidants, and most people don't get enough of it in their diet. Even people who get enough Vitamin C can benefit from higher doses to reduce the effects of toxic exposures."

Vitamin E

You can name vitamin E for "excellent" when it comes to keeping you young. Recently, Yale researchers found that Tuscan residents 65 years and older who ingested foods with vitamin E on a daily basis had better physical functioning. The thinking is that this has to do with antioxidants, which prevent muscle or DNA damage, which can lead to the development of atherosclerosis and other conditions. The study, which appeared in the *Journal of the American Medical Association*, reported that participants got their vitamin E through the diet, approximately 15 mg a day of alpha-tocopherol, a component of vitamin E. This is roughly equal to the Recommended Dietary Allowances (RDA) for men and women 14 years and older. Foods you may want to choose to add vitamin E to your diet include almonds, hazelnuts, sunflower oil and seeds, olive oil, spinach, broccoli, and tomato sauce. Vitamin C works synergistically with vitamin E by recycling oxidized vitamin E, further boosting its antioxidant benefits.

natural news

The ongoing *Nurses' Health Study* (NHS), established in 1976, showed that women who had the highest level of vitamin E had the lowest rate of death from heart disease.

Coenzyme Q10

Coenzyme Q10 (CoQ10) is also an important antioxidant, and most people don't get enough of it, says Dr. Janson. "It's critical for the production of energy at the cellular level." After the age of 40 or so, our production of CoQ10 declines. So taking supplements of CoQ10 can be even more beneficial for prevention of cardiovascular disease and for brain preservation.

Flavonoids and Carotonoids

Flavonoids and *carotonoids* also act as potent antioxidants. Some of the best sources of these plant compounds are legumes (beans), soy, white grapes, cranberries, apples, onions, garlic, tea, tomatoes, and celery. Red wine contains the flavonoid resveratrol, which research shows makes the immune system younger and provides anticancer effects. Certain flavonoids found in hops and beer have potent antioxidant activity exceeding that of red wine, tea, or soy, according to the Linus Pauling Institute at Oregon State University.

Pick yourself a yellow, red, orange or dark green leafy vegetable, like a carrot, cantaloupe, sweet potato, tomato, kale, or watermelon, and you'll be rewarded with the benefits of carotenoids, antioxidants full of vitamin A, and, specifically, beta carotene. These nutrients play a big role in keeping your immune system healthy and keeping you young. Although the carotenoids lutein (found in spinach, broccoli, and kiwis) and zeaxanthin (found in leafy greens and tangerines) can't be used to make vitamin A, they do enhance eye health and are thought to help prevent cataracts and macular degeneration. Higher lutein levels have also been associated with thinner artery walls, making them less prone to blockages. Like lutein and zeaxanthin, lycopene isn't used to make vitamin A, but it's another beneficial carotenoid that may have anticancer properties; you'll find it in tomato products, watermelon, and guava.

def•i•ni•tion

Flavonoids (or bioflavonoids) are compounds found in fruits, vegetables, and certain beverages that have beneficial biochemical and antioxidant effects. They have been reported to have antiviral, antiallergic, antiplatelet, anti-inflammatory, antitumor, and antioxidant activities.

Carotenoids make certain vegetables yellow, orange, or red. The body can make some carotenoids, like beta carotene, into vitamin A. All carotenoids are antioxidants.

Protect Your Genes with Fruits and Veggies, Too

As we've seen, the antioxidants in fruits and vegetables are potent protection when it comes to aging. Well, they're also one of the best ways to nourish, protect, and keep our genes young. We may not think about it but as we age, our genes, which are made up of DNA and determine whether we have blue eyes or brown or whether we are short or tall or have red or blond hair do, too. When this happens it leads to sagging skin, aching joints, age spots, memory problems, and a weakened immune system. As we've seen, the good news is cell damage is reparable and aging can be reversed. "Nourishing our bodies, our cells, and our genes is extremely important if our goal is to 'live long and prosper,' a heart-felt salutation from Mr. Spock of the *Star Trek* TV series," says Vincent Giampapa, MD, F.A.C.S., one of the founders of the American Academy of Anti-Aging Medicine (A4M), the first president of the American Board of Anti-Aging Medicine, and author of *The Gene Makeover: The 21ˢᵗ Century Anti-aging Breakthrough.*

For gene protection, ideally, we should aim for 8–10 servings a day of fruits and vegetables. That's because the pigments that color fruits and vegetables come from antioxidants and other phytonutrients that boost your defenses against genetic damage and enhance genetic expression.

Yellow, orange, red, and green foods protect your genes, while purple, blue, black, and magenta foods help to repair our genes. White, pale yellow, and reddish brown foods help to build DNA. The more you eat, the better off you are. Dr. Giampapa recommends focusing on foods from the following color groups:

- **Yellow, orange, bright red (carotenoids):** Carrots, lettuce, spinach, tomatoes, avocados, kiwi, lemons, cayenne, cinnamon, turmeric.

- **Green/white (sulfur compounds, isothiocyanates, indols):** Asparagus, broccoli, cauliflower, arugula, radishes, sprouts, onions, leeks, garlic

- **Purple, blue, black (phenolics, flavonoids):** Blueberries, cherries, raspberries, strawberries, eggplant, beets, green and black tea, red and white wine, cinnamon, ginger, peppermint.

- **Tan (phytosterols, phytoestrongens, fiber, saponins):** Brown rice, millet, whole-wheat breads, amaranth, couscous, wild rice, all beans, soy nuts, tofu, brown mushrooms, green peas, almonds, peanuts, walnuts, nut butters.

- **White/pale yellow, reddish brown (proteins, omega–3 fatty acids, omega–6 fatty acids):** Chicken, cottage cheese, eggs, tofu, turkey, low-fat milk, soy milk, almond milk, rice milk, canola oil, macadamia nut oil, olive oil.

Sugar Slows You Down

Can too much sugar make you age faster? Yes. Although sugar, as glucose, is important in providing the major source of energy for metabolism, when sugar is joined (oxidized) with free radicals, it coats the surface of proteins and prevents them from functioning properly. Scientists call this process glycation. "Collagen is the most plentiful protein in your body and the one most affected by glycation," says Dr. Giampapa. "Skin, blood and lymph vessels, joints, tendons, ligaments, and internal organs are comprised of collagen." Most aging conditions (like those that follow) are linked to glycation. These are all good reasons to avoid sugar when you can.

- Memory loss: Sugar coating of brain neurons (brain cells)

- Depression: Disruption of the brain's neurotransmitter function

- Reduced ability to handle stress: Damaged cortisol receptors

- Hormone imbalances: Increased unbound or free cortisol

- Skin wrinkling and sagging: Collagen glycation

- Impaired immune function: Damage to thymus gland, lymphatic tissue, and immune cells

- Allergies, leaky gut syndrome, irritable bowel disorders, and other digestive issues

Healthy Aging Secrets from Around the World

What do the Okinawans in Japan, the Sardinians in Italy, and the Seventh-Day Adventists in Loma Linda, California, have in common? According to a study published in *National Geographic* magazine in 2005, it looks like they've all tapped the Fountain of Youth. Okinawans eat more soy, like tofu; Seventh-Day Adventists eat more nuts; and Sardinians eat more olive oil. Even though there are differences in their diets, the similarity is that the composition of their diets tends to be high in antioxidants, healthy fats, proteins, and carbs that are low on the glycemic index. (The glycemic index, or GI, ranks carbohydrates according to their effect on our blood glucose levels.) We'll talk more in a minute about the specifics of how these diets promote longer, healthier lives, and how you can incorporate their practices into your diet and lifestyle.

For instance, Okinawa leads the pack, with a life expectancy of 78 years for men and 86 years for women. The Okinawan diet is just that much healthier in plant compounds and antioxidants, and it's that much lower in calories. If you take your cue from their practices, you can increase your own vitality and longevity!

Cut Your Calorie Intake

Okay, we know it's tough to control your portions. One of the biggest problems is that we often keep eating after we are technically "full." That's because it takes a while for the brain to catch up with the stomach—about 20 minutes or so. But limiting your calories by waiting out your hunger until your brain can catch up can help you avoid excess calories and pounds. The Okinawans, who were studied extensively for 25 years for *The Okinawa Program: How the World's Longest-Lived People Achieve Everlasting Health—And How You Can Too*, make it a habit to eat until they are just 80 percent full.

Why is this important? Bradley Willcox, M.D., a clinical scientist and geriatrician at the Pacific Health Research Institute at the University of Hawaii in Honolulu and co-author of *The Okinawa Program*, explains: "Calorie restriction is the one consistent way of extending the limit of life span. Studies show that this has remarkable health consequences, since the more calories we eat, the more we burn, and the more free radicals we create. Less damage to internal organs means they wear out slower." Put that way, it's kind of like putting fewer miles on your car. Make sense?

This doesn't mean you have to go around feeling hungry all day long. Far from it. It just means you need to avoid foods that are "calorie-dense," as Dr. Willcox puts it, meaning those that are high in fat and sugar. The Okinawan diet is very low in calorie density—so despite only 1,800 calories a day—compared to diets in the United States, which might consist of 2,500 or 3,000 calories, the amount of food is the same (2–3 pounds). The Okinawans render these remarkable stats by choosing foods that are high in water and fiber, and low in fat, which makes them naturally low in calories. Such foods as veggies and tofu promote satiety, that full feeling.

natural news

Grape seed extract (GSE) can help you get smart by protecting your brain against future age-related dementia, according to a recent study at the University of Alabama at Birmingham. The antioxidants in polyphenols such as those in grape seed may protect vulnerable organs, like the brain, shifting oxidation away from proteins and lipids in cells or tissues. More study is needed to show how much GSE is optimal for overall brain health.

Eat Ten Vegetables and Fruits Daily

Okay, we admit, getting 10 servings of fruits and vegetables does seem like a lot. But look how you benefit. As we've seen previously, fruits and veggies are the main sources of dietary antioxidants, and more antioxidants means less cell damage from those nasty free radicals the body does create. When we have less free-radical damage, our bodies are able to "run" longer. So the more we eat, the better off we are.

The Okinawans and the Sardinians grow much of their own food, further boosting its nutritional value. We can do this, too, if we live in climates that are garden-friendly. If you don't want to get your hands dirty, stop off at that farmer's market you pass every day (you know you want to), or your local veggie stand, and stock up. If you eat two servings with each meal and four fruit snacks, you'll be tipping the antioxidant scales in your favor.

Choose Low-Glycemic Index Carbohydrates

One of the worst things you can do (diet wise) is eat a piece of white bread. That's right, you heard us. White bread is a high-glycemic carbohydrate, which means it's converted into glucose in your body in a flash. Okay, so you may get a quick jolt of energy, but you'll pay for it with a crash soon afterward. Same goes for sugar, sugary snacks, refined grains like white rice, and even fruit juice. Worst of all, it will leave you wanting more, which means more calories.

A better strategy, and one employed by the Okinawans, is to substitute these lightweight carbs with carbohydrates that have substance and are much more filling. In Okinawa this might be sweet potatoes or brown rice, but these foods could also be other foods like whole-grain bread, whole-wheat pasta, and fruits and vegetables that pack a fiber punch.

Reduce Proteins

Meat, meat, meat. Most Americans love their meat—so much so that the dinner plate is usually full of protein, with little room for vegetables. To change this, says Dr. Willcox, use the three-fourths rule and fill only a quarter of your plate with animal protein. Fill the rest with luscious vegetables and leafy green salads, and you'll approach the

20 percent marker that Okinawans aim for in their meat consumption. The Seventh-Day Adventists take it one step further and don't eat red meat at all. They also nix tobacco and alcohol.

Choose Fats Wisely

When you choose which foods to eat, aim for a diet that is 25 percent fats, to keep your immune system and arteries young. Fats on the good team include soy (favored by the Okinawans); olive oil (used by the Sardinians); canola, safflower, and sesame oil; and avocados and peanuts. Omega-3 fatty acids, mostly found in coldwater fish like cod, mackerel, and salmon (and fish oil supplements), and flaxseed oil, can help keep your brain and cardiovascular and immune systems young. Natural grazing methods for sheep in Sardinia mean higher concentrations of heart-healthy omega-3s and conjugated linoleic acid (CLA) in foods.

Start reading labels so you know to avoid foods that are heavy with saturated fats, the main cause of high dietary cholesterol. You find saturated fat in animal products like meats, butter, cheese, and other dairy products. Also on the no-no list are trans fatty acids, which are rampant in margarine and baked goods like those cookies and donuts. You'll also find them at just about every drive-through window in the United States.

Go Nuts!

When it comes to between-meal snacks, we can also learn from these groups of long-lived people. Researchers at Loma Linda University found that one of the factors in Seventh-Day Adventists' longevity was the fact that they eat a small serving of nuts five to six times a week. The Nurses Health Study linked regular nut consumption (five servings a week—of 5 oz.) to a lower risk of heart disease, from 35 to 50 percent.

Nutrient-dense nuts are a good source of vitamin E, which we mentioned before. The fact that they have high quantities of antioxidants may be one reason they are thought to reduce the risk of heart disease. Nuts raise HDL, or so-called "good cholesterol," while lowering LDL, so-called "bad cholesterol," likely by helping keep arteries clear of plaque. Although nuts do contain fat, it's the good kind—monounsaturated, found in foods like olive oil.

To go nuts, choose almonds, walnuts (they also have omega-3 essential fatty acids, which are good for you, too), hazelnuts, and macadamia nuts. Four or five servings of nuts a week may also help lower blood pressure, according to the DASH (Dietary Approaches to Stop Hypertension) guidelines.

It's The Best Medicine

Want to stay young? Try laughter or hasya yoga, a growing trend in the United States, India, and other countries. Not only does laughter yoga reduce stress, it also boosts immune health. In fact, studies have shown that 20 seconds of a good, hard belly laugh is worth three minutes on the rowing machine. Laughter yoga is part of a growing trend in the United States, India, and other countries.

Try these exercises from Laughter Yoga creator Madan Kataria, a family physician from India to get you started:

◆ **Hearty laughter:** Laughter by raising both the arms in the sky with the head tilted a little backwards.

◆ **Greeting laughter:** Joining both the hands and shaking hands with at least four or five people in the group.

◆ **Milk shake laughter:** Hold and mix two imaginary glasses of milk or coffee and pour the milk from one glass into the other by chanting "Aeee …," and then pour it back into the first glass by chanting "Aeee …" Then, everyone laughs while making a gesture as if they are drinking milk. For more information visit www. laughteryoga.org.

Get Physically and Emotionally Fit

Besides watching what you eat (and growing it, if you like), you need to get moving to stay young. Yes, this means getting off the couch! One study in the Archives of Internal Medicine showed that you can turn back the clock 10 years by being physically active on a daily basis!

According to a recent review of studies from the Netherlands, aerobic exercise can also give the 50-and-over crowd a boost in brainpower just when they need it most.

Experts say you need three main types of physical activity to keep fit— aerobic or cardiovascular exercise, strength training, and balance-flexibility. In Okinawa, people tend to engage in those activities as part of their daily lives, says Dr. Willcox, co-author of *The Okinawa Program.* "They're mostly hard-working mountain farmers, as are Sardinian shepherds, so they get strength training through moving their muscles, and they walk a lot, which is aerobic. Okinawans also engage in things like traditional dance that has movements very similar to tai chi (a Chinese practice of slow, fluid movements) that develops flexibility and balance. We can use these lessons to improve our own health."

Commit, for example, to 20 minutes a day of brisk walking, tai chi movements, or gardening, as the Okinawan elders do. For strength training, use medium-weight dumbbells and do a couple reps each morning and night. Yoga also increases strength along with flexibility and balance.

Learn How to Handle Stress Better

Stress can be one of the biggest factors in aging. Untreated stress can exacerbate or even cause chronic illness and lead to high blood pressure and heart attacks. That's because when we feel stressed it triggers what is known as the "fight or flight" response. "It increases blood pressure, metabolism, heart rate, breathing, blood flow to your muscles, and brain waves," says Herbert Benson, M.D., director emeritus of the Benson-Henry Institute for Mind Body Medicine at Massachusetts General Hospital. "The body goes into a hyper state preparing for running or fighting."

The opposite of the fight-or-flight response is the Relaxation Response, created by Dr. Benson, which is a medically proven method of stress reduction that helps to break the train of everyday worrisome thoughts. The Relaxation Response not only works while you're doing it by, among other things, blocking the stress hormones adrenalin and nor-adrenalin, but it also has beneficial long-term effects by lowering blood pressure and making you feel calmer and more in control. It also can lower blood pressure and make you less anxious and depressed. There is even evidence that it affects the brain, causing brain cells to get thicker, perhaps improving memory. You can trigger the Relaxation Response with these two simple steps. It's best to practice this for 10–20 minutes once or twice daily:

1. Sit in a comfortable place and repeat a word, sound or phase like "one" or "peace."

2. When other thoughts come to mind, disregard them and come back to the repetition.

For more information on the Relaxation Response visit www.mbmi.org.

De-Stress Like the Okinawans

When Dr. Willcox and his colleagues were doing research in Okinawa, they discovered that residents have their own unique approach to stress reduction. There they have a wonderful expression that really exemplifies their approach to life and illustrates the fact that they are able to handle stress so well. The phrase "Nan kuru nai sa" means "Don't worry, it'll work out." "They're survivors," says Dr. Willcox. "They tend to let stress roll off their back. What we can do is to learn some of those coping strategies like meditation and using positive affirmations—for example, 'I am a good person. I love and accept myself for who I am'—to restructure the way we think about things and react to them."

"Many Okinawans have *ikigai*, which roughly translates to 'that which makes one's life worth living,'" says Dr. Willcox. "It's the reason they get up in the morning. One centenarian who's 102 has two prize bulls; for another, it might be her religion; for another, it's her sweet potato garden." This belief also acts as a buffer against stress and diseases like hypertension.

"There is a larger social network in Okinawa than you see in most places," says Dr. Willcox. "People look out for each other. There's a real connectedness there." One of the ways that people connect in Okinawa is by forming mutual support groups called Moai. "People will bring a little money, and whoever needs it most that month will get it. They talk about problems and just have fun together." The Sardinians have strong social networks, as do the Seventh-Day Adventists. To connect in your own life, start with your immediate family. You can also join or start a self-help group or a club, use e-mail to connect, take up a sport, or volunteer.

natural news

Increasing oxygen in the body is the best anti-aging formula available, and it is as simple as breathing, says Stephen Hartman, the director of professional training and association at the Kripalu Center for Yoga & Health in Stockbridge, Massachusetts. "Increased oxygen boosts the immune system that fights off colds, flu, and viruses. It triggers the metabolism and helps us digest our food and burn calories more efficiently. Increased oxygen in the body helps the body detoxify from poor diet, stress, and adrenalin. Oxygen in the system produces endorphins that act like natural antidepressants. So how do you get more oxygen? Breathe! I recommend taking a breathing break in the same way someone might take a smoking break. Take five minutes every couple hours to go outside and breathe deeply. When you are driving in your car or working at your computer and notice that you are barely breathing, continue to do what you are doing, only take deep, deliberate inhales for as long as possible. You will feel the positive effects and increase in energy immediately."

Benefits of Qigong

Qigong (*qi* [*chi*] means "energy" and *gong* [*kung*] means "a skill or a practice") started more than 5,000 years ago when Chinese scholars, studying the workings of the universe, concluded that everything is energy. Qigong teaches that sickness results from too much or too little energy in different parts of the body. Qigong practice is designed to help you redirect the flow of energy in your body to regain energy balance and regain or maintain optimal health and wellness.

Qigong exercises can help restore normal body functions in people with chronic conditions like hypertension, cardiovascular disease, aging, asthma, allergies, neuromuscular problems, and cancer. The main conclusion from many studies is that qigong exercise helps the body to heal itself. In this sense, qigong is a natural anti-aging medicine. You can read more about qigong in Chapter 5 or visit www.SpringForestQigong.com.

natural news

Want to stay young? Try cat's claw. No, don't alert PETA! This is just an herb that comes from a large, woody vine with hook-like thorns. This natural remedy for aging should be considered an essential part of any supplement program, says Dr. Giampapa. That's because the bark of the cat's claw plant contains compounds known as Carboxyl Alkyl Esters, which are the most potent form of natural compounds that increase DNA repair. The minimum daily dosage should be between 150—200 mg. a day.

Natural Rx

CoQ10: 400 mg. A good brand is www.vitalineformulas.com.

Selenium: 100–200 mcg daily

Vitamin A: 5,000 IU

Vitamin C: 500–1,000 mg daily, two times a day

Vitamin E: 400 IU

Zinc: 15–50 mg daily

Heart Disease

A heart beats 80,000 to 100,000 times and pumps approximately 2,000 gallons a day—and it weighs just 11 ounces and is about the size of a fist. This vital organ will beat two billion to three billion times over your lifetime and will pump 50 million to 65 million gallons of blood. Its main job is to deliver oxygen and blood to cells throughout the body. The heart pumps blood to the lungs, where it receives oxygen, the critical nutrient for cells. The blood then comes back to the heart and is pumped to all the different organs of the body, to provide them with oxygen and other nutrients.

Most of the heart consists of muscle, or myocardium, sandwiched between two thin protective layers, the epicardium (the outer layer) and the endocardium (the inner layer). Heart cells are connected to neighboring cells through a series of junctions. They also merge during development, so they have multiple nuclei. The merged cells and conjunctions between the cells allow the electrical signals to pass between the cells of the heart.

Unlike our biceps, another form of striated (skeletal) muscle, the cardiac muscle works through electrical impulses instead of through our own conscious effort. In the crudest sense, the heart is a muscle like any other muscle: it can contract and relax. But unlike all your other muscles, it does it on its own, automatically, all the time.

Eating Heart Smart

To be heart smart, we need to eat right, not smoke, exercise, consume alcohol in moderation, and reduce stress as much as possible. Good nutrition for the heart involves a diet low in saturated fat, high in mono- and polyunsaturated fats and fiber (to manage cholesterol), and high in antioxidants like vitamins C and E. Garlic also reduces cholesterol and improves circulation. Bad nutrition for the heart is a diet high in saturated fats and transfatty acids—the partially hydrogenated oil found in packaged cookies, crackers, baked goods, and fast foods.

The American Heart Association's new dietary guidelines set out four basic goals:

1. Eat a varied and healthful diet.

2. Avoid weight gain and maintain an appropriate body weight.

3. Get your blood pressure to a normal level.

4. Keep your cholesterol at a desirable level.

Recently, researchers at the Boston University School of Medicine and the Karolinska Institute in Sweden looked at the medical histories for more than 24,000 women. Following these lifestyle practices cut their heart attack risk by up to 92 percent!

1. Drink a moderate amount of alcohol—no more than a half a glass of wine a day.

2. Eat a healthy, balanced diet. Focus on fruits, veggies, whole grains, fiber, fish, and legumes.

3. Exercise each day. Take a 40-minute walk. Choose one day each week for an hour or more of strenuous activity.

4. Keep your weight under control. Make it your goal that your waist size is 85 percent or less than your hip size.

5. Don't smoke. If you do smoke, quit. After one year of not smoking, your risk drops dramatically.

The Importance of Supplementation

While lifestyle changes can obviously play an important role (a 92 percent reduction in heart attack risk is pretty great, right?), supplementation is important, too, especially when medications typically given for heart disease, high cholesterol, and high blood pressure tend to deplete the body of the very nutrients it needs in order to have normal heart function. For example, cholesterol-lowering drugs called statins can deplete B vitamins, which help keep the nervous system calm and keep the heart from getting overexcited. Supplements in the form of plant sterols (more on these in a minute), herbs, and other nutrients can help fill the gap and boost heart health.

Niacin: The Natural Cholesterol Buster

Niacin, called nicotinic acid (vitamin B₃), was first discovered to reduce cholesterol in 1955. It works in the liver, where the body produces most of its cholesterol to lower so-called "bad" cholesterol and raise "good" cholesterol. It also reduces triglycerides.

Until recently, using niacin caused flushing, an itchy reddening of the skin. But now sustained-release formulations prevent this side effect. The best currently on the market is Niamax, which has been thoroughly researched for safety and efficacy at the University of Minnesota. You can also find the same formulation in Endur-acin, either in drug stores or online at www.endur.com.

Beware of and avoid products labeled as "No Flush Niacin" that contain either niacinamide or inositol hexanicotinate. Neither has any benefit in lowering cholesterol, regardless of claims that they can do so.

natural news

The ongoing Nurses' Health Study (NHS), established in 1976, showed that women who had the highest level of vitamin E had the lowest rate of death from heart disease.

Don't use niacin if you have liver damage, abuse alcohol, or have gout. Ask your doctor to test your liver enzymes when measuring your cholesterol levels (with a simple blood test) to make sure your liver is properly handling the niacin.

Plant Sterols

Natural compounds called plant sterols, found in fruits, vegetables, whole-grain products, cereals, nuts, and vegetable oils, are key to heart health. Plant sterols resemble cholesterol in their chemical nature and block it from being absorbed into the body. The FDA has now approved plant sterols, concentrated naturally in the seeds and oils of plants, to be added to a wide variety of foods, such as orange juice, dairy substitutes, cheese, granola bars, bread, and cereal, as one way to lower cholesterol.

Plant sterols are a class of natural fatlike plant compounds with chemical structures similar to cholesterol so that they block its usual absorption. The overall effect in clinical studies has been an average "bad" (LDL) cholesterol decline of 8 to 15 percent, with total cholesterol falling by 10 percent. "It's a wonderful addition to restrictive diets because it's a whole variety of foods to eat to add to the benefit of cholesterol reduction," says Dr. Joseph Keenan, professor of family medicine at the University of Minnesota. The American Heart Association guidelines recommend 1 to 2 g of plant sterols a day, but even if you are a vegetarian, this is a hard number to meet.

"Basically, every one of us needs to take a supplement to get what we really need to make a difference in cholesterol," says Dr. Keenan, who also holds a joint professorship in the University of Minnesota School of Food Science and Nutrition. "For folks with mild cholesterol problems, adding foods with plant sterols to the diet can keep them from going on a drug." Eat plant sterols with your main meal for the best cholesterol-lowering effect. (This is not recommended for pregnant women.) You can also take plant sterols as a supplement. To have a significant cholesterol-lowering effect, you need to consume 800 mg daily. For more information and a complete plant sterol product listing, visit www.corowise.com.

You can also take an immediate-release phytosterol supplement that goes to work virtually as soon as you swallow it at the start of a meal. You can find it at www.endur.com as EP Immediate Release Phytosterols. Take two 450 mg tablets at the start of two major meals daily. Taking these supplements daily can bring total cholesterol levels down by as much as 10 percent and the "bad" LDL cholesterol down by up to 14 percent, as shown in clinical trials.

natural news

Fiber is good for reducing our risk of heart disease, but almost half of us don't eat any whole grains, says Janet Bond Brill, Ph.D., R.D., the author of *Cholesterol Down: 10 Simple Steps to Lower Your Cholesterol in 4 Weeks Without Prescription Drugs*. To reduce your risk of heart disease, up your fiber consumption to 25 to 30 g daily. To do this, eat at least five portions of fruits and vegetables, and two or three portions of whole-grain breads or cereals. "Starting off the day with a bowl of steel-cut oatmeal, which is the least processed oatmeal, a whole grain, and a good carbohydrate, is the best and easiest thing you can do to protect your heart," says Dr. Brill. "People who eat whole grains or high-fiber food have much less risk of heart disease. For more information, visit www.CholesterolDownBook.com.

Coenzyme Q10

Heart-friendly coenzyme Q10 (CoQ10), or ubiquinone, is a fat-soluble, vitaminlike substance that is involved in energy production in every cell. This important nutrient supports heart and blood vessel function, protects against congestive heart failure, and acts as important antioxidant. It also helps repair some of the deformity of the *mitral valve*, which separates the upper and lower chambers of the left side of the heart. Beverly Yates, N.D., the author of *Heart Health for Black Women: A Natural Approach to Healing and Preventing Heart Disease*, enthuses, "I can't say enough about CoQ10. Each cardiac cell has approximately 4,000 mitrochondria where CoQ10 is processed. The mitochondria of the cells is the powerhouse, the energy source. If someone is at high risk, if they are stressed or aging, if they have already had a heart attack or stroke, they would do well to take 100 to 300 mg a day."

CoQ10 is naturally present in a variety of foods, as well as in supplements. It's particularly high in organ meats such as heart, liver, and kidney, as well as in beef, soybean oil, sardines, mackerel, and peanuts. For many, a supplement can be the easiest way to add this nutrient.

D-Ribose

D-ribose, a naturally occurring carbohydrate, is also excellent for restoring energy production in the cell, especially when it comes to the heart. A study in the medical journal *European Journal of Heart Failure* in 2003 showed that D-ribose improves diastolic function (when the heart relaxes after it contracts) and quality of life in congestive heart patients. Congestive heart failure is a chronic condition in which the heart fails to pump blood effectively. You can get D-ribose in supplement form.

Folic Acid

The name *folic acid* was derived from the Latin word *folium*, which means "leaf." A vitamin of the B-complex group, it is very important for maintaining normal homocysteine (an amino acid) levels. Too much homocysteine in the blood is related to higher risk of coronary heart disease. An elevation of homocysteine can also damage muscles and predispose blood factors to form clots rather than to inhibit them.

Research shows that when homocysteine levels rise, so does the risk of heart disease and heart attack. The Physicians' Health Study (1990), which involved almost 15,000 doctors, found that men who had homocysteine levels 12 percent above average had 3.4 times the risk of heart attack than men with low levels, regardless of other risk factors for cardiovascular disease.

If you have elevated homocysteine levels, you can correct that with folic acid and vitamins B_6 and B_{12}. Eat dark, leafy greens like spinach and kale, along with brewer's yeast, black-eyed peas, wheat and rice germ, liver, soy flour, lentils, soybeans, kidney beans, lima beans, navy beans, and legumes. If you can't get enough (and most people don't), add a supplement or two or three.

natural news

Garlic has been called nature's aspirin. Like aspirin, garlic works to keep the blood thin, which can be a good thing when you want to avoid heart attacks and stroke, says Dr. Brill. "Garlic is also the basis of the Mediterranean style of eating, which is the best way to eat for taste and heart health, and protecting your arteries as well."

Omega-3 Fatty Acids

The body uses omega-3 fatty acids to synthesize prostaglandins, substances that mediate many chemical processes in the body and are important for the structure and function of cell membranes. They reduce the tendency for blood platelets to stick together, thus reducing blood clots, and they are beneficial in preventing hardening of the arteries and heart attacks.

Although the highest source of omega-3 fatty acids is chinook salmon and sockeye, Atlantic and pink salmon are also high in this substance, as are tuna, mackerel, sardines, lake trout, anchovies, herring, blue fish, and sable fish. Salmon, trout, and tuna containing omega-3 fatty acids have been shown to lower high blood homocysteine levels.

For the prevention of coronary artery disease, try to eat at least three fish meals a week. Many studies show that regular consumption of fish—just a portion a week of salmon, for example—that has very high amounts of omega-3 fatty acids can reduce your risk of heart attack by up to 30 percent.

Supplementation with fish oil from fatty, deep-water ocean fish, like haddock, flounder, sole, tuna, and salmon, works just as well. Researchers at the Agency for Healthcare Research and Quality recently confirmed that long-chain omega-3 fatty acids, found in fish or fish oil supplements, reduce the risk of heart attack and other problems related to heart and blood vessel disease. Plus, when you substitute foods high in omega-3 fatty acids like fish, you increase your polyunsaturated fat intake and decrease your intake of foods high in saturated fats.

Flaxseed oil is one of the few nonanimal sources of omega-3 fatty acids. It's wonderful for the heart, but it's also a good source of fiber. Just be sure to grind flax seeds in a coffee grinder to break the seal; otherwise, you won't get the benefit from the omega-3.

Vitamin E

It's difficult to get enough vitamin E from foods like vegetable oils, nuts, and green leafy vegetables. Vitamin E as an antioxidant (prevents damage from free radicals) reduces heart risk, but you can't reach optimal levels from diet alone. Look for a vitamin E supplement that contains all eight isomer forms, four tocotrienols and four tocopherols. Take it the way it occurs in nature.

Soy

Proclaimed "nature's wonder food" by many dietitians and health professionals, soy was endorsed in 2000 by the Food and Drug Administration. Isoflavones, a class of phyto or "plant" estrogens found in soy protein (called genistein and daidzein), help reduce your risk of heart disease by making blood vessels less prone to forming plaque and by lowering total and LDL (bad) cholesterol. Soy also helps inhibit platelet aggregation (keeping the blood thin).

If you are increasing your soy intake and eating it instead of animal protein, you're increasing your monounsaturated fat as you are decreasing saturated fat intake. As with eating more fish, it's a double benefit. Soy also has all the amino acids that your body needs, typically found only in animal products such as eggs, chicken, fish, beef, and milk. You can enjoy the benefits of soy by eating it or taking a supplement of soy protein isolate with isoflavones.

natural news

Recently, researchers at Cedars-Sinai Medical Center found that green tea leaf catechins, powerful antioxidant compounds, inhibit the development of new plaque deposits. (Oxidation is the initial step in atherosclerosis formation, and antioxidants prevent this from happening.) The heart-protective benefits of tea start with drinking just one to two cups a day. Black tea contains compounds known as catechins, which are converted to theaflavins, which reduce total cholesterol levels and the risk of heart disease. If you aren't a tea lover, use supplements that contain tea extracts.

Sip Sherry

Sherry, like red wine, contains antioxidants called polyphenols. Animal studies show that sherry can help decrease total cholesterol and raise HDL (good) cholesterol following moderate intake. Aim for one drink a day for women and two for men.

Pick a Pomegranate for Heart Health

If you want to boost heart health, the Harvard Men's Health Watch suggests you pick a pomegranate. Two studies showed that neck artery thickness decreased and cardiac blood improved when men drank pomegranate juice. The antioxidant power of phytochemicals from pomegranates also helps to prevent so-called bad cholesterol (LDL cholesterol) from damaging blood vessels. Antiplatelet actions of the juice could also help prevent artery-blocking blood clots.

risky remedy!

Pomegranate juice may interact with medications you are taking. If you have any questions, check with your doctor first.

Chocolate Reduces Heart Attack Risk

A taste of chocolate can help your heart. Research shows that 2 tablespoons of dark chocolate cut heart attack risk by half by making blood platelets less sticky, which means they are less likely to form a blood clot. Aspirin has a similar effect in the body. Researchers are not sure which chemical in cocoa reduces platelet stickiness, but think it may be in the group of chemicals called flavonoids. More research needs to be done, but for now, eating dark chocolate in moderation is fine.

natural news

Hibiscus flower extract can help your heart, according to a new study in the *Journal of the Science of Food and Agriculture*. That's because hibiscus is chock-full of antioxidants that can help lower bad cholesterol, just like red wine and tea. The extract has the potential to be useful in the prevention and even treatment of a number of cardiovascular diseases in which cholesterol plays a major role. Look for it soon at a health food store near you.

B Vitamins

We've talked about vitamin B_3 and niacin, but vitamins B_6 and B_{12} and folic acid are also important for heart health. All of these play a vital role in the maintenance of normal homocysteine levels, which have been very clearly associated with an increased risk of heart attack and stroke. As a general rule of thumb, take 500 mg a day for each of the B vitamins. Let your urine be your guide, says Dr. Yates. "Until you have seen your urine be bright yellow, you haven't gotten enough B vitamins. Once you get to that yellow threshold, you can start to back it down. B vitamins are water soluble, so if you get too much, it's not going to hurt you."

It's also smart to eat foods rich in B vitamins, like spinach, broccoli, asparagus, lentils, garbanzo beans, and black-eyed peas.

natural news

Studies clearly show that people who are physically active have a significantly reduced risk of heart attack. Aim for 30 minutes a day of physical activity, not exercise, like walking, working in the house, gardening, and mowing the lawn. The good news is, it doesn't have to be 30 minutes all at one time. You can break it up into three 10-minute or six 5-minute segments and still get 75 to 85 percent of the cardiovascular benefit.

Heart-Smart Herbs

To many natural practitioners, hawthorn (Crataegus oxycantha) is the most important general heart herb. "Hawthorne helps with the heart regulation in terms of both rhythm and rate, and actually nourishes cardiac tissue specifically," says Dr. Yates. "It helps strengthen and fortify it." In traditional herbal medicine, it's known as a tonic. It keeps cholesterol from being deposited in the walls of the arteries and improves the blood supply to the heart by dilating the coronary arteries. Additionally, hawthorn is *antiarrhythmic* and promotes antioxidant actions by increasing blood flow in the peripheral blood vessels.

Hawthorn's flavonoids (beneficial antioxidant compounds found in fruits and vegetables) protect small capillary vessels from free-radical damage and help make vessels less susceptible to damage by strengthening their structure. It can even help with *congestive heart failure*. Hawthorne actually increases the force of the contractions of the heart muscle so it can squeeze blood out more effectively.

Clinical trials in Europe have confirmed the effectiveness and safety of hawthorn extracts in early congestive heart failure, mild angina, arrhythmia, and hypertension, as well as recovery from heart attacks.

def•i•ni•tion

Arrhythmia, or irregular beat, is any variation from the normal rhythm of the heartbeat.

Congestive heart failure is a special cardiac circumstance that refers to the inability of the heart to effectively pump enough blood.

The **mitral valve** separates the left atrium from the left ventricle of the heart.

The Benefits of Qigong

Qigong (*Qi*, or *chi*, means "energy," and *gong*, or *kung*, refers to a skill or a practice) started more than 5,000 years ago when Chinese scholars studying the workings of the universe concluded that everything is energy. Qigong teaches that sickness results from too much or too little energy in different parts of the body. Qigong practice is designed to help you redirect the flow of energy in your body to regain energy balance and regain or maintain optimal health and wellness. Several studies show that this practice helps those with heart disease.

In a 30-year study with stroke and hypertensive patients who had both drug therapy and qigong, the group that practiced qigong 30 minutes twice a day decreased by about 50 percent the incidence of total mortality, mortality due to stroke, and morbidity due to stroke. At the end of 30 years, 86 patients survived in the qigong group and 68 survived in the control group. These results clearly show that qigong has significant potential for preventing strokes and extending life. In another study, when aged hypertensive patients practiced qigong for a year, cardiac output increased and heart energy and blood circulation improved.

Natural R_x

Alpha lipoic acid: 200–600 mg.

Arginine: 300 mg daily. Helpful for the blood vessels and for keeping the blood supply to the heart really strong.

B-complex vitamin: As directed.

Black tea extract: 300 mg daily.

CoQ10: 400 mg daily. www.Vitalineformulas.com

EP Immediate Release Phytosterols: Two 450 mg tablets at the start of two major meals daily. www.endur.com.

Folic acid: 400 mcg daily.

Garlic: Three to five cloves daily or equivalent in capsule, 200–300 mg.

Green tea: Tea: 1 TB. per cup of tea, 3 cups daily. Extract: 300 mg daily.

Hawthorne: 100–200 mg.

Magnesium carbonate: 900 mg daily.

Magnesium citrate: 300–400 mg.

Niamax: As directed. You can also find the same formulation in Enduracin either in drug stores or online at www.endur.com.

Omega-3 fatty acids, combined EPA and DHA: 1,000 mg daily.

Plant sterols: 400 mg twice daily.

Sherry: One drink daily for women, two daily for men.

Taurine: 200–300 mg. Helpful for the blood vessels and for keeping the blood supply to the heart really strong.

Vitamin B_6: 500 mg daily.

Vitamin B_{12}: 500 mg daily.

Vitamin C: 200–2,000 mg daily in divided doses.

Vitamin E: 400–800 IU daily, as mixed tocopherols and tocotrienols. Vitamins C and E work well together to protect against free-radical damage, a leading cause of heart disease.

Heartburn

Heartburn is aptly named, since it feels like you have a fire in your stomach. That burning, painful, feeling can strike because of stress or certain foods, can occur when you're sleeping or while you're exercising, and can accompany diabetes, unstable blood sugar, or a hiatal hernia.

If you experience heartburn often (more than two times a week), you may have gastroesophageal reflux disease (GERD). You get GERD when the muscles in your esophagus don't close like they should. This means the contents of your stomach, including undigested food and bile (yikes!), can flow back up into your esophagus, irritating it.

Putting Out the Fire: Foods to Avoid

As we said, certain foods can cause heartburn to occur more often than others. The worst culprits are foods that have a high fat or acid content. For this reason, orange juice and lemonade are on the list, as are chocolate and potato chips. The National Heartburn Alliance uses a red, green, and yellow coding system to help heartburn sufferers gauge whether they should eat certain foods. Red means you should generally avoid the food, as with macaroni and cheese. Yellow means you can consume it, but be careful, as with low-fat cottage cheese; and green means it's okay to eat, as with extra-lean ground beef. It can be helpful to become a diet detective and use a food diary to pinpoint which foods affect you most. You can find more information at www. heartburnalliance.com.

natural news

You may have heartburn because you don't have enough stomach acid, not because you have too much! It sounds crazy, but it's true. "The confusing part is that having too much acid and having too little can create the same symptom of heartburn," says Brenda Watson, C.N.C. and author of *The Fiber 35 Diet*. "The problem is, heartburn is treated with over-the-counter antacids and acid-blocking medications, but these should be used only as short-term remedies. The unfortunate thing in this country is that people take them for years. If we don't have enough acid, we can't absorb key nutrients, like B_{12}, calcium, magnesium, and zinc."

Digestive Digest

To get digestion off to a good start, first drink an 8- to 10-oz. glass of room-temperature water 30 minutes before a meal, says Watson. The lining in your stomach is made of mucous, which is 90 percent water. But the average person is dehydrated, so drinking water starts mucous production before you eat, and you'll have less of a chance of heartburn. But avoid drinking too much water with meals. Don't have more than a glass of water with any meal, because this dilutes the enzymes generated by saliva.

Next, take the time to chew your foods well, since digestion starts in the mouth. Watson explains that chewing thoroughly smashes the food enough that when it gets down to the stomach and small intestine, enzymes have enough surface area so they can extract nutrients. "If you don't chew well, it's much harder for nutrients to be absorbed by the body. It can also set you up for heartburn."

Digestive Enzymes to the Rescue

When it comes to proteins, you may want to turn to the digestive aid betaine hydrochloric acid (HCl). Betaine HCl supplements the stomach's own production of HCl, or stomach acid. This is important, says Watson, because when you don't have enough HCl, undigested protein passes through your digestive tract and creates toxicity in the body. Digestive enzymes like those found in tropical fruits, such as bromelain from pineapple (which reduces tissue irritation) and papain from papayas (which soothes the stomach), can provide help in digesting proteins as well.

Don't Be Bitter! Okay, Go Ahead

Okay, given the choice, we probably wouldn't chose to eat something bitter. But it can make sense if you have heartburn. That's because bitter herbs like dandelion can help improve digestion, sending a message to the stomach to produce more acid and to the pancreas to produce more digestive enzymes. When this happens, we're able to digest our food more easily. Deglycyrrhizinated licorice can also help calm the digestive tract.

natural news

Broccoli sprouts can eliminate H. pylori (a bacteria that can infect the stomach and lead to heartburn, ulcers, and even stomach cancer)— at least temporarily, according to researchers at William Beaumont Hospital in Michigan.

So getting in the habit of either making yourself a nice cup of dandelion tea or chewing licorice 20 minutes before you eat can help you avoid bouts of heartburn.

Say Hello to "Friendly Bacteria"

Most of us take more antibiotics than we should. This can mean that the good bacteria in our digestive tract get depleted. That's because when we take an antibiotic, it wipes out the good with the bad. But even if you don't often take antibiotics, adding probiotics or "friendly bacteria" to your daily routine can be a good move when it comes to digestive health. Both acidophilius bifidus, which works mainly in the small intestine, and lactobacillus, which works mainly in the large intestine, help restore a healthy lining to the intestinal tract. This can improve digestion, lead to improved

natural news

A special kind of acupuncture may help prevent that upset stomach, according to new research in the *American Journal of Physiology—Gastrointestinal and Liver Physiology*. This needle-free therapy may reduce the relaxation of a certain muscle in the esophagus, which keeps digestion moving along the way it should.

immunity, and promote overall good health. Probiotics help B vitamins absorb better, too. You can take them as supplements in capsules, tablets, and powders, and in foods like yogurt.

Natural R_x

Acidophilus bifidus: 10 billion microorganisms twice daily.

Aloe (aloe vera liliaceae): One capsule of 50–300 mg daily for a maximum of seven days. Soothes intestinal tract.

Betaine hydrochloric acid (HCl): As directed.

Bromelain: As directed.

Chamomile: Tea, 1 TB. per cup of water, 4 cups daily.

Dandelion bitter herb: Tincture, ½ tsp., 40 drops, or 2.5 mL three times daily; tea, 1 TB. per cup of water, 3 cups daily. Stimulates digestion.

Gentian bitter herb: ¼ tsp., 20 drops, or 1.3 mL 10–20 minutes before meals three times daily. Stimulates salivation and the secretion of stomach acid; aids digestion.

Ginger bitter herb tea: 1 TB. per cup of water, 4 cups daily. Stimulates digestion.

Lactobacillus: 10 billion microorganisms twice daily.

Licorice: Chew deglycyrrhizinated licorice 400–1,200 mg 20 minutes before meals. Soothing to the intestinal tract.

Papain: As directed. Soothing effect on the stomach and aids in protein digestion.

Slippery elm (ulmus rubra) tea decoction: 1 TB. per cup of water, 2–3 cups daily; soothes the intestinal system; fibrous bark contains large quantities of a gentle laxative that assists elimination.

Hemorrhoids

Hemorrhoids can be a pain in the you-know-what. Hemorrhoids are a swelling or inflammation of veins in the rectum or anus. External hemorrhoids are outside the rectum and are sometimes painful and inflamed. Internal hemorrhoids occur inside and usually aren't painful, but they may bleed when irritated.

You can get hemorrhoids from strained bowel movements during constipation or diarrhea, prolonged periods of sitting, obesity, and a couch-potato lifestyle. A family history can also influence whether you'll get hemorrhoids. Hemorrhoids are an equal-opportunity offender in half of men and women by the age of 50, although if you are pregnant, you are more likely to have them. Usually, your symptoms will disappear within a few days. While you have hemorrhoids, natural remedies can help you feel better.

Boosting Fiber in the Diet

No one wants to talk about constipation, but it can be a huge factor when it comes to hemorrhoids. If you have to strain to go, this just puts more pressure you-know-where. This is why it's important to build more fiber into your diet. One easy rule of thumb is to increase the amount of fruits and veggies and whole grains. You can start looking at labels on foods and make it your new goal to consume 25 to 30 g of fiber a day.

You may also be dehydrated, so up your water consumption to the recommended eight glasses a day. Exercise, particularly yoga, can help, too, by stimulating the bowel to get moving.

Topical Herb Treatments

You'll find witch hazel in many over-the-counter products that treat hemorrhoids. That's because this unassuming shrub has astringent properties that also make it ideal for soothing and healing hemorrhoids. Native Americans knew the therapeutic properties of the bark, leaves, and twigs of the witch hazel bush for a variety of conditions and passed on this knowledge to the early settlers.

The astringent properties in witch hazel come from substances called tannins, which you'll also find in your favorite cup of tea. They tighten the "veins" in your hemorrhoids and relieve the swelling and pain, too.

Butcher's Broom

Butcher's broom also has a long history of use for hemorrhoids. The active ingredient in butcher's broom, ruscogen, has both anti-inflammatory and vein-constricting properties. When you apply it topically as an ointment, it helps tighten blood vessels, shrink swollen tissues, and ease itching. Horse chestnut cream can help, too, thanks to a natural compound known as aescin, which eases swelling and inflammation. Other astringent herbs that can be applied topically in cream or tea form include white oak bark, yarrow, comfrey, plantain, and raspberry.

Neem Oil

Known in India as "The Divine Tree," the bark, leaves, and oil of the neem tree have antibacterial, anti-inflammatory, and astringent properties. A widely used ayurvedic remedy, neem oil has been touted for its medicinal properties for over 5,000 years. Applied topically, neem oil promotes healing while easing the itching and the pain of hemorrhoids.

natural news _____

Agatha M. Thrash, M.D., the co-founder of Uchee Pines Lifestyle Center in Seale, Alabama, suggests these remedies to ease the discomfort of hemorrhoids:

♦ Use a cold or hot compress of an astringent such as goldenseal tea.

♦ Maintain knee-chest position five minutes twice daily.

♦ Use a very mild laxative to stimulate easy bowel movement. The laxative may be prune juice, mild senna tea, or very mild licorice tea.

♦ Avoid standing for long periods.

Hydrotherapy

Sitz baths several times a week can help take the fire out of hemorrhoids. If you don't have a bathtub, you can even buy a plastic sitz bath that will fit over your toilet for less than $20 at your drugstore. The idea is to soak the lower half of your body in a soothing bath to encourage healing. You can do this for up to 20 to 30 minutes; keep the water warm or alternate cold and warm sitz baths every few minutes. Gently pat the area dry when you finish.

If you want to add healing herbs, try Motherlove's Sitz Bath. This herbal mix contains certified organic or ethically harvested (in a way that avoids depleting the land) wild crafted witch hazel leaf, yarrow (heals and slows bleeding), uva ursi (an astringent herb that reduces swelling), and sea salt in a muslin bag you add to a sitz bath. Not only can you reuse the herbs, but you can also use it as a compress. Need a sitz bath to go? Sitz Bath Spray contains witch hazel leaf, yarrow, uva ursi, and healing lavender. Find both at www.motherlove.com.

dial your doc _____

If you see bleeding from your rectum or blood in your stool, talk to your doctor. Bleeding can be a symptom of other digestive diseases, including colorectal cancer.

Natural Rx

Bioflavonoid complex with rutin, daflon, hesperidin: As directed.

Calendula: Cream, apply topically.

Comfrey: Cream or tea, apply topically.

Motherlove Sitz Bath (www.motherlove.com): As directed.

Neem oil: Apply topically.

Plantain: Cream or tea, apply topically.

Raspberry: Cream or tea, apply topically.

Rutin: As directed.

Sitz Bath Spray (www.motherlove.com): As directed.

Vitamin C: 200–2,000 mg daily in divided doses.

Witch hazel: Apply topically.

Yarrow: Cream or tea, apply topically.

High Blood Pressure (Hypertension)

You may have high blood pressure and not know it. One in three Americans do—65 million of them. Because high blood pressure has no warning signs or symptoms, it's easy to miss this condition, which is why it's known as the "silent killer." You need to be even more vigilant if you've got a family history of high blood pressure, you are over your ideal weight, or you have prehypertension. Changing your diet, losing weight, and getting active can also help control and prevent high blood pressure. Natural remedies can be very helpful at getting your numbers in line as well.

def•i•ni•tion

Prehypertension means you are at risk for high blood pressure. If your blood pressure is between 120/80 mmHg and 139/89 mmHg, you may want to make lifestyle changes now to prevent high blood pressure later.

What the Numbers Mean

Blood pressure is simply the pressure of blood against the walls of your arteries. The pressure is caused by the heart as it pumps the blood through your arteries, and the arteries as they resist the flow. If your blood pressure is higher than it should be, you have high blood pressure. We measure blood pressure in millimeters of mercury (mmHg). The top number (say, 120 over 80) is systolic blood pressure (the most important number for those who are 50 or older), which indicates arterial pressure as the heart beats, while the bottom or lower number, diastolic pressure, is the pressure between beats while the heart is at rest. When you have high blood pressure—say, 140/90 mmHg or higher—also known as hypertension, it increases your risk of heart disease, including heart attack and stroke.

Changing Your Diet

Make a DASH (Dietary Approaches to Stop Hypertension) for good health! Research shows the DASH diet (www.dashdiet.org) reduces both systolic (top number) and diastolic (bottom number) blood pressure. In fact, the DASH diet has been shown to lower blood pressure in just two weeks! It's also been shown to reduce LDL (low-density lipoprotein) cholesterol, or so-called "bad" cholesterol. With DASH, you'll get all the key nutrients for lower blood pressure, like potassium, calcium, and magnesium. It's also rich in fruits, veggies, low-fat or nonfat dairy, whole grains, lean meats, fish, poultry, and nuts and beans.

A 2008 study in the *Archives of Internal Medicine* showed that women who eat diets similar to the DASH diet have a lower risk of coronary heart disease and stroke. Those who had better DASH scores (based on eight food and nutrient components—fruits, vegetables, whole grains, nuts and legumes, low-fat dairy, red and processed meats, sweetened beverages, and sodium) had lower risk. For more information on how to put this to work for you, visit www.dashdiet.org.

Eat More Fiber

You are what you eat. And if you eat a high-fiber diet, you can lower your blood pressure and even improve healthy blood pressure levels, according to a study in the *Journal of Hypertension*. Researchers at the Tulane University School of Medicine came to this conclusion after analyzing data from 25 clinical trials with almost 1,500 participants. When people ate 7.2 to 18.9 g of fiber a day (read your labels for guidance on how much you are eating), it significantly reduced systolic blood pressure by 5.95 mmHg and diastolic blood pressure by 4.20 mmHg. You can also take fiber in supplement form.

natural news

Flavonoids, antioxidants found in green tea, improve blood vessel health. So says a study in the *Journal of the American College of Nutrition*. Boston University and Swiss researchers discovered this benefit of green tea, which appears to help blood vessel cell function.

Enjoy Cocoa

Chocolate can actually help high blood pressure. Research shows that diets high in flavonoids, which are antioxidants that are contained in chocolate are good for cardiovascular function. One study published in *The Journal of the American College of Cardiology* showed that cocoa helped improve vascular functioning in diabetics. Another review of data in *The Journal of Nutrition and Metabolism* in 2006 suggests that cocoa and chocolate exert beneficial effects on cardiovascular risk by lowering blood pressure. "According to studies, eating chocolate can absolutely help lower blood pressure," says Dr. Lucille. "Nibble on dark chocolate in moderation, a small square or two a day of at least 70% cacao. A little goes a long way."

Tomato Supplements

Four dietary supplements, including Lyc-O-Mato, an all-natural tomato lycopene complex, have been clinically shown to lower blood pressure as well as prescription medications, without the side effects. Each Lyc-O-Mato capsule contains the active ingredients that it would take three to five cooked tomatoes every single day to achieve!

Lycopene, an antioxidant found in the sauce of cooked tomatoes, alone won't do the job. Look for Lyc-O-Mato on labels.

Grape Seed Extract

Like wine, grape seed extract has powerful natural plant compounds called polyphenols that act as antioxidants. Research shows polyphenols consumed as foods or supplements can be beneficial when it comes to reducing the risk of cardiovascular diseases. In fact, when scientists at the University of California in Davis looked into the benefits of grape seed extract, they found that it helped to lower systolic blood pressure by 12 mmHg and diastolic blood pressure by 8 mmHg in folks who had metabolic syndrome. This means they have several conditions at once, including high blood pressure, extra weight, not enough HDL (or "good") cholesterol, and insulin resistance. Pretty impressive!

You'll find this specially formulated grape seed extract sold in a number of products, as MegaNatural BP grape seed extract. Ordinary grape seed extract products are good antioxidants but will not lower blood pressure. Visit www.polyphenolics.com to find more information.

Omega-3 Fatty Acids

Omega-3 fatty acids from coldwater fish like salmon, herring, sardines, and mackerel can lower blood pressure, too. Omega-3 fatty acids appear to reduce the resistance to surges of blood flow to the arteries, which improves performance of the left ventricle, the muscular pump. As a result, arteries are more flexible and the heart muscle is more powerful, both of which improve blood flow and reduce blood pressure. If you don't like fish, one good supplement brand is called Nordic Naturals, and you can even get lemon-flavored cod liver oil!

L-Arginine

L-arginine is an amino acid, a natural substance in the body and one of the building blocks of proteins. It's helpful for high blood pressure because it's converted into nitric acid, and this helps dilate blood vessels, resulting in increased blood flow and—you guessed it—lower blood pressure. Research shows if you add more L-arginine to the vascular endothelial cells through supplementation, you get more nitric acid. The best way to benefit is to keep a constant level in your bloodstream. You'll find sustained-release L-Arginine made by the Endurance Products Company at www.endur.com.

Coenzyme Q10

Coenzyme Q10 (CoQ10), or ubiquinone, is an antioxidant found in every cell that is involved in energy production. The problem is, as we age, we manufacture less of this necessary nutrient needed for basic functioning. Statin drugs used to lower LDL (or "bad") cholesterol can lower our supply, too. Some people with hypertension have low blood levels of CoQ10, so it can make sense to supplement with this nutrient to improve energy metabolism.

This is especially important to the heart muscle. A small study in the *European Heart Journal* in 2006 showed that CoQ10 improved functioning in people with advanced chronic heart failure. Studies also show it can help with symptoms like swelling and shortness of breath, and improve quality of life. If you have any questions, check with your doctor first. You can find CoQ10 at your health food store or at www.vitacost.com.

Qigong

Numerous studies have found that by simply slowing your breathing to 10 breaths per minute or less for just 15 minutes a day, you can dramatically reduce high blood pressure without the need for medication. "Most folks breathe between 15 and 20 breaths per minute," says Gary Rebstock, co-author with Master Chunyi Lin of *Born a Healer* about Lin's journey, and the creator of Spring Forest Qigong, a type of qigong practice. "Breathing that rapidly keeps you from utilizing your full lung capacity." In fact, most folks use only about 60 percent of their lung capacity, which means that at any given moment, 40 percent of the air in your lungs is stale air. (Doctors call this functional residual capacity.) "Energy breathing expands your lung capacity and dramatically increases the exchange rate of oxygen, which, of course, is the body's primary fuel," says Rebstock.

Here's how to slow your breathing using a qigong method. Even just five minutes can make a big difference in the way you feel. Try it right now and see!

Qigong energy breathing:

1. Sit or lie in a comfortable position. Smile to relax your mind and body.

2. Place the tip of your tongue gently against the roof of your mouth and breathe through your nose in slow, gentle, deep breaths. Picture in your mind that you are connected to the limitless energy of the universe.

3. As you breathe in, gently pull your lower stomach in a little. Imagine you are using your entire body to breathe. Feel the air flowing into every part of your body.

4. As you breathe out, let your stomach out and visualize any tiredness or stress, pain or sickness, or doubt or worries changing into smoke. Visualize it shooting out of your body to the ends of the universe.

5. To end your energy breathing session, take one final slow, gentle, deep breath. Slowly open your eyes, rub your hands together palm to palm, and then gently massage your face, running your fingertips gently up each side of the bridge of your nose to your forehead, then out and down to your chin in a circular motion several times.

For more information, visit www.SpringForestQigong.com.

Qigong exercises can also help restore normal body functions in people who have high blood pressure. Long-term studies of hypertensive patients who practiced Yan Jing Yi Shen Gong for 30 minutes twice a day showed significant benefits in lowering blood pressure. (This qigong is claimed to be especially valuable for therapeutic purposes and

natural news

If you're going to improve your blood pressure, you need to get active. Just lace up those sneakers, head out the door, and walk for 40 minutes most days of the week. Why not take your dog along? You'll both benefit!

delayed senility. The qigong exercise consists of a combination of sitting meditation and gentle physical movements that emphasizes a calm mind, a relaxed body, and regular respiration.)

Ah, Aromatherapy!

Aromatherapy can reduce the impact of stress by inducing relaxation and, therefore, supporting lower blood pressure, says holistic aromatherapist Jade Shutes, B.A., Diploma AT. Try her stress-buster remedy to ease tension.

Stress-buster remedy:

> 14 drops ylang ylang oil
>
> 5 drops roman chamomile oil
>
> 20 drops mandarin/tangerine oil

Blend the essential oils in a small amber bottle. You can then place 4 to 5 drops in a full-body soothing bath, or place 10 drops in 1 oz. of apricot kernel (or other vegetable oil). Massage the neck and shoulders as needed, or simply open the bottle and smell as needed throughout the day.

Learn to Relax

Biofeedback is a great way to learn to relax and lower blood pressure naturally. A new do-it-yourself biofeedback program called Healing Rhythms, created by Deepak Chopra, M.D.; Dean Ornish, M.D.; and Andrew Weil, M.D., can be helpful for stress reduction. You can find it at www.wilddivine.com.

Natural R$_x$

Calcium: 800–1,200 mg daily.

CoQ10: 100–300 mg daily. www.vitalineformulas.com.

Folic acid: 400 mcg daily.

Garlic: Eat two or three cloves daily. Real garlic is better than supplements.

L-arginine: As directed.

Lyc-O-Mato: As directed. www.lycored.com.

Magnesium: 500–700 mg.

MegaNatural BP grape seed extract: As directed. www.polyphenolics. com.

Olive leaf extract: As directed.

Omega-3 fatty acids: 1,000 mg.

Potassium: 4.7 g daily.

Salt substitute: To taste.

Hypoglycemia

If you have hypoglycemia, or low blood sugar, it means your blood glucose (blood sugar) levels aren't where they should be. Functional hypoglycemia, which we're talking about here, occurs when cells in the pancreas respond to the rise in blood glucose levels (like when you eat something with a lot of sugar in it) by oversecreting insulin to reduce blood sugar. When this happens, your blood sugar takes a nosedive and the brain becomes deprived of optimal levels of glucose. (Glucose is the primary fuel for the brain, so low levels of it affect the brain first.) This impacts your ability to function both mentally and physically, leaving you with headaches, brain fog, dizziness, and fatigue. It can also affect your mood, making you irritable.

When your body is in what it perceives as an emergency state, the fight-or-flight state, because blood sugar levels are falling, the adrenals are also stimulated to make the stress hormones adrenaline and corti-sol, to block the insulin's effect and keep your blood sugar where it needs to be. When this happens repeatedly, it takes its toll on the adrenals and they can't make normal amounts of cortisol and DHEA (Dehydroepiandrosterone). As a result, you become chronically depleted, exhausted, and fatigued.

You can do a simple self-test for hypoglycemia by noticing whether your symptoms go away when you eat something that has protein or complex carbohydrates in it. But there are also several tests for hypo-glycemia, including glucose tolerance tests that measure insulin and adrenaline levels. If you are hypoglycemic, you may find relief in the right diet and nutrients.

Keep Your Furnace Stoked

When you have hypoglycemia, keeping your blood sugar stable is most important. It's critical not to miss or delay meals. Begin with breakfast. Yes, eat breakfast. Don't skip it! Throughout the day, eat six small meals or three meals and three snacks so that you're spacing out your food.

Try not to go more than five or six hours without eating. This will help your body maintain good blood sugar control more easily.

Choosing the Right Foods

Besides eating at the right time, it's important to choose the right foods. If you have hypoglycemia, when you start to feel shaky, you may feel like eating sweets because this type of carbohydrate is absorbed into the bloodstream and digested pretty much immediately. Avoid this inclination. That's because this quick fix is not a long-term solution. In fact, you'll feel your blood sugar dipping again quite soon. This yo-yo effect can eventually lead to more serious problems down the road, like diabetes.

To avoid the up-and-down roller coaster of hypoglycemia, eat complex carbohydrates and protein instead. When you choose a snack, for example, pick those with protein or protein and fat. Snacking on crackers and cheese, for example, will sustain you a lot longer than eating a low-fat cracker by itself. Other good snacks that contain protein include nuts and seeds.

If you have the right balance of protein and complex carbohydrates, insulin can do its job of pushing sugar into cells and lowering your blood sugar. You make it more difficult for the body to do what it does normally if you are loading up on sweets.

When it comes to sweets, why not try a piece of fruit, like an apple? (Avoid fruit juice, because without the fiber, it's too much of a sugar rush.) If you must indulge that sweet tooth, do so after a well-balanced meal. Avoid caffeine as well, because it can cause the same symptoms as low blood sugar. Avoid or limit alcohol. If you do drink, make sure you do so with food.

The Benefits of Fiber

Eating high-fiber foods and whole grains as part of a whole-food diet is also essential to good blood sugar control. That's because fiber helps slow the absorption of carbohydrates so glucose is released into the system more slowly. Water-soluble forms of fiber also increase a cell's sensitivity to insulin, preventing oversecretion and improving the uptake of glucose by the liver and other tissues. All of this keeps blood sugar on an even keel. Good sources of fiber include legumes, oat bran, nuts, seeds, psyllium seed husks, pears, apples, dried beans, and most vegetables.

Taking doses of specific nutrients that support the adrenals throughout the day is a great way to ease the symptoms of hypoglycemia. Beverly Yates, N.D., a naturopathic doctor and founder of the Naturopathic Family Health Clinic in Mill Valley, California, says that when folks do an adrenal tune-up, often the hypoglycemia disappears. Start with these doses at breakfast and repeat them at lunch and snack time. Use the timer on your watch or cell phone to remind you to take these nutrients regularly:

- Holy basil: 100–200 mg
- Ashwanganda: 100–200 mg
- Panex ginseng: 100–200 mg
- Vitamin C: 500 mg

Other Nutrients That Regulate Blood Sugar Levels

One of the key nutrients for hypoglycemia control can be chromium, which is important for the proper functioning of insulin and, in turn, proper blood sugar control. It also aids in the metabolism of carbohydrates and proteins. Without chromium, insulin's action is blocked and glucose levels are elevated. Studies show that a chromium deficiency may be an underlying contributing factor in the tremendous number of U.S. cases of hypoglycemia, diabetes, and obesity. In one double-blind crossover study of eight female patients, reported in the medical journal *Metabolism* (1987), 200 mcg of chromium (as chromium chloride) given twice daily for three months alleviated hypoglycemia symptoms and improved the results of glucose tolerance tests.

Other vitamins are also essential for effective carbohydrate and glucose metabolism. The herb gymnema, along with biotin, zinc, and magnesium, helps stabilize blood sugar levels, minimize blood sugar swings, and allow people to go longer between meals because they don't get as hypoglycemic. B-complex vitamins improve carbohydrate metabolism, and vitamin C enhances adrenal function, so supplementing with these nutrients makes sense as well.

Margot Longenecker, N.D., a naturopathic doctor who practices in Branford and Wallingford, Connecticut, recommends glutamine, an amino acid, to help with carbohydrate cravings. "I like it in a powder form. You can also put it under your tongue, and it can work more instantly if you are experiencing a dip." Biotin also helps reduce sugar cravings.

Handling Stress Better

Stress can undermine your efforts to maintain good blood sugar control. That's because when you get stressed, you're less likely to eat properly, which exacerbates the symptoms of hypoglycemia. That's why it's important to find stress-reduction techniques, such as yoga, deep breathing, and meditation, that work for you. (You'll find more information about these practices in Chapter 5.) Reducing stress also improves adrenal function, an added plus that can ease low blood sugar.

Getting enough exercise is another important part of any hypoglycemia treatment and prevention plan. Regular exercise improves many aspects of glucose metabolism, including enhancing insulin sensitivity and improving glucose tolerance in existing diabetics. Some of the effects of exercise on blood sugar control may stem from the fact that exercise increases tissue chromium concentrations. Aim for one hour of exercise five days a week.

dial your doc

After making changes, if you don't improve in a month, check with your health care practitioner. You may want to be tested for such conditions as food allergies, candidiasis (yeast infection), and hypothyroidism (underactive thyroid), which may mimic hypoglycemia.

Natural Rx

Ashwanganda: 100–200 mg three times daily.

B-complex vitamin: As directed.

Biotin: 3–30 mcg daily.

Chromium: 200 mcg three times daily with meals.

Ginseng: 100–200 mg three times daily.

Glutamine: 500–1,000 mg daily in divided doses under the tongue.

Gymnema: 400 mg daily.

Holy basil: 100–200 mg three times daily.

Magnesium: 300–700 mg daily.

Multivitamin and mineral: As directed.

Vitamin C: 1,500 mg daily in divided doses. Use ascorbic forms of vitamin C or try a chewable; Emergen-C has a light form, so there is less sugar. To do a self-test to see if you are getting enough vitamin C, look at your urine. Once it starts getting a saturated yellow, you can begin to back off your levels and take less—say, 1,000 mg or less to bowel tolerance.

Zinc: 15–50 mg daily.

Insomnia

Sleep is essential to our health and well-being, but often it's one of the first things we sacrifice in our 24-7 world. According to the National Sleep Foundation, 50 million Americans suffer from sleep deprivation. We need between 7 and 9 hours of sleep, but this seems like pie in the sky for most of us, who average 6.7 hours of sleep a night.

You may also toss and turn once you hit the sack due to disorders like sleep apnea, when you stop breathing during sleep, sleep walking, or restless legs syndrome. This means that, even though you are technically "asleep," you don't awake refreshed. If you feel anxious or depressed, or suffer from chronic pain from, say, arthritis, this can also interfere with sleep. Add this to a life spent on the run, fueling up on caffeine, tobacco, and sugar and no wind-down routine once we near bedtime, and most of us are in the sleep debt zone.

You may have trouble sleeping once in a while or it may become a pattern. Either way, natural remedies can provide relief. More than 1.6 million U.S. adults are estimated to use complementary and alternative therapies to treat insomnia or troubled sleeping, according to a new national survey published in the *Archives of Internal Medicine*. You can put these to work for you, too.

dial your doc

Do you snore? If you do and awaken feeling tired, you may have sleep apnea. Other signs you may have it? Feeling really sleepy, feeling depressed, or having high blood pressure. If you think you may have sleep apnea, talk to your doctor, who may refer you to a sleep specialist or sleep disorder physician to help you deal with it more effectively. For mild sleep apnea, you may want to try a dental device. For those with a more severe condition, a pneumatic splint can help prevent the airway from collapsing at night.

Why We Need Those ZZZ's

Strangely, no one is quite sure why we need to sleep. One theory is that we need it to restore energy, recharging our batteries on a daily basis. Our sleep is regulated by what is known as the circadian biological clock located in the hypothalamus deep in the center of our brains. This 24 hour "clock" responds to daylight by keeping us alert and to darkness by making us sleepy. Not getting enough sleep can impact the entire body, including the immune system and cardiovascular system, and can even contribute to obesity. In some cases, a lack of sleep can lead to gastrointestinal problems such as irritable bowel syndrome, gastritis, and ulcers. Sleep deprivation can also lead to car accidents. According to the National Sleep Foundation, more than 100,000 sleep-related vehicle crashes occur each year.

Insomnia also affects our concentration, productivity, and mood. According to the National Sleep Foundation (NSF), one in three people are so sleepy that it interferes with their daily activities. You've probably felt the effects of a lack of sleep when you need to get something important done, like finishing that report at work, participating in a company meeting, or being there for your kids after school.

natural news

Good sleep is essential to memory and learning. Why? Think of your brain like a camera, says Helene Emsellem, M.D., Director of the Center for Sleep & Wake Disorders in Chevy Chase, Maryland, and author of *Snooze...or Lose!* As you go throughout your day, your brain is "taking pictures" and storing information. "When we sleep, our brain has the time to process this new information, make connections, and form memories." In this way, we literally learn while we sleep. Cool, huh?

Reasons You Can't Sleep

Usually, there's more than one reason why you can't seem to get the proper amount of sleep. The top four are caffeine, nicotine, alcohol, and sugar. It's easy to reach for caffeine, whether it's in coffee, tea, or soda. But did you know that it is also present in over-the-counter medicines used to treat headaches and menstrual discomfort? For this reason, it's important to monitor how much caffeine you are actually ingesting over the course of the day.

On average, it takes three to five hours for caffeine to leave the body, but if you think caffeine is impacting your sleep, try stopping six to eight hours before bedtime. Like caffeine, nicotine is another stimulant, so avoid it before bedtime. And while you may think a drink will relax you and enable you to get to sleep more quickly, it will disturb the quality of sleep you have overall, leaving you less than refreshed.

Avoiding the wrong foods can also help you rest better. It can be smart to skip foods that contain the amino acid tyramine, like cheese, ham, sausage, and bacon, because they discourage the production of serotonin, which can aid sleep. If your stomach gives you trouble, avoid vegetables in the nightshade family, such as eggplant and bell peppers, since they can cause indigestion. Nightshade veggies can also increase inflammation and pain for arthritis sufferers, which can interfere with sleep. You'll want to limit foods with lots of sugar, too, as these will only rev you up and then lead to a crash when they are quickly metabolized, leaving you with low blood sugar. Finally, if you think you have food allergies, you may want to be tested so you can avoid foods that trigger symptoms.

natural news

If you've accumulated a sleep debt, it's tempting to try to "catch up" on the weekends, but this doesn't really work. Instead, you end up giving yourself jet lag, says Joyce Walsleben, Ph.D., Associate Professor of Medicine at the Sleep Disorders Center at the NYU School of Medicine. "You may as well have gone to Paris by the time the weekend is over because you can't fall asleep. It becomes an ongoing cycle." But it's one you can break. She suggests adding 15 minutes of sleep each night for a week, then another 15 minutes for the next week or so, by either going to bed earlier or staying in bed later. These minutes add up to more rest for you.

Foods and Herbs to Send You to Dreamland

It's a tradition: every Thanksgiving you have a turkey. Once you've eaten it, you want to take a nap. Why? Because it contains tryptophan, a natural sleep chemical that modulates and deepens sleep. But did you know you can find it in other foods year-round, like tuna, whole-grain crackers or bread, nut butter, bananas, dates, and figs? This makes them ideal snacks for about an hour before bedtime.

Get your ZZZ's Naturally with Valerian

Relaxing valerian is a handy herb to have when sleep eludes you. Ancient Greeks and Romans knew of its medicinal powers, and even Hippocrates touted its healing properties. Valerian is known as a nervine, which means it is soothing to the nervous system, so it's a natural for insomnia and is good for anxiety as well. The German equivalent to the FDA, what is known as German Commission E, has documented no known side effects for valerian. So unlike prescription medicines, it is not considered habit forming and doesn't interfere with normal sleep stages like REM (rapid eye movement). This means you'll wake up feeling less groggy and more alert.

A study in the medical journal *Pharmacology, Biochemistry and Behavior* that involved 128 volunteers who were given valerian extract resulted in a statistically significant improvement in the time required to fall asleep.

Passionflower

Passionflower is especially helpful for pain from aching muscles, since it depresses nerve function that can disturb sleep. This nervine, a natural tranquilizer and sedative, can also help stop those chattering thoughts in your head that can keep you awake at night. Europeans have long found it useful to ease the jitters, so much so that the German Commission E has approved passionflower for those who have trouble sleeping and for worry and anxiety. Since it isn't a narcotic, you don't need a prescription, nor do you need to worry about it becoming habit forming. Just take it as you feel you need it for rest and anxiety.

Kava Kava

You've probably heard about kava kava's anti-anxiety properties. For this reason, it can also help ease insomnia. Once you feel calmer, it's easier to drift off to dreamland. Make sense? If you are taking other anti-anxiety medications, check with your doctor first.

Chamomile Tea

Finally, one of the simplest herbal remedies is a nice cup of chamomile tea. Chamomile soothes jangled nerves and improves digestive function. It gently relaxes the nervous system and has a mildly sedating effect. A cup of tea can be just the thing to send you off to Dreamland.

Vitamins and Minerals

Sure, you can get your tryptophan in turkey and other foods, but you can also take vitamins to induce the same effect. Vitamins B₃ (niacin) and B₆ (pyridoxine) both help trigger tryptophan and serotonin, two of the body's natural sleep chemicals. It's best to take them in the morning, though, so they don't overstimulate the body's deep sleep cycle (REM) and disturb your sleep. Just what we don't want!

Calcium and Magnesium

Other supplements you can add to your sleepy-time list include calcium and magnesium. That's because magnesium has muscle-relaxing effects, relieving leg cramps, and calcium is calming and slightly sedating. In fact, both supplements affect the same part of the brain that sleeping pills do. To get the most benefits of these sleep savers, take 500 mg of calcium and 400 mg of magnesium right before you go to bed.

 natural news

To get your calcium easily, Dr. Walsleben suggests calcium chews like Viactiv. "You get the benefit of 500 mg of calcium carbonate and 100 IU of Vitamin D. It can also satisfy your cravings for sweets. Most chews have only 15 to 20 calories per cube."

Melatonin

Melatonin, a hormone produced in the brain by the pineal gland from tryptohan, is our signal for when it's time to go to bed and when it's time to wake up. Think of it like an internal alarm clock. Levels are highest just before we go to sleep. When it is dark, we produce more melatonin; when it is light, we produce less. Because of this, we think melatonin is linked to circadian rhythm and other processes in the body. As we get older, we produce less melatonin, so supplementing with it for occasional insomnia can help. As a rule, you should take it about two hours before bedtime. It's best to take this product under a health practitioner's care.

natural news

When sleep eludes you, it may be time to hit the tub. Agatha M. Thrash, M.D., co-founder of the Uchee Pines Lifestyle Center, recommends a neutral bath, which means filling a tub full of water at a temperature between 92°F and 96°F. Step in and soak for 10 to 50 minutes, letting your mind relax. When you're done, gently dry yourself off and return to bed in a calm state of mind.

Ah, Aromatherapy!

One of the best ways to induce sleep is to use the power of aromatherapy. Holistic aromatherapist Jade Shutes, B.A., Diploma AT, and founder of the East West School for Herbal and Aromatic Studies in Willow Spring, North Carolina, recommends these remedies for insomnia:

Aromatic insomnia bath:

> 5 drops lavender
>
> 3 drops Roman chamomile
>
> 2 drops mandarin

Place drops in ½ cup of whole milk or 1 tablespoon honey. Add to your bath once you are in the bath.

Sleep well spritzer:

> 5 drops lavender
>
> 5 drops mandarin
>
> 3 drops Roman chamomile
>
> 2 oz. water

Combine essential oils and water in a 2-ounce bottle with a spray top. Shake before each use. Spritz pillows and the bedroom with the aromatic spritzer right before going to bed.

Flower Power

Bach Flower Remedies (see Chapter 5) are made from a "sun tea" of specific wildflowers or trees known for their healing properties, then diluted (similar to homeopathic remedies, in that regard). They work to balance negative emotions, freeing the body's energy to heal itself. You can take the remedy under the tongue, or add a few drops to a glass of water and sip it. Nancy Buono, a Bach Foundation Registered Practitioner (BFRP) and Director of Bach Flower Education, recommends these Bach remedies to help with insomnia. For more information, visit www.bachflowereducation.com.

Behavior	Bach Flower Remedy
Thoughts interrupt sleep and keep spinning in the mind, keeping you awake at night	**White Chestnut,** to calm the mind and release repetitive thoughts
High-energy, driven people are so wound up and high-strung that it is difficult to fall asleep	**Vervain,** to unwind and relax

Exercise Instead of Counting Sheep

Yes, we know it's hard to get off that couch. But exercise can make a big difference in how well you sleep. Recently, Stanford researchers put this theory to the test by putting sedentary men and women with sleep problems on a new program of moderate exercise. The results? After just 16 weeks, they went to sleep twice as fast and slept 40 minutes longer each night. Think this could work for you?

One thing to be aware of, however, is that you shouldn't exercise too close to bedtime. That's because exercise raises your body temperature. This leads to a fall in temperature five or six hours later, which makes falling asleep easier. But if you exercise too close to bedtime, you'll be too revved up to go to sleep. Instead, exercise for at least 20 minutes, five or six hours before bedtime, three or more times a week.

Seven Tips for a Good Night's Sleep

1. Go to bed and get up at the same time.

2. Consume less or no caffeine; avoid alcohol and nicotine.

3. Drink fewer fluids before going to sleep.

4. Avoid heavy meals close to bedtime—but don't go to bed hungry, because this tends keep you awake. An ideal snack is half a turkey sandwich or milk because it contains L-tryptophan, which makes you sleepy.

5. Exercise regularly, no later than three hours before bedtime. Exercise raises your body temperature and delays the onset of sleep.

6. Establish a wind-down routine, like soaking in a hot tub, listening to relaxing music, or reading.

7. Don't take the laptop to bed. New research shows that the brightness of the computer screen can reset your body clock, wake you up, and make it more difficult to go to sleep.

For more information, visit the National Sleep Foundation's website at www.sleepfoundation.org.

Natural R$_x$

Calcium: 500 mg. Muscle relaxant; calms nerves. Use with magnesium for best effect.

Chamomile (matricaria recutita): Nerve tonic; relaxes and tones the nervous system; good for digestive upset. Tincture (1:5, 45 percent alcohol): 3 mL three times daily. Juice: 10 mL twice daily in water before meals. Tea: 1–2 cups after meals and before bed.

Kava kava (piper methysticum): One 180–210 mg capsule (standardized to 30 percent kavalactones) 30–60 minutes before bed.

Lavender tincture (1:5, 45 percent alcohol), 2.5 mL three times daily. Relieves mild anxiety and depression.

Lemon balm (melissa officinalis): Sedative; good for nervous insomnia, headaches, and digestive upsets. Tincture: ½ tsp., 40 drops, or 2.5 mL daily. Tea: 1 TB. per cup of water, 2–3 cups daily.

Magnesium: 400 mg. Acts as a muscle relaxant; calms nerves; good with calcium.

Melatonin: 0.03–3 mg in the evening.

Pasque flower tincture (1:5, 25 percent alcohol): 1 mL (about 20 drops) in warm water 30 minutes before bedtime. If insomnia continues to be a problem, see your health care professional.

Passionflower (passiflora incarnata) tincture: ½ tsp., 40 drops, or 2.5 mL three times daily. Tea: 1 TB. per cup of water, 3 cups daily. Strong calming herb.

Valerian (Valeriana officinalis): Improves quality of sleep; beneficial to nervous system; an anti-anxiety agent. Tincture (1:5, 25 percent alcohol): for tenseness, restlessness, and irritability; up to 5 mL three times daily. As an aid to sleep, 5–10 mL 30 minutes before bedtime. Tea: Add 2 tsp. dried root to 1 cup water, bring to a boil, simmer five minutes, and strain—drink three times daily or before bed.

Vitamins B_3 and B_6: Helps induce the body's natural sleep chemicals, tryptophan and serotonin; supports central nervous system. B_3, 10–35 mg daily; B_6, 2–200 mg daily.

Irritable Bowel Syndrome

One in five Americans has irritable bowel syndrome (IBS), one of the most common gastrointestinal disorders affecting the colon, or large bowel. If you are one of them, you know the uncomfortable abdominal cramping it causes. You also know you can alternate between diarrhea one day and constipation the next, and experience bloating and gas. No one knows for sure what causes IBS, but it could be that the muscles in the bowel are just extra sensitive and can be affected by emotional upset and the foods we eat. Whatever the reason, IBS affects almost twice as many women as men.

IBS has a very strong link to stress, says Greg Nigh, N.D., L.Ac., who practices at Nature Cures Clinic in Portland, Oregon (www.naturecuresclinic.com). "It's a self-feeding loop. Stress causes IBS, and the symptoms of IBS cause stress. IBS can be very limiting in daily activities. People feel like they're not healthy, which can be stressful, especially if they haven't had any significant health problems before. When they get stressed about their health, that stress causes more symptoms." To begin to heal the symptoms of IBS, diet is the first place to start.

Changing Your Diet

If you have IBS, your digestion is compromised. Dr. Nigh says, "If you don't have enough acid in your stomach, this leads to problems with digesting proteins and absorbing nutrients. If you don't digest your proteins, then those undigested proteins get down into the lower bowel, where they start to putrefy, which leads to inflammation in the bowel." (Read on to "Digestive Help" for more information.)

The foods we eat can also cause inflammation in our gut. Lowering the burden of inflammation by changing what we eat can help the healing process.

Foods to Avoid

If you have IBS, you'll want to avoid certain foods that stimulate or irritate the gastrointestinal tract. This means avoiding foods high in fat, like chocolate, or caffeine, like coffee and diet sodas (carbonated drinks are also aggravating to the bowel), since these cause the bowel to contract, and the bowel is already overstimulated. Nix sugar-free foods like sorbital, and alcohol, too. Since you'll be feeling gassy and bloated, it's a good idea to minimize foods like beans, cabbage, and peas as well. Allergies to foods like wheat, dairy, and corn can also contribute to IBS, but this factor can be overlooked. To determine which foods affect you most, go on an elimination diet by avoiding offending foods for two weeks and see how you feel.

The Benefits of Fiber

Fiber is critical, says Dr. Nigh. "Fiber cleans the gut out and creates an environment that helps healthy bacteria to grow." Certain kinds of fiber, like beta glucan, a kind of fiber derived from oats, is also very good at absorbing toxins and carrying them out of the body. In addition, it can be helpful to take a tablespoon or two of flaxseed powder, a soluble fiber that helps to lower cholesterol.

Fiber is also found in foods such as whole-grain breads and cereals, beans, and fruits and vegetables such as apples, peaches, broccoli, raw cabbage, and raw carrots. But don't be too gung-ho. Instead, begin to add foods with fiber to your diet a little bit at a time, to let your body get used it. Too much fiber can cause cramping and gas—just what you don't want.

dial your doc

You can try an elimination diet—Dr. Nigh has written an eBook to help with this, which can be found at www.naturecuresclinic.com—or doctors can run blood tests to look for foods you are allergic to. Blood tests will show antibodies for foods you might be allergic to that are triggering your IBS.

Herbal Help

Soothing peppermint oil can be just the thing to calm down an overactive digestive tract that alternates between constipation and diarrhea. This is because peppermint oil acts as a muscle relaxant. Using peppermint oil that has enteric coating is important because it keeps the oil from being absorbed in the stomach. Instead, it moves to the small intestine and the colon, where it is released for maximum benefit. According to a study reported in the *Journal of Digestive Liver Disease*, when volunteers with IBS took Mintoil peppermint oil (two enteric-coated capsules twice daily) for four weeks, their symptoms improved.

In another study reported in the *American Journal of Gastroenterology*, when 52 patients took a capsule of enteric-coated peppermint oil capsules (Colpermin) three to four times daily, before meals, for a month, 79 percent experienced relief from abdominal pain and 29 percent were pain free! So you may want to consider trying this. German Commission E, Germany's counterpart to our FDA, thinks so, too, as it has approved this remedy for the treatment of irritable colon.

Often in Germany, clown's mustard (Iberis amara) or wild candytuft is used together with peppermint oil to treat the symptoms of IBS. In the medical journal *Advances in Therapy* (2003), an overview of research done on a brand of clown's mustard called Iberogast showed its soothing therapeutic effects on the gastrointestinal tract. Iberogast also contains eight other herbs, including chamomile, milk thistle, and licorice, for digestive health. You can try peppermint oil and clown's mustard together or one at a time to see what works for you.

natural news

A study in the *Journal of Alternative and Complementary Medicine* shows that one or two tablets of a standardized turmeric extract taken daily for eight weeks may improve IBS. About two thirds of all the subjects in the study reported an improvement in symptoms after treatment, and there was a favorable shift in bowel pattern.

Digestive Help

Digestive enzymes like bromelain (which comes from pineapples) can help with digestion and normalize bowel function. You take them with your meal, to help you digest your food.

Research also shows that probiotics, or "friendly bacteria," dietary supplements with beneficial yeasts and bacteria, are promising therapies in IBS. Probiotics may ease the inflammation associated with IBS and help restore normal local immune function. "Everyone should take probiotics every day, for the rest of their life," says Dr. Nigh. "Hundreds of different strains of bacteria live in our gut that are healthy, so no supplement will have them all. The main ones to look for are acidophilus and bifidus, and these can be purchased together. People who have irritable bowel can take 100 billion a day. It's an enormous dose, but that's the dose needed for irritable bowel. For general health, anywhere from 4 billion to 10 billion is a daily dose."

Learn to Relax

Since IBS can be aggravated by stress, learning how to relax can help. One of the most useful tools is biofeedback. A new do-it-yourself biofeedback program called Healing Rhythms, created by Deepak Chopra, M.D.; Dean Ornish, M.D.; and Andrew Weil, M.D., can be helpful for stress reduction. You can find it at www.wilddivine.com.

Quite a bit of research also has focused on the therapeutic effects of hypnosis on IBS. In fact, 16 studies with hypnosis showed an improvement in all the major symptoms of IBS, improving them by half. Overall, the response rate to hypnosis treatment is 87 percent. Anxiety and depression also improve after treatment with hypnosis.

Bust a Yoga Move

Research at British Columbia Children's Hospital in Vancouver, British Columbia, has shown that adolescents aged 11 to 18 with IBS can benefit from yoga. The yoga intervention consisted of a one-hour instructional session, demonstration, and practice, followed by four weeks of daily home practice guided by a video. The adolescents in the study who found yoga helpful said they'd continue to use it to manage their IBS symptoms at home.

Ah, Aromatherapy!

Holistic aromatherapist Jade Shutes, B.A., Diploma AT, owner of the East West School for Herbal and Aromatic Studies (www.TheIDA.com) in Willow Spring, North Carolina, recommends this remedy to ease IBS:

Soothe the belly oil:

> 1 oz. vegetable oil (such as apricot kernel or sunflower oil)
>
> 6 drops peppermint
>
> 5 drops ginger
>
> 10 drops lavender

Massage the abdominal area and lower back two times daily or as needed.

Natural R$_x$

Acidophilus bifidus: 100 billion daily. For general health: 4 billion to 10 billion daily.

B complex: 50–100 mg daily with extra B$_5$, pantothenic acid; 100 mg daily for stress.

Bromelain: 500 mg three times daily with meals.

Calcium polycarbophil: As directed. Brand name Equalactin. Can help with alternating diarrhea and constipation, and abdominal discomfort.

Clown's mustard (Iberis amara): Herbal combination tincture: 20 drops after meals three times daily.

Fennel seed (Foeniculum vulgare): Tea, 1 TB. per cup of water, 3 cups daily after meals.

Ginger root (Zingiber officinale): Tea, 1 TB. per cup of water, 3 cups daily after meals.

Iberogast: As directed.

L-glutamine: As directed. An amino acid can help nourish the lining of the gut; a small percentage will get anxious from taking this—if so, discontinue.

Magnesium: 200 mg two to three times daily.

N-Acetylcysteine (NAC) capsules and tablets: 600–1,200 mg daily. Good antioxidant.

Peppermint oil, enteric coated: 1–2 capsules three times daily after meals, or 0.6 mL daily.

Jet Lag

You've been planning your trip for months and can't wait to leave your everyday life behind and get on the plane. But have you thought about how you'll feel once you land? To make sure you feel your best with minimal jet lag, it can be smart to do your homework. This can mean everything from making sure your sleep bank is full of restful slumber before you go, to taking along helpful remedies that can ensure you hit the ground running!

Before You Leave

Since *jet lag* is more likely to occur when you cross more than two time zones, start acclimating yourself a few days before. If you are traveling east to Europe, say, go to bed an hour earlier; if you are heading west to Hawaii, make it an hour later. In addition to rearranging your bedtime, it can make sense to head to the store for these helpful remedies!

Take Your Vitamin C!

One of the best vitamins to help reduce jet lag and help the body handle stress is antioxidant-packed vitamin C, says Brigitte Mars, author of *The Desktop Guide to Herbal Medicine.* Mars also suggests packing "green foods" with lots of nutrients (especially if safe veggies won't be available) like spirulina or blue-green algae. Bring a multivitamin as well to cover you for any kind of nutritional deficiencies you may have while traveling. (Let's face it, we don't always eat the way we should when we are away from home.)

def•i•ni•tion

Jet lag occurs when the body's clock gets out of sync when traveling across one or more time zones by plane. That's because the daylight and darkness hours are different than what you're used to.

No Jet Lag in a Bottle

No Jet Lag is a homeopathic remedy designed to let you go from point A to point B with a minimum of discomfort (see www.nojetlag.com). The ingredients in No Jet Lag include Arnica montana and Bellis perennis, which are good for tension and sleeplessness; Chamomilla and Lycopodium, which ease stress and anxiety; and Ipecacuanha, which lessens dehydration and nausea.

You can take No Jet Lag with any other medication. Like other homeopathic remedies, it's most effective when taken separately from food and drink, but it has been specially formulated so that it may, if necessary, be taken in association with food and/or drink.

Another natural remedy that can help you get acclimated once you arrive is Cerebral Tonic Pills called Bu Nao Wan, a Chinese Patent Formula. "Bu Nao Wan pills contain Schizandra berries, Jujube dates, and goji berries, among other herbs which help improve memory, concentration, fatigue, and insomnia," says Mars. You'll find them in a natural foods store or a Chinese grocery store, or at www. healingherbsofchina.com.

If You Feel Queasy When Traveling

While the ipecacuanha in No Jet Lag is good for nausea, you may also want to pack some candied ginger. You can find this in your local health food store along with Newman's Own Organics Ginger Mints (www.newsmansownorganics.com). Another nausea solution is Sea-Band Anti-Nausea Ginger Gum (www.sea-band.com).

To Stay Regular

To make sure your bathroom breaks remain the same, Mars suggests bringing along raw dehydrated flax seeds and alfalfa tablets. Both of these will help prevent traveler's constipation. You'll also want to up your water intake.

To avoid spending most of your vacation in the bathroom with diarrhea, try to ward off intestinal complaints by taking an acidophilus supplement a week before leaving and during the trip, to help establish those friendly bacteria in your gut, says Mars. If you have diarrhea, she suggests Ume concentrate made from umeboshi plum in pills or paste, or charcoal capsules.

Nancy Eagles, a chartered herbalist whose website is www.iannaherbs. com, suggests this Slippery Elm Balls recipe for diarrhea:

> 3 TB. slippery elm powder
>
> 2 TB. honey
>
> 1 tsp. ginger powder

Mix together and form into balls the size of a thumbnail. Roll in slippery elm powder or sugar. Allow to dry. Store in a mint tin.

When you have diarrhea, it's also very important to guard against dehydration. Eagles suggests combining 1 teaspoon salt plus 1 teaspoon sugar in 1 cup of warm water and sipping it.

To Be Calm

In this day and age, we all know that traveling can be stressful. So the one thing you want to be sure to pack is your Rescue Remedy, a combination of five Bach flower essences that are known for their healing properties. Rescue Remedy works to balance negative emotions, calming you and helping you handle situations with more ease. You can even give it to your pets to ease traveling trauma!

Either take Rescue Remedy under the tongue (4 drops) or add it to a small glass of water and sip it. Rescue Remedy comes in a spray and in pastilles (small medicinal pills), too. For more information, visit www. rescueremedy.com.

Nancy Buono, a Bach Foundation Registered Practitioner (BFRP) and director of Bach Flower Education, also recommends the Bach remedy Walnut for jet lag to help you adjust to a new time zone, diet, and climate. You can take the remedy under the tongue or add a few drops to a glass of water and sip it.

Aromatherapy can also help erase stress and ease the effects of jet lag. "Geranium and lavender essential oils are superb for jet lag because of their balancing effects," says holistic aromatherapist Jade Shutes, B.A., Diploma AT.

Shutes recomends this remedy for jet lag:

Combine four drops geranium with five drops lavender into a 1-oz. bottle of sunflower or apricot kernel vegetable oil. Massage on the hands, neck, face, and shoulders. You can also take a bath with this blend by simply adding four drops geranium and four drops lavender to the bath water after you are in the bath.

Once You Are on the Plane

Keep drinking. And we don't mean martinis when there is too much turbulence. We are talking about water, H_2O, so you don't get dehydrated. "Drinking one glass of water for every hour in flight is ideal," says Mars. "One of my favorite ways of staying hydrated is to bring cucumbers along." Make yourself at home. If your tootsies smell dandy, feel free to take off your shoes and put in ear plugs and wear an eye mask to create a quiet zone for yourself. You may also want to bring along a light blanket and an inflatable neck pillow. Try to sleep, if you can, as this will help ease jet lag. But do make it a point to move. "Sitting in one position too long without stretching can not only make you stiff, but it can also lead to problems like blood clots," says Mars.

Call ahead to order a healthy meal. You can go natural by ordering vegetarian, vegan, or even gluten-free meals. Make it a point, too, to bring healthy snacks with you, like an apple or low-fat mozzarella sticks or cashews or pistachio nuts.

Adjusting to Your New Time Zone

When you get on the plane, start by putting yourself in the mind-set of your destination. First, change your watch to "local time." When you arrive, stay awake, if you can, until your normal bedtime. If you must nap, limit it to an hour or so, or you may have trouble catching those zzzz's at night. If caffeine tends to cause insomnia, monitor your intake and limit drinking coffee and diet sodas to early in the day, if possible.

Since exposure to full-spectrum light tells the pineal gland in the brain, which regulates our sleep-wake rhythm, to reset its internal clock, make it a point to get outside every day. At night, the pineal gland produces melatonin, which induces sleep. So if you need help sleeping, choose a natural melatonin supplement of 0.03 to 3 mg in the evening before retiring.

Natural Rₓ

Asian ginseng: One 100-mg capsule, containing 4 to 7 percent ginsenosides, twice daily. Helps the body adapt to jet lag.

Betaine hydrochloride: As directed. Can help you adjust to new foods in your diet.

Cerebral tonic pills: 4–6 tablets three times daily; www.healingherbsofchina.com.

Charcoal: Two capsules, as directed. www.kirkmanlabs.com.

Electrolyte powder: As directed. For dehydration after diarrhea.

Ginger tincture: ½ tsp., 40 drops, or 2.5 mL three times daily. Capsules: 300 mg twice daily. You can take syrups and chewable gum as well.

Melatonin: 0.03–3 mg in the evening.

Multivitamin: As directed.

No Jet Lag homeopathic remedy: One tablet of No Jet Lag at the time of each take-off, another tablet every two hours in flight, and another tablet after each landing, including at intermediate stops. During long flights, the two-hour intervals may be extended if the user is sleeping. www.nojetlag.com.

Qing Hao (artemisia annua herb): As directed. www.chineseherbsdirect.com.

Rescue Remedy: As directed.

Ume concentrate: Pills or paste, as directed.

Vitamin C: 200–500 mg daily.

Walnut flower essence: As directed.

Menopause

They call it "the change," and it brings plenty of them. If you're in menopause, you know all about the hot flashes, mood swings, and brain fog. With the ovarian production of estrogen and progesterone decreasing, other "changes" or symptoms of menopause can include weight gain, loss of libido, night sweats, and achy joints.

Women can also become more sensitive to pain, says Pamela Hannaman, N.D., a naturopathic physician in Richmond, Virginia. "Neurotransmitters in the brain have a lot to do with at what level we start perceiving pain. It's all related to serotonin. During menopause, our pain threshold changes because our serotonin levels start to diminish. We have less resilience to pain. We feel it sooner and we feel it more intensely."

Women may also experience more emotional ups and downs. Being in menopause may mean you don't see a real reason why you're feeling blue or lethargic. Things can be going great in your life, but you might feel somewhat depressed because of neurotransmitter changes. This may be due to the shift in ratio between estrogen and progesterone, which can also cause insomnia.

You're officially in menopause if you haven't had your period for one year. Once you are, it may be smart for you to take advantage of the myriad benefits natural remedies offer to promote general well-being and improve the specific symptoms of menopause. This is especially important since the conventional treatment for many menopausal symptoms has been hormone-replacement therapy, which has been associated with serious health risks.

Looking into "the Change"

Because of the hot flashes and other symptoms that can be inconvenient, it can seem like menopause is a condition, but it's actually a natural transition that every woman experiences. The more we see it that way, the easier it will be. "The biggest thing is to honor and understand how natural a process it is," says Holly Lucille, N.D., a naturopathic physician and author of *Creating and Maintaining Balance: A Woman's Guide to Safe, Natural Hormone Health.* "But menopause has become the catchall for all the stressors and changes—physically, mentally, or emotionally—that women are experiencing at that time." That's why, if you have symptoms, they deserve a deeper look.

The Importance of Adrenal Support

When it comes to easing the transition of menopause, one of the best strategies is to support the adrenal glands. In the body's wisdom, it has designed the adrenal glands to be a back-up source of estrogen and progesterone after menopause. Think of the adrenal glands as a bridge out of the reproductive years to the post-reproductive years.

When the production of hormones begins to change in menopause, the adrenal glands are there to keep the body stable. That's why addressing adrenal health is one of Dr. Lucille's first approaches in dealing with menopausal symptoms. First, she says, make sure you have a blood sugar–stabilizing diet. Eat small, frequent meals throughout the day so your blood sugar doesn't go up and down. (For more tips about how to eat for stable blood sugar, see the section on hypoglycemia.) If you don't eat, rapidly falling blood sugar levels can stimulate the adrenal glands to release stress hormones like adrenaline and cortisol to block insulin's effect and keep blood sugar stable. When this happens repeatedly, it takes its toll on your already depleted adrenals, and they can't make normal amounts of cortisol and DHEA (Dehydroepiandrosterone). As a result, you become chronically depleted, exhausted, and fatigued. Eating regular small meals and snacks with protein prevents this process.

Making space for rest, relaxation, and repair is also important for adrenal health, says Dr. Lucille. "We can have big, busy lives if we weave in times and places where we can unburden, like taking more baths or being out in nature."

Detox to Ease Symptoms

Menopause symptoms can result when the body is overburdened with toxins. For Dr. Lucille, hormone health is enhanced by a whole-body cleanse. "If you throw away the diagnosis of menopause and you listen to women, sometimes the symptoms are those of toxicity in the body." When you think about a cleanse, you may think of that funny skit on *Saturday Night Live* about a cereal named Colon Blow, but that's not how it works, says Dr. Lucille. "There are a lot of misconceptions about cleansing. I say it's not fasting or colon blow. It's assisting your own body's ability, which may be overburdened by toxicity. I view it as rebooting your computer. When you clean things out and decrease toxicity, you increase vitality."

For an easy do-it-yourself cleanse, Dr. Lucille recommends Enzymatic Therapy Whole Body Cleanse (www.enzy.com). This is one of the only companies in the nutraceutical business registered as an FDA-standard pharmaceutical-grade manufacturing facility. It is also organically certified. The Whole Body Cleanse is a simple two-week program that uses a soothing herbal blend to support detoxification for the whole body, including the intestines, liver, gall bladder, and circulatory and lymphatic systems. Milk thistle is part of the mix, to help eliminate toxins and support liver function. Visit www.enzy.com for more information.

Natural Support for Transitional Times

These herbal remedies can be very supportive in the menopausal transition. They can help to relieve common symptoms such as hot flashes, mood changes, and overall hormonal balance. Using them can help you move through this "change" in your life more smoothly and easily.

Black Cohosh

If you have hot flashes, suffer night sweats, and feel just plain irritable, reach for black cohosh, one of the most relied-upon menopause remedies. This member of the buttercup family has been well studied for its safety and effectiveness. "Black cohosh continues to have an incredible safety profile," says Dr. Lucille, who likes to use Remifemin, a specialized black cohosh extract. "It has actually been shown to help prevent breast cancer." Dr. Lucille refers to a recent study (2007) conducted at the University of Pennsylvania School of Medicine and reported in *The International Journal of Cancer*, which shows that Remifemin, a specific formulation of black cohosh, lowers the risk of breast cancer by as much as 60 percent. This is encouraging, given the recent reports of risks regarding hormone-replacement therapy (HRT). Remifemin is safe particularly for women who should not take estrogen, say researchers. For more information on this product, visit www.enzy.com.

natural news

Like black cohosh, some foods are high in naturally occurring plant sterols (similar in chemical formula to estrogens), so it can make sense to add them to your diet. They include apples, cherries, olives, plums, anise seed, wheat germ, food yeast, whole grains, garlic, barley, corn, parsley, oats, rice, wheat, sage, coconut, carrots, peanuts, yams, soybeans, alfalfa leaf tea, licorice root tea, and foods of the nightshade family (bell pepper, paprika, pimentos, eggplant, potatoes, and tomatoes).

Dong Quai

Another natural remedy for hot flashes is dong quai, a small, fern-leafed (it looks like parsley), aromatic plant that comes from China. Second only to ginseng in popularity there, this phyto, or plant, estrogen has mild estrogenic effects that are well worth noticing. Basically, the plant compounds in dong guai help by occupying estrogen receptor sites, thereby blocking estrogen from being absorbed. Since they are far less potent, this means less stimulation for the body and fewer symptoms. In fact, because phytoestrogens are a mild form of estrogen, they actually help balance out the overall effect of estrogens, helping you to feel more, well, normal. You can take dong quai as a supplement or buy the root crowns (they are aromatic, with a celerylike flavor) and put them in chicken soup.

natural news

For relief from hot flashes, Dr. Lucille also recommends vitamins C and E and hesperidin, a citrus flavonoid that helps maintain vascular integrity. Together with C, it's a kind of bioflavonoid complex. In addition, she recommends gamma oryzanol, a compound that comes from rice bran oil. "Research shows that it reduces hot flashes. It was used in the 1960s and is now popular again."

Chaste Tree

The Mediterranean is not only a good inspiration for diets and vacations. It's also home to the chaste tree (vitex agnus-castus) plant. This medicinial herb has small, dark, peppercorn-like fruits and was well known to ancient Greek physicians like Hippocrates, the father of modern medicine, who used it as a treatment for injuries and inflammations. Today it's used for hormonal balance, helping to increase the level of progesterone while reducing the level of estrogen. Shifting this balance can help relieve the symptoms of menopause, including mild anxiety, nervousness, and sleeplessness. For many practitioners, it's the number-one progesteronic herb to use.

natural news

Menopause is a huge endocrinological shift, but it is also a mental, emotional, and spiritual one. "It is a metamorphosis; you are changing and there is a very natural pull inward," says Dr. Lucille. Practices like yoga and meditation can help you go inward and understand more about yourself as you ease into this new phase of your life.

Homeopathic Remedies

To ease hot flashes and night sweats, try these homeopathic remedies. Take three pellets as needed five times daily:

- ◆ Belladonna
- ◆ Calcarea carbonica
- ◆ Cimicifuga (black cohosh)
- ◆ Gelsemium
- ◆ Lachesis

The homeopathic remedy Pulsatilla can ease emotions during hormonal changes. Take three pellets as needed five times daily.

Ah, Aromatherapy!

Holistic aromatherapist Jade Shutes, B.A., Diploma AT, recommends creating an aromatic spritzer for relief from hot flashes:

Hot flash spritzer:

1. In a spritzer bottle, add 4 oz. water (or 2 oz. lavender hydrosol and 2 oz. rose hydrosol).

2. Add 10 drops cypress, 4 drops rose, and 3 drops peppermint essential oil.

3. Shake before use.

4. Spritz the face, neck, and shoulders as needed. (Avoid the eyes, as irritation will occur.)

To soothe emotions, Jade recommends making a natural menopausal remedy.

Menopausal massage oil:

5 drops Neroli

10 drops Mandarin

1 oz. vegetable oil, such as apricot kernel or sunflower oil, or unscented lotion or cream

Blend ingredients and massage on the shoulders, neck, and face, or apply onto the whole body after a shower.

To find essential oils, visit www.leydenhouse.com or www.naturesgift. com.

Flower Power

Bach Flower Remedies (see Chapter 5) are made from a "sun tea" of specific wildflowers or trees known for their healing properties, then diluted (similar to homeopathic remedies, in that regard). They work to balance negative emotions, freeing the body's energy to heal itself. You can take the remedy under the tongue, or add a few drops to a glass of water and sip it. Nancy Buono, a Bach Foundation Registered

Practitioner (BFRP) and Director of Bach Flower Education, recommends these Bach remedies to help with the changes menopause brings. For more information, visit www.bachflowereducation.com.

Condition	Bach Flower Remedy
Poor self-image; feel old, ugly, fat; self-disgust	**Crab Apple,** to cleanse and purify both the body and your outlook
Emotions are raging and out of control; body also feels out of control	**Cherry Plum,** to restore rational feelings and a sense of calm control
Hot flashes	**Walnut,** to assist the body in adapting to the changes

The Menopause Formula

Using the General Menopause Formula, created by Agatha M. Thrash, M.D., founder of the Uchee Pines Lifestyle Center in Seale, Alabama, daily can help ease menopausal symptoms. Here's how to make it:

1. Boil 4 cups water.

2. Add 1 to 3 teaspoons black cohosh (use the smaller amount if it causes a headache) and 1 teaspoon licorice powder.

3. Simmer gently for 20 minutes.

4. Pour the entire mixture into a container and steep 30 minutes with 1 teaspoon each of red raspberry leaf, alfalfa leaf, and catnip leaf.

5. Drink throughout the day.

natural news

When you go through menopause, estrogen is the dominator, so natural progesterone creams may help. Use them for just three months at a time while you work on your diet, exercise, and added nutrients. A company that creates good products for women over 40 is Emerita. Dr. Lucille recommends its progesterone cream, called Progest, because it's natural and paraben free. For more information, visit www.emerita.com.

Natural R~x~

Alfalfa (medicago sativa): Rich in minerals. Contains phyto (plant) estrogens and makes a gentle substitute for estrogen after menopause. Tea: 1 TB. of leaves per cup of water, 3 cups daily.

B-complex vitamin: As directed.

Belladonna homeopathic remedy: Three pellets as needed five times daily.

Black cohosh: Capsules and tablets standardized to 2.5 percent triterpene glycosides: 40 mg twice daily. Consider Remifemin. Good for hot flashes and depression during menopause; relieves muscle pain and headaches; eases fatigue and mood swings; increases vaginal lubrication; regulates hormones to stop irregular bleeding. Use at least two to three months to see results.

Calcarea Carbonica homeopathic remedy: 3 pellets as needed five times daily.

Chaste tree (Vitex agnus-castus): As directed. For menopause, take at least three to six months to see results. Different brand formulations are available, including Agnoly and Femicur.

Cimicifuga homeopathic remedy: Three pellets as needed five times daily.

Dong quai (Angelica sinensis), also called tang-kuei: Capsules and tablets: 100–200 mg daily. Relieves menopausal symptoms such as hot flashes; strengthens blood and female reproductive organs.

Enzymatic Therapy Whole Body Cleanse: As directed. www.enzy.com.

Evening primrose capsules: 500 mg three times daily.

Gelsemium homeopathic remedy: 3 pellets as needed five times daily.

Lachesis homeopathic remedy: 3 pellets as needed five times daily.

Motherwort (Leonurus cardiaca): Tea, 1 TB. of leaves per cup of water, 3 cups daily. Effective for menopausal anxiety, exhaustion, nervousness, and heart palpitations; treats headaches, dizziness, and irritability.

Multivitamin and mineral: As directed. Doctor's Choice for 45 Plus. www.enzy.com.

Oat grass (Avena sativa) tincture: ½ tsp., 40 drops, or 2.5 mL three times daily. Take daily for menopausal symptoms, two weeks per month for premenopausal problems. Relaxes nervous system, reduces fatigue; can help fight osteoporosis through its rich calcium content.

Pulsatilla homeopathic remedy: 3 pellets as needed five times daily.

Vitamin B5: 250 mg twice daily.

Vitamin C: 200–2,000 mg daily in divided.

Migraines

If you've ever had a migraine, you'll never forget it. Over 30 million people in the United States—three quarters of them women—know the knifelike, throbbing pain of a migraine. You may feel migraine pain in the forehead, temple, ear, or jaw, or around the eye, but it's usually on one side at a time. You'll probably have other symptoms, too, like being overly sensitive to light, sounds, and smells.

Ooh, My Head

According to Hilary Garavaltis, ayurvedic practitioner and dean of curriculum for the Kripalu School of Ayurveda at the Kripalu Center for Yoga and Health in Stockbridge, Massachusetts, in ayurvedic medicine, headaches come in three types:

Vata: A throbbing, shooting headache usually located at the base of the skull. It is present more at dawn or dusk and is usually associated with constipation or indigestion. Vata-aggravating factors include hearing too much noise and stimulation, having too many things happen too quickly, and traveling. The recommended solution is to take pacifying measures, such as seeking a quiet, calm environment; ingesting warm liquids and foods; and putting a warm cloth on the base of the skull.

Pitta: An intense, sharp, penetrating headache in the temporal region, often accompanied by nausea. It is often present at midday or midnight and is due to excess heat or sun, or acid indigestion. The recommended solution is to get out of the heat and lie down in a quiet, dark, cool place with a cool cloth. Drink something cooling and not too stimulating. Apply sandalwood paste to the temples and forehead area. If indigestion is chronic, see your health care practitioner.

Kapha: A slow, dull, achy headache in the front of the head and in the sinus area. It is often present in midmorning or midevening. The recommended solution is to use Nasya oil to break up congestion and create a better flow. Warm steam with eucalyptus can help to decongest and open up the area. Avoid foods like dairy and wheat. Choose warm, moist, well-cooked foods. Withdraw to a warm environment and take time to be calm and quiet. Do not overstimulate yourself.

About half of migraine sufferers experience what is known as the pro-drome, a phase that is also a warning that a headache may be coming. This is when chemical changes are going on in the brain 12 to 24 hours before the attack. During the prodrome, it's common to have food cravings for things like chocolate, experience constipation or diarrhea, feel blue or tired, have incredible surges of energy, and need to urinate more frequently.

Twenty percent of sufferers experience an "aura," or visual disturbance, which is a warning signal usually 30 minutes before the headache strikes. Symptoms of the aura can include blurry vision, flashing lights, hallucinations, tingling, or numbness of the face. Once you have a migraine, it can last from 4 to 72 hours.

Most migraine sufferers are between ages 20 and 45. Migraines run in families, so if your parents have migraines, chances are you will, too. *Tension type headache* is the second-most-common type of headache. The two other types are *sinus* and *cluster* headaches.

def•i•ni•tion

Tension type headache is the second most common type of headache. Often triggered by stress, it usually feels like you have a vise around your head. You won't experience the migrainelike symptoms of nausea or sensitivity to light, noise, or smells. Supplements that can bring relief include Valerian root.

Sinus headache means pain and pressure in the sinus area. Often migraine sufferers have sinus aggravation or irritation that seems like a sinus headache, but the migraine is the underlying cause of the pain. Once the migraine is treated, they feel better.

Cluster headaches are brief but painful headaches that last 15 minutes to 2 hours on either side of the head, often accompanied by red, watery eyes. They occur every day or multiple times a day for about two weeks to two months, and then spontaneously go away. Capsaicin cream, (the active component of cayenne pepper) can help ease cluster headaches by inhibiting the production of what is known as substance P.

The Headache Diet

Certain foods are no-no's for migraine sufferers. Caffeine, chocolate, soy, red wine, aged cheeses, sourdough bread, onions, citrus fruits, guar gum, and monosodium glutamate (MSG) can all be triggers. So can fermented, smoked, and salted foods that contain tyramine, a compound produced from the natural breakdown of the amino acid tyrosine, because they cause blood vessels to dilate, which can cause migraines. Keeping track of what you eat and the reaction you have can help you avoid these foods in the future. You can also get a copy of a tyramine-free diet from the National Headache Foundation by calling 1-888-NHF-5552 (1-888-653-5552).

You can use food to help ease headaches, too. If you are prone to early-morning headaches, Fred Freitag, D.O., associate director of the Chicago-based Diamond Headache Clinic, suggests having a piece of fruit before you go to bed. "The fructose will help stabilize blood sugar. You can also cut up fruit and eat it throughout the day."

Antimigraine Supplements

When it comes to supplementing with the right nutrients, one of the best places to start is with magnesium, because it relaxes the blood vessels in the brain. Sometimes it can help to stop a headache before it starts. A new migraine remedy, called Migralex (www.migralex.com), contains 75 mg of aspirin and 500 mg of magnesium. If you have a migraine, you can take one to two pills three to four times a day as needed. For prevention, take one pill a day.

Headache Relief Formulas

Alexander Mauskop, M.D., author of *What Your Doctor May Not Tell You About Migraines*, recommends MigreLief, which contains magnesium, B2, and feverfew. You take one tablet in the morning and the evening with a meal. You should see results in 30 to 90 days. You can find more information about it at www.migrelief.com. You also can try a formulation called Migravent, which also contains butterbur. Studies show that butterbur is effective at helping to prevent migraine headaches. (More about butterbur in a minute.) Or you may want to try each nutrient separately to see how they work for you.

Feverfew

When we want to be toned, we go to the gym. When we want our blood vessels to be toned, we take feverfew. Doing so can help treat and prevent migraines, because when blood vessels dilate, due to substances like serotonin and histamine, migraines can result. Many studies show that taking feverfew as a dried leaf capsule can be effective when it comes to migraine intervention. A review of recent research regarding feverfew was published in the medical journal *Public Health Nutrition* (2000), which reported that this herb is effective and safe when it comes to preventing migraines. Just be sure to buy high-quality supplements, especially when it comes to nutrients like feverfew, to ensure botanical integrity. If you are pregnant, don't use feverfew.

Vitamin B₂

Here's another supplement to put on your to-take list: vitamin B_2 or riboflavin. Studies show its preventive power. When 55 participants in a study reported in the medical journal *Neurology* (1998) took 400 mg of B_2 daily for three months, most of them cut their migraine attacks by half. You may see results in only two months, say researchers.

Butterbur

An oft-used herbal remedy for pain and fever, today butterbur (Petasites hybridus) is widely used to prevent migraines because of its anti-inflammatory properties. In fact, two thirds of participants in a study reported in the medical journal *Headache* (2005) had more than a 50 percent reduction in migraine attacks when they took butterbur extract. Feverfew does contain liver-toxic compounds, so it's important to choose a butterbur rhizome extract in which these have been removed correctly. One of the best brands, called Petadolex, is made by Weber & Weber. You can find it at www.betterhealthinternational.com.

risky remedy!

Pregnant women should not take herbal supplements for their migraines. Even though herbs come from nature, they still have chemicals that may have an effect. More research needs to be done to know exactly what that may be.

CoQ10

A study in the medical journal *Cephalalgia arch* shows that coenzyme Q10 (CoQ10) is an effective preventive treatment for migraine headaches. Thirty-two patients (26 women, 6 men) with a history of migraines were treated with coenzyme Q10. Sixty-one percent of patients had a greater than 50 percent reduction in the number of days with migraine headache. Best of all, there were no side effects.

The Power of Water

It sounds too simple to work, but drinking water may help to "head off" a migraine attack. "Some patients report that if they drink a couple of glasses of water, they can often forestall a headache coming on," says Joel Saper, M.D., founder and director of the Michigan Head Pain & Neurological Institute. "It's not that they're dehydrated; it's that the physiology of the body changes when you add pure water, and that change may in some way trigger a switch that turns off or prevents the headache."

When you do get a migraine, it's time to put your head on ice. Grab two ice packs and put one on the area where it hurts the most and one on the back of the neck, says Dr. Freitag. Also, putting an ice pack on your head and a hot water bottle or flaxseed pack (warmed in the microwave) on your feet can be helpful, since your head is throbbing and your body is chilly. Or try taking a hot bath with an ice pack on your head. Doing both at the same time is a natural remedy that addresses two problems at once.

Easing Nausea

Sometimes a smell can trigger a migraine or, if you already have one, make you nauseous. Migrastick, which is a rollerball stick that contains essential oils of lavender and peppermint, can help relieve nausea by blocking bad smells that bother you. In addition, it has pain-relieving properties, which means you can apply this cooling remedy to your temples, forehead, or nape of the neck—wherever it hurts! In a small open clinical trial in 2001, 91 percent of participants were satisfied with Migrastick's effectiveness in reducing the number, length, and

intensity of migraine attacks. You can find more information at www.
migrastick.com.

Another remedy that works for nausea is eating soda crackers and sipping cola over crushed ice. "The caffeine also has a prokinetic effect
on the gut. It helps reverse gastric statis and helps get the gut moving
again," says Christine Lay, M.D., a neurologist at the Headache
Institute at St. Luke's–Roosevelt Hospital Center in New York. If you
like ginger ale for nausea, choose a natural brand, because some contain
the preservative sodium benzoate, which can actually be a trigger for
migraine. Candied ginger (you can find this at your health food store)
can also work to ease nausea.

Ah, Aromatherapy!

Holistic aromatherapist Jade Shutes, B.A., Diploma AT, recommends
these remedies to ease headache pain:

Migraine-buster gel:

> 5 drops peppermint
>
> 3 drops lavender
>
> 1 TB. aloe vera gel

Mix all in a small bowl. Apply to the temples and the back of the neck.
Be sure to wash hands after applying. *Avoid the eye area!*

Tension type headache–buster oil:

> 1 oz. apricot kernel or sunflower vegetable oil
>
> 5 drops lavender oil
>
> 3 drops peppermint oil

Massage on the temples, neck, and shoulders.

Relief Tips

Sleep can help, too. After you take some remedies, try to get a half-
hour of solid rest, says Dr. Frietag. "It gives the medicine a chance to
work, and if you fall asleep even for a short period of time, that can stop

a migraine cold. We don't know how sleep does it, but it is one of the most powerful ways to stop a migraine."

After your headache is gone, be easy on yourself. Think of it as a time to rest and replenish yourself. Rehydrate yourself—aim for a quart and a half a day, says Dr. Frietag—and replenish necessary B-complex vitamins that help curb migraine headaches. For more information, visit the websites www.headaches.org, www.migraines.org, and www. achenet.org.

Just Relax

Incorporating relaxation and tension-relieving practices like progressive relaxation, belly breathing, biofeedback, yoga, acupressure, and acupuncture into your life may help relieve and prevent headaches. Try one or a few of these on for size.

Progressive Relaxation

Start with your face. Contract all the muscles for a moment and then relax. Move on to the shoulders and all the different muscle groups of the body in succession, from head to toe.

Belly Breathing

To relieve the tension and stress that can bring on tension headaches and aggravate migraines, try this belly breathing exercise created by Dennis Lewis, author of *Free Your Breath, Free Your Life*. "Our belly is one of the major areas that get tight and tense when we are under a lot of stress," says Lewis. "And this greatly affects our internal organs, our breath, our energy, and our overall health." This exercise will help you relax. "When we open our belly and allow our diaphragm to move deeper down into our abdomen on inhalation, and farther up to squeeze our lungs and support our heart on exhalation, it has a powerful influence on our respiration, on the way we breathe, and on our lives."

1. Lie down comfortably on your back on your bed, a mat, or a carpeted floor. Position yourself with your feet flat on the floor and your knees bent (pointing upward). Simply follow your

breathing for a minute or two with your attention. See if you can sense which parts of your body your breath touches.

2. Continue to follow your breathing as you rub your hands together until they are very warm.

3. Put your hands (one on top of the other) on your belly, with the center of your lower hand touching your navel. Watch how your breathing responds. You may notice that your belly wants to expand as you inhale and retract as you exhale. Let this happen, but don't try to force it.

4. If your belly seems tight, rub your hands together again until they are warm and then massage your belly, especially right around the outside edge of your belly button. Notice how your belly begins to soften and relax.

5. Now rub your hands together again until they are warm and put them on your belly again. Watch how this influences your breath. Do not try to do anything. Simply watch and enjoy as your belly begins to come to life, expanding as you inhale and retracting as you exhale.

6. If your belly still seems overly tight and does not want to move as you breathe, press down with your hands on your belly as you exhale. Then as you inhale, gradually release the tension. Try this several times. Notice how your belly begins to open more on inhalation.

7. When you are ready to stop, be sure to sense your entire abdominal area, noting any special sensations of warmth, comfort, and energy.

8. Spend a few minutes allowing these sensations to spread into all the cells of your belly, all the way back to your spine.

(The Belly Breathing Practice is taken from Dennis Lewis' website, www.authentic-breathing.com and is used with his permission. Dennis Lewis is the author of *The Tao of Natural Breathing* and the audio program *Natural Breathing*.

Do-It-Yourself Biofeedback

Research shows that biofeedback can also be helpful for migraines. By using a do-it-yourself biofeedback program like Healing Rhythms (www.wilddivine.com), created by Deepak Chopra, M.D.; Dean Ornish, M.D.; and Dr. Andrew Weil, M.D., you can learn to lower your stress levels, which may help reduce the incidence of tension headaches as well.

Bust a Yoga Move

A new study in *Headache* (2007) showed the effectiveness of yoga therapy in managing migraines without auras. Seventy-two patients with migraines without auras were randomly assigned to yoga therapy or a self-care group for three months. At the end of the study, headache frequency, severity, pain, and associated depression and anxiety were all significantly lower in the yoga group compared to the self-care group.

Acupressure and Acupuncture

Acupressure, a kind of traditional Chinese medicine that's based on the same ideas as acupuncture, may help. "I've had patients do acupressure on the acupuncture point between the thumb and index finger, called Large Intestine 4, during the aura and not get their headache," says Robert A. Duarte, M.D., Director of the Long Island Jewish (LIJ) Pain and Headache Treatment Center in Manhasset, New York, and a certified acupuncturist. "It's not 100 percent, but it's an option."

Research shows that acupuncture can be a safe and effective natural treatment for the relief of tension-type headaches. One theory is that the practice releases endorphins, the feel-good chemical in the body. From the Traditional Chinese Medicine point of view, it is thought to relieve the stagnation of chi, or energy, in the body.

A recent study in the medical journal *Complementary Therapies in Medicine* (2007) indicates that acupuncture provides 50 to 80 percent relief to people with acute or chronic pain, so it may help migraine sufferers, too.

dial your doc

If your headaches have gotten worse over days and weeks, you've never had headaches before (especially if you are over 50), or the headaches come on suddenly and don't go away, call your doctor. Other warning signs include weakness, numbness, or a change in your hearing, sight, memory, personality, or cognitive abilities. Also contact your doctor if your headache is accompanied by a stiff neck, a rash, nausea, vomiting, a fever, breathing problems, or a head injury.

Natural R$_x$

Alpha lipoic acid: 600 mg.

Butterbur: 50–100 mg twice daily with meals.

Capsaicin: Apply topically as directed.

CoQ10: 300 mg.

Feverfew: 50–100 mg of feverfew extract daily.

Ginger: Tincture, ½ tsp., 40 drops, or 2.5 mL three times daily; tea, 1 TB. per cup of water, 3 cups daily; capsules, 300 mg twice daily.

Magnesium: 500 mg.

Migralex: 1–2 pills three to four times daily as needed; for prevention, take 1 pill daily.

MigraLief: As directed.

Migrastick: As directed.

Migravent: As directed.

Omega-3 essential fatty acids: 1,000 mg EPA/DHA.

Valerian root: For tension headache, capsules and tablets: 250–400 mg daily; tincture, ½ tsp., 40 drops, or 2.5 mL three times daily.

Vitamin B$_2$: 400 mg.

Vitamin B$_{12}$: 1,000 mcg daily.

Nausea

Ugh, nausea! Two of the most common causes of nausea are motion sickness and morning sickness. In fact, about half of pregnant women experience morning sickness, a combination of nausea, headache, and dizziness, during their first few months of pregnancy, or the first trimester, as the uterus expands and hormones surge.

Motion sickness occurs when you hit the road or sea or air and travel in cars, trains, boats, and planes. Nausea is caused by conflicting messages caused by changes in position involving the middle or inner ear that controls balance. Children suffer more from motion sickness than adults.

Ginger

When it comes to herbal remedies for nausea, ginger should be your first line of defense. That's because ginger is a natural alternative to settle the stomach and reduce nausea, whether you have morning sickness or motion sickness. Many studies have shown that it's as effective as antinausea medicines. A review of five studies including a total of 363 patients published in the medical journal *Evidence Based Nursing* in 2006, for example, found that ginger was even an effective means for reducing post-operative nausea and vomiting.

One of the most soothing ways to use ginger to ease nausea is to brew a nice pot of ginger tea with fresh ginger root first thing in the morning. That way, you can sip three to four cups of tea throughout the day or refrigerate it, if you prefer it cold. Many health food stores also have dried ginger, and it's gently candied with just a little bit of crystallized sugar on it. Take it with you when you're on the go or traveling. Sea-Band Anti-Nausea Ginger Gum can also be helpful (for more information, visit www.sea-band.com). You might also take one or two capsules of ginger root powder one to four times daily for morning sickness. Powdered red raspberry leaves or alfalfa herb may be taken in capsules, too.

natural news

Stock your kitchen cabinet with a variety of teas that soothe nausea so they are there when you need them. Besides ginger, you can choose sweet basil, peppermint, catnip, raspberry leaf, sage, black horehound, cinnamon, and mint. (Mint oil actually helps relax the smooth muscle of the digestive tract and helps ease nausea.) Licorice tea can be especially helpful for morning sickness. Sip the teas hot or cold, as desired, and as often as necessary.

Homeopathic Help

Homeopathic remedies are a plus when it comes to motion sickness. Try Borax (good for airplane travel) and Cocculus (for a car or a boat) to help motion sickness when you are on the move. You can also try Hyland's Motion Sickness formula, which contains Tabacum (for headache with nausea), Petroleum (nausea and dizziness), and Cocculus indicus (dizziness and nausea) and Nux vomica (sour stomach). Nux vomica is also helpful for morning sickness when taken alone. You can find Hyland's Motion Sickness in your health food store or visit www. hylands.com/products/motionsickness.php.

You can also take Trip Ease, a safe and natural homeopathic remedy for treating motion sickness. Trip Ease has no side effects, and you can take it with other medications. Like other homeopathic remedies, it's most effective if you take it before you eat or drink. You'll find it at www.caprx.com.

Acupressure Hits the Spot

A review of various studies published in the *Journal of Alternative and Complementary Medicine* showed that applying pressure to the acupressure point known as P6 can be beneficial for nausea and vomiting. To access what is known at the Nei Kuan acupressure point, aim for a spot 2 inches below the wrist between the two tendons. (For more information, visit www.acupuncture-acupressure-points.com/acu-point-P6.html.) You can also buy wristbands that will apply pressure to this same area. The knitted elastic Sea-Band, for example, has been proven in studies to be effective in easing nausea and vomiting.

It works by applying pressure with a plastic stud to the P6 point. The band is free of side effects and can be worn as needed. Kids can use it, too. The Sea-Band is sold in drug chains and pharmacies around the world.

But the P6 pressure point isn't just useful when you are traveling. A study in the *Journal of Advanced Nursing* in 2007 showed that the Nei Juan acupressure point was a useful treatment for pregnant women who were experiencing a severe form of morning sickness known as Hyperemesis gravidarum that features excessive nausea and vomiting.

Ah, Aromatherapy!

If you know you have motion sickness and are about to board a plane, go on a boat, or take a long car ride, holistic aromatherapist Jade Shutes, founder of the East West School for Herbal and Aromatic Studies in Willow Spring, North Carolina, recommends that you have a bottle of peppermint and/or ginger essential oil handy. When the feeling of motion sickness arises, simply take out the bottle of peppermint or ginger essential oil and take a few deep breaths (breathing in through the nose and out through the mouth). Or place a couple of drops in a cotton ball and waft it under the nose. Peppermint oil also comes in capsule form that you may find helpful to calm your digestive tract. One brand is Pepogest (www.evitamins.com).

dial your doc

If you are pregnant and you have any questions about whether these remedies are right for you, contact your doctor.

Natural Rx

For morning sickness:

Alfalfa: Powdered capsules four times daily.

Arsenicum homeopathic remedy: As directed.

Catnip: Tea, 1 tsp. in a cup of water three times daily.

Choline: 500–1,000 mg daily.

Ginger: Tea, 1 TB. in a cup of water three times daily.

Ginger root powder: 1–2 capsules, one to four times daily.

Magnesium: 400 mg in the morning.

Methionine: 1,000 mg daily.

Mint: Oil, as directed; tea, 1 tsp. in a cup of water three times daily.

Nux vomica homeopathic remedy: As directed.

Peppermint capsules: As directed.

Red raspberry leaf: Powdered capsules four times daily; tea, 1 tsp. in a cup of water three times daily.

Sage: Tea, 1 tsp. in a cup of water three times daily.

Sweet basil: Tea, 1 tsp. in a cup of water three times daily.

The Sea-Band: As directed. www.sea-band.com.

Vitamin B_6: 25 mg two to three times daily. Helps break down increased hormones.

Vitamin C: 250 mg two to three times daily.

Vitamin K: 50–80 mcg daily.

For motion sickness:

Charcoal tabs: As directed.

Cocculus homeopathic remedy: As directed.

Ginger: Tea, 1 TB. in a cup of water three times daily.

Ginger essential oil: As directed.

Ipecacuana homeopathic remedy: As directed.

Magnesium: 500 mg.

Nux vomica homeopathic remedy: As directed.

Peppermint essential oil: As directed.

The Sea-Band: As directed.

Trip Ease: As directed.

Vitamin B_6: 100 mg.

Osteoporosis

You don't have to be old to get osteoporosis, although it seems like this condition, which means "porous bones," goes hand in hand with adding more candles to your birthday cake. Yes, it's true that, as we age, it's more of a challenge to keep our bones in shape. "Bone is living tissue," says Holly Lucille, N.D., a naturopathic doctor who practices in Los Angeles and the author of *Creating and Maintaining Balance: A Woman's Guide to Safe, Natural Hormone Health.* "It works like construction crews and demolition crews. Unfortunately, as we age, the demolition crew is working harder than the construction crew, as more bone is broken down than replaced." Gradually, osteoporosis thins and weakens bones to the point that they become fragile and break more easily, usually in the hip, spine, and ribs.

When women go through menopause, the lack of estrogen production and protection makes our bones more vulnerable. Smoking, caffeine, alcohol, and carbonated soda, which leach calcium from our bones, can weaken our skeletons, as can conditions like irritable bowel syndrome. Dr. Lucille has seen a rise in the number of cases of osteoporosis. "Women in my practice who have had hysterectomies and have been on hormone-replacement therapy have severe osteoporosis. It's also on the rise for men."

But back to the good news: even as we get older, because our bones are living tissue, they are constantly replenishing and renewing themselves. This means we can be proactive about bone health by choosing the right nutrients and exercise. Since bone is made up of calcium, protein, and other minerals, getting enough calcium and other important nutrients can help protect bones by slowing bone loss. Weight-bearing exercises can help by stimulating bone cell formulation. Following is more information on how to bone up for good health!

According to *Osteoporosis: A Guide to Prevention and Treatment, a Special Health Report from Harvard Medical School,* research shows that drinking four or more cups of coffee can increase your risk of breaking a bone by boosting calcium excretion. Too much animal protein may also cause calcium to leach from your bones. This is a good reason to head in a vegan direction, eating less meat and more vegetarian products.

Foods with Calcium

We all know that calcium is a key nutrient when it comes to preventing osteoporosis. Milk and other dairy products are the richest sources of calcium, but you don't have to go high fat to get the nutrients you need. There are low-fat substitutes for everything from milk to yogurt to cheese to ice cream, and many are fortified with vitamin D as well. You can also find calcium in sardines, peanuts, firm tofu, spinach, calcium-fortified orange juice, and salmon.

Maintaining the Right Balance

Your body functions best at a certain *pH*, which is an *alkaline* environment. If your body becomes too *acidic*, it will turn to your bones, where calcium is stored, so it can maintain a more neutral, beneficial balance. So make it a point to include alkaline foods in your diet, such as cruciferous vegetables like broccoli, green leafies like spinach, asparagus, garlic, watermelon, Brussels sprouts (if you dare!), and alfalfa sprouts. You can also use a green food to help maintain an alkaline balance.

For more information about the foods to add and avoid concerning pH and osteoporosis, visit www.essense-of-life.com/info/foodchart.htm or www.thewolfeclinic.com/acidalkfoods.html. You can buy a simple kit at any health food store to test your pH.

def•i•ni•tion _____

> **pH** is potential of hydrogen and measures the acidity or alkalinity of substances. The pH range is from 1 to 14, with 7 being neutral. The higher the pH of a food or liquid is—say, 7 or greater (papayas)—the more **alkaline** it is. The lower the pH of a food or liquid—say, less than 7 (think cranberries)—the more **acidic** it is.

Supplemental Remedies

Although foods rich in calcium and vitamin D are the first line of defense, our busy 24×7 lifestyle often means we skimp on these nutrients. In this case, supplements that you can find at your health food store can be a tremendous help. A recent analysis of past studies published in the scientific journal *The Lancet* showed that using calcium, or calcium in combination with vitamin D, can help prevent fracture and osteoporotic bone loss. Calcium citrate is a very absorbable version of calcium. You can also build better bones with Floridix Calcium-Magnesium, which contains zinc and vitamin D, which act as co-factors for improved absorption. You can find more information about it at www.florahealth.com.

While you're bone-building, add vitamin K to your arsenal, a nutrient that helps osteocalcin, a protein in the body bind calcium to bone. It also helps retain calcium in the bones. Research published in *The American Journal of Clinical Nutrition* showed that low intake of vitamin K increased the risk of hip fractures in women.

Because of our diet and our compromised food supply, it's just as important to make sure you get micronutrients that strengthen bone, like boron, copper, manganese, molybdenum, strontium, and silicon, which promote higher bone density. A study in the *New England Journal of Medicine* showed, for example, that when postmenopausal women with osteoporosis took calcium, vitamin D, and strontium, they reduced their risk of vertebral fractures by 49 percent. Dr. Lucille recommends a supplement called Osteo Prime Plus, made by Enzymatic Therapy, a blend of all these nutrients and more, plus a form of vitamin K (K_2, or menaquinone) that is used in Japan as a drug to increase bone density and decrease fracture risk. A review of studies on vitamin K₂ showed that, overall, this nutrient reduces hip, vertebral, and nonvertebral fracture. You can find it at www.vitanetonline.

Dr. Lucille also recommends Enzymatic Therapy's Doctor's Choice for women ages 45 and over as a high-potency vitamin and mineral adjunct. "It also contains digestive enzymes, which is important because those naturally decrease as we get older. Adding them can help the absorption of the minerals we need to fend off osteoporosis. That's why I love it for women of this age."

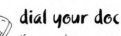

dial your doc

If you take anticoagulants like warfarin (Coumadin), keep your vitamin K intake consistent, since this nutrient affects blood clotting. If you take an anticoagulant, discuss with your doctor before taking vitamin K.

natural news

Why do we need vitamin D for bone health? It helps us to absorb calcium. How do we get it? One of the best ways is to step outside. To get vitamin D safely from the sun, aim for 10 to 15 minutes with hands, face, and arms exposed two to three times a week. However, many people also have trouble getting enough vitamin D during the winter months, when sunlight is limited. You can find vitamin D in foods like salmon, mackerel, egg yolks, milk and fortified juices, breakfast cereals, and soy milk. But if your diet is less than ideal, take a supplement to close the gap.

Exercises That Keep Bones Strong

To keep bones strong, you've got to get off the couch. Aim for some type of exercise for one hour five times a week. Weight-bearing exercises done three to four times a week with light weights (2 to 5 pounds) can help keep bones strong and slow the rate of bone loss. But did you know you can also do yoga to help avoid osteoporosis? In yoga, you are bearing the weight of your own body to keep your bones in better shape. You can read more yoga exercises and resources in Chapter 5.

Tai chi, a 2,000-year-old practice that originated in China as a form of self-defense, can, like yoga, strengthen your bones and help you improve your balance, which may help you avoid falls and reduce the chances you'll have a fracture. Since tai chi involves a series of postures or movements done slowly and methodically, it is often described as "meditation in motion." Doing tai chi on a regular basis can help strengthen you in body, mind, and spirit.

Tasty Bone-Boosting Snacks

Why not get creative and make building bones delicious? Judy Stone, CN, M.S.W., a certified nutritionist and author of *Take Two Apples and Call Me in the Morning: A Practical Guide to Using the Power of Food to Change Your Life!*, recommends these snacks and routines that are good for your bones:

Make a smoothie. Mix 3 rounded teaspoons of vanilla whey protein powder, ½ cup of low-fat milk, ⅓ cup of frozen blueberries, 1 teaspoon flaxseed oil, ¼ teaspoon lemon extract, and ice in a blender. Blend on high until texture is smooth. Or grab a ready-made smoothie with over 120 mg or 10 percent of calcium.

Have a lassi. "People who live in hotter climates know the art of creating cooling, refreshing drinks," says Stone. "A mango lassi, a yogurt-based drink, is an Indian delight that boosts your calcium intake, too." To make it, peel two mangos, and cut the soft fruit off the seed and put in a blender. Add 1½ cups low-fat plain yogurt, 3 cups cold water, 2 teaspoons sugar, ½ teaspoon cardamom, a pinch of salt, and ice. Blend until ice is crushed in blender.

Pop a calcium chew. Satisfy that sweet tooth with a chew called Viactiv, for example, which contains calcium and vitamins D and K. The chews come in chocolate and caramel flavors.

Use amaranth. A grain that's calcium rich, amaranth can be used or substituted for wheat or grains like couscous, used in the Middle Eastern grain dish tabouli to boost its nutrient punch. You can find it in most natural food stores.

Create a calcium-rich salad. Use grains like rice, barley, and quinoa (soak them overnight before cooking, to deactivate phytic acid, which can block calcium absorption) with lightly steamed, calcium-rich vegetables like raw bok choy for crunch and flavor, along with chicken, turkey, and shredded cheese. You'll get the calcium, fiber, and protein you need.

Add zest with arugala and watercress. Great on sandwiches and in wraps and salads, these greens have a mildly peppery flavor and contain bone-building calcium.

natural news

Improve lactose tolerance and calcium and vitamin D levels by starting with small amounts of foods that contain lactose, and gradually increase to determine your tolerance. Include lactose-containing foods as part of a meal or a snack, to make them easier to digest; choose calcium-rich foods that are lower in lactose, such as aged cheeses like Swiss, Colby, Parmesan, and cheddar; and try dairy foods like yogurt and buttermilk that are made with active cultures and are easier to digest. Look for the National Yogurt Association's seal "Live and Active Cultures" on the carton.

Natural R$_x$

Boron: 200 mg.

Calcium citrate: 1,200 mg daily.

Enzymatic Therapy's Doctor's Choice for 45+: As directed.

Evening primrose oil: 1 TB. daily; take with fish oils and calcium to decrease bone turnover.

Iprislavone: 600 mg.

Isoflavones: 1,000 mg daily. Found in soy. Helps build bones.

Magnesium: 300–700 mg daily.

Oat grass: ½ tsp., 40 drops, or 2.5 mL three times daily; tea, 1 TB. per cup of water, 3–4 cups daily; can help fight osteoporosis through its rich calcium content.

Omega-3 essential fatty acids from fish oil: 3 g EPA daily, 3 g DHA daily.

Osteo Prime Plus by Enzymatic Therapy: As directed. www. vitanetonline.

Strontium: 200 mg three times daily; take it on an empty stomach.

Vitamin D: 800 IU.

Vitamin K: 700 mcg.

Peptic Ulcer

If it were a soap opera, you'd call it *The Pain and the Churning*, because that's what an ulcer feels like. Normally, when we eat something, hydrochloric acid (HCl) in the stomach breaks down our food into digestible elements, while mucous and bicarbonate ions protect our stomach lining. We need this digestive aid, as gastric juices are extremely corrosive.

But when the stomach lining is affected by things like stress, NSAIDs (nonsteroidal anti-inflammatory drugs) like aspirin and ibuprofen, allergies, smoking, and diet, it can lead to painful peptic ulcers. A gastric ulcer occurs when stomach acid actually wears a hole in the stomach lining. A duodenal ulcer occurs in the upper part of the small intestine, next to the stomach. Ulcers are also often caused by the bacteria Helicobacter pylori (H. pylori). The symptoms of ulcers can also include nausea, gas, bloating, and even weight loss.

def•i•ni•tion

Helicobacter pylori, or H. pylori, is a bacteria that is one of the most common causes of ulcers. It weakens the protective coating of the stomach or duodenum. Antibiotics are used to treat this infection.

1-2-3 Testing

You can find out if you have H. pylori bacteria through a blood test that looks for antibodies, or a breath or stool test. If you do have an infection, you may also need tests like the upper GI (gastrointestinal) series; this involves taking x-rays of your stomach and duodenum. Sometimes a biopsy is needed. Once you have a diagnosis, your doctor will probably prescribe antibiotics for a week or two, along with an acid-controlling medication. You may also find it helpful to use natural remedies in conjunction with conventional methods to speed recovery.

Healing Herbs

When it comes to natural remedies for ulcers, begin with licorice root. This anti-inflammatory remedy stimulates the mucous layer in the stomach to rebuild, which is just what you want when it is feeling unprotected. This is due to its effect on the hormone secretin, which influences mucous production. A compound in licorice called glycyrrhetinic acid can elevate blood pressure, but a method was devised to remove it, kind of like decaf coffee. Licorice without this component is called deglycyrrhizinated (or DGL) licorice. If you take 1000 to 1,500 mg of DGL licorice between meals or 20 minutes before meals, you may notice a big difference in how you feel. Research shows it can be as effective as prescription antacids like Zantac in treating the symptoms of peptic ulcers.

Mastic Gum

This centuries-old gastrointestinal aid comes from the Greek pistachio tree, which produces a gum resin. (You can also eat it as a rock candy!) Studies show mastic gum helps wipe out the H. pylori bacteria that can cause peptic and duodenal ulcers. In fact, 80 percent of volunteers in a study reported in the medical journal *Clinical and Experimental Pharmacology and Physiology* had symptom relief from peptic ulcers. Get it at your health food store or visit www.modernherbalist.com.

Slippery Elm

When the mucous in the lining of your stomach and duodenum isn't all that it could and should be, reach for a demulcent herb like slippery elm. This soothing herb contains mucilage, a gelatinous compound that coats the digestive tract and relieves peptic ulcer pain. You can find USDA organic slippery elm bark powder at www.herbspro.com.

Antibacterial Herbs

Think cause and effect. If your ulcer is caused by H. pylori, a bacteria, you'll want to put antibacterial herbs to work for you in addition to taking antibiotics. These include goldenseal, Oregon grape, and bayberry.

Foods That Can Help

Think *F* for fiber when it comes to ulcer care. Choosing veggies like rhubarb and aloe vera, along with pectin (from apples) and psyllium (from supplements), may reduce your risk of developing an ulcer in the first place and, if you already have one, may heal it. Focus on foods containing flavonoids, like yams, cranberries, onions, and green tea, because these nutrients can help keep the growth of H. pylori in check.

Grab That Juicer!

Raw cabbage juice is especially effective in helping to heal ulcers. Research shows that drinking a liter of fresh cabbage juice throughout the day helps heal ulcers in less than 10 days! We think this is because cabbage contains high amounts of glutamine, which help make up the compounds that protect the stomach and duodenum. You can also take glutamine as a supplement.

Keep Your Furnace Stoked

When you have an ulcer (or are prone to them), it's essential to keep your stomach from getting too empty. "Eating four or five small meals a day ensures that the GI lining is coated and, therefore, protected from excess acid," says Barbara S. Silbert, D.C., N.D., a naturopathic doctor practicing in Bethel, Vermont. "Not eating after 5 P.M. can help, especially if people are eating late out of stress."

Don't drink beverages that can irritate the lining of the stomach or increase acid production. (You've already got enough of that!) Top culprits include coffee (with or without caffeine), alcohol, carbonated beverages, fruit juice, and milk—yes, milk. Milk used to be considered beneficial, and you may still think drinking it will coat your stomach and make it feel better, but milk actually promotes gastric acid production. It's also important to cut back on spicy and fatty foods, which can aggravate ulcers.

natural news

Research shows that probiotics (friendly bacteria) can help treat peptic ulcers, too. A new study published in the *American Journal of Gastroenterology* compared the effect of following the usual "triple therapy" used to treat H. pylori, two antibiotics and an acid blocker (like ranitidine, Zantac or famotidine, Pepcid), to using triple therapy plus a probiotic and a compound from cow's milk that has antibacterial, immune system–boosting properties (bovine lactoferrin).

Eight weeks after the end of treatment, H. pylori tests were negative in 92 percent of those who added the lactoferrin and probiotic, but in only 76 percent of those treated with triple therapy alone. The regimen with lactoferrin and probiotic also caused fewer side effects, occurring in only 9.5 percent of the people who used the lactoferrin and probiotic, compared with 40.6 percent of those who received triple therapy alone. The latter experienced side effects including nausea, diarrhea, a metallic taste in the mouth, headache, and abdominal pain, a nice bonus.

Ancient Chinese Secret

The Chinese medicine Wei Yao is an effective stomach medicine for those who have peptic ulcers, says Deborah Wiancek, author of *The Natural Healing Companion.* "It helps with acid regurgitation, neutralizes excess stomach acid, and reduces stomach pain, gas, and stomach distention." You can find it at Chinese or Korean grocery stores.

A recent Chinese study also showed that acupuncture can be effective in the treatment of peptic ulcer by improving stomachache and increasing appetite. Researchers concluded that the practice has a reliable therapeutic effect on peptic ulcers.

Learn to Relax

Making relaxation and stress reduction a regular part of your routine is important if you suffer from a peptic ulcer. Alternative therapies like yoga, qigong, meditation, flower essences, and aromatherapy can all be helpful (see Chapter 5 for more information on all of these practices), as can biofeedback. A new do-it-yourself biofeed-back program called Healing Rhythms, created by Deepak Chopra, M.D.; Dean Ornish, M.D.; and Andrew Weil, M.D., can be helpful for stress reduc-tion. You can find more at www. wilddivine.com.

dial your doc

Don't take a chance. Peptic ulcers will get worse if they aren't treated. Call your doctor right away if you have sudden sharp pain that doesn't go away; black, bloody stools; or vomit that is bloody or looks like coffee grounds.

Natural Rx

Acidophilus bifidus: 4 billion to 10 billion daily.

Bayberry tincture: ½ tsp., 40 drops, or 2.5 mL three times daily.

Evening primrose oil: 1 TB. daily; preliminary research suggests that gamma linolenic acid (GLA) from evening primrose oil (EPO) may have anti-ulcer properties.

Glutamine: 500 mg four times daily.

Goldenseal: Capsules and tablets, 100 mg three times daily for a maxi-mum of two weeks.

Licorice (Glycyrrhiza glabra/deglycyrrhizinated): 1,000–1,500 mg of DGL between meals or 20 minutes before meals.

Mastic gum: As directed.

Omega-3 fatty acids: 1,000 mg daily. 1 TB. flaxseed oil daily. in animal studies, treatment with omega-3 fatty acids reduced the risk of ulcers caused by NSAIDs.

Oregon grape: Capsules, 100 mg three times daily.

Slippery elm: As directed.

Vitamin C: 500 mg three times daily.

Vitamin E: 400–800 IU daily. In animal studies, vitamin E has a pro-tective effect on gastric mucosal injury induced by H. pylori infection.

Wei Yao: 3 pills two to three times daily.

Zinc: 15–50 mg daily. May help cure ulcers.

Poison Ivy and Poison Oak

Ah, the great outdoors! Nothing is better than getting out in nature. But sometimes nature gets *you* when you wander too close to poison ivy and poison oak.

To avoid contact with these plants, it's very important to know how to identify them. Here's a basic rundown of how to do that. Poison ivy is a woody vine, a trailing shrub on the ground, or a free-standing shrub that produces urushiol, a skin irritant that causes an itchy rash. Normally found in wooded areas and around lakes and streams in the East and the Midwest, poison ivy normally has three almond-shaped leaves and grayish-white berries. The leaves are green in the summer and red in the fall, with yellow or green flowers.

Poison oak grows from New Jersey to Texas as a low shrub. Western poison oak, along the Pacific coast, grows to 6-foot-tall clumps or vines up to 30 feet long. The three oaklike leaves have clusters of yellow berries. Poison oak, like poison ivy, contains urushiol, which causes an allergic reaction. For pictures of these potent plants, visit www.poison-ivy.org and www.poisonivy.aesir.com.

If you do come in contact with urushiol from poison ivy or poison oak, wash the area right away; shower or take a bath within 5 to 10 minutes. It's also important to realize that you can get poison ivy and oak from garden tools that were sitting in poison ivy or oak, or from clothes that were in contact with these plants. If you have any doubt, wash your clothes as well.

If you do get poison ivy or poison oak, a rash will begin to appear one to two days later. The area will become red and swollen, small blisters will begin to form, and the rash will start to itch. Typically, this lasts about a week. To speed healing and soothe symptoms, we have some natural cures for you.

Herbs and Remedies to Take the Itch Away

You may not know it, but if you get poison ivy or poison oak, there's usually a remedy growing within 100 feet! Brigitte Mars, author of *The Desktop Guide to Herbal Medicine*, recommends gumweed (grindelia species), jewelweed, and plantain as wonderful plant remedies for poison ivy. "You just have to pick them, chop them up, and apply them to the area that's been affected." If you're not feeling quite so bold, you can find formulas that contain these herbs and other beneficial ones at your local health food store and apply them to affected areas to help calm the itch and help the toxins pass through your system more quickly.

For itching and oozing poison ivy and oak, Mars suggests making a paste of baking soda and apple cider vinegar. You can also make a paste from oatmeal. Leave it on until you shower or take a bath, and apply again.

Poison ivy soap from companies like Burt's Bees (www.burtsbees.com) can help as well. To help cleanse toxins internally, try burdock root and red clover tea, 3 or 4 cups a day.

The homeopathic remedy Rhus toxicodendron, which is homeopathic poison ivy (remember, like treats like), can often stimulate the immune system to minimize any outbreaks. You can take it if you have been exposed to poison ivy or if you know you're going to be walking through it. You can find this at your health food store.

Take a Bath

Epsom salts and baking soda baths may be helpful if you have poison oak and poison ivy. To give your skin an oatmeal bath, either use a prepared product or use this method from Barbara Close, the founder of Naturopathica in East Hampton, New York, to soothe inflamed skin:

1. Put ½ cup of rolled oats in a washcloth. Tie the end with a rubber band.

2. Fill a sink with warm water.

3. Squeeze the ball into the sink to create oat milk.

4. Splash it over the affected areas.

Natural R_x

Burdock root: Tea, 1 TB. per cup of water, 3 cups daily.

Calamine lotion: As directed.

Gumweed (grindelia species): Apply topically.

Juleweed: Apply topically.

Plantain: Apply topically.

Red clover: Tea, 1 TB. per cup of water, 3 cups daily.

Rhus toxicodendron homeopathic remedy: As directed.

Premenstrual Syndrome

If you're a woman, you know all about premenstrual syndrome (PMS), that time of the month when you feel like another woman has taken control of your body. You know the one: moody, anxious, irritable, angry, and so tired, not to mention depressed. She also may have tender breasts and food cravings that are out of control. Chocolate, anyone?

You may also feel like grabbing a big cup of joe. That's right. When you have PMS, you may want caffeine even more, but as a side effect, it can promote breast tenderness and, in some cases, fibroid cysts in the breast. In addition, you may crave refined carbohydrates, white flour, sugar, and alcohol. This lack of fiber impacts the body's ability to remove excess estrogen. If constipation becomes chronic, it can make PMS even worse because the liver can't process estrogen as well and levels can build up. A deficiency of potassium can also play a part in PMS by influencing the kidneys' ability to maintain proper fluid volume.

natural news

"Our cycle in a less stimulated society is matched up with the moon, a lunar cycle," says Holly Lucille, N.D., a naturopathic doctor and author of *Creating and Maintaining Balance: A Woman's Guide to Safe, Natural Hormone Health* (www.allheallucille.com). "Cycle, by definition, means it changes, it cycles, it's not a steady straight line where our moods and our personality stays the same. There are normal variations, but anything that is made more magnified or acute, in terms of the symptoms, like painful breasts, isn't considered normal or desirable."

That's why if you have PMS, it's important to take a look at the body as a whole, everything from what you eat to how you handle stress.

Natural Nutrients

Besides avoiding sugar, caffeine, refined carbs, and alcohol, it's smart to add a quality multivitamin to your daily to-do list. Studies show that women who take a good multivitamin have fewer symptoms of PMS than women who don't. Vitamin B₆ should definitely be in the mix, since often women are on birth-control pills that can cause a deficiency of this important nutrient (along with folic acid); this can then lead to depression during PMS and menstruation. Iron is also important, since women may become anemic and tired during the menstrual cycle. Calcium and magnesium, which is a smooth muscle relaxant, can help reduce cramps. Look for vitamin E, too, a known antioxidant that also reduces breast tenderness and helps with insomnia.

Another essential PMS nutrient is flaxseed oil, a great source of alpha linolenic acid, a type of omega-3 fatty acid. When you grind up flax seed (you can get flax seed and a grinder at the health food store) you'll release lignans, which help bind up free estrogen in the body. "It's actually very estrogen protective if you're trying to balance hormones," says Keri Marshall, N.D., a naturopathic doctor whose practice, Makai Naturopathic (www.makainaturopathic.com), is in Dover, New Hampshire. Flax seed is also a great source of fiber that can help ease constipation and move hormones out of the body. (Avoid seeds and nuts if you have irritable bowel syndrome.) When you grind flax seeds, you also get a fresh release of the oil on the spot. This can be helpful, as flaxseed oil can tend to go rancid pretty quickly. This way you can grind flax seeds and sprinkle them into your yogurt and smoothies whenever you want to.

Flax seeds also contain phytoestrogens (estrogenlike plant-based substances) that help regulate periods by balancing out estrogen levels. How? Phytoestrogens bind to estrogen receptor sites in the body, blocking stronger estrogens. In the body's infinite wisdom, you just metabolize out the excess estrogen. Gamma linoleic acid, which is found in borage oil, black current oil, and evening primrose oil, increases what is known as Prostaglandin E-1 in the body. This helps reduce inflammation and relieves breast tenderness, cramps, and headaches associated with PMS and menstruation. Taking vitamins C and B₆, magnesium, and zinc also helps the body use gamma linoleic acid more effectively. This helps reduce inflammation in the body around the time of PMS, which can reduce excessive cramping. A good source of gamma linoleic acid from evening primrose oil and omega-3 essential fatty oils is Nordic Naturals Omega Woman formula. You can find it at your health food store.

natural news

If you have chronic constipation, you may want to look into cleansing the liver and colon to ease PMS. "When your liver is working really well, you're less likely to get PMS," says Deborah Wiancek, N.D., author of *The Natural Healing Companion*. To cleanse the liver, Dr. Wiancek uses liver herbs such as milk thistle, dandelion root, and licorice. Foods that detoxify the liver include beets, artichokes, carrots, garlic, and ginger.

Colonics are the next step she takes to cleanse the body. "They can be especially helpful for women who have long-term problems with constipation because toxins are building up in the colon. Liver herbs will remove the toxins in the colon, and if you're constipated, you want to get rid of them right away. The two go hand in hand." If this sounds like it might be for you, it's best to see a trained health practitioner to make sure you are doing it properly.

Pretty Important PMS Herbs

The Ancient Greeks knew the power of the chaste tree berries. when it came to that time of the month. You can think of chaste tree, or Vitex agnus castus, as the balancing herb. That's because it helps PMS by both increasing progesterone and keeping estrogen under control, which is responsible for the many symptoms of PMS. This means it will help you feel more balanced, too. A study in the medical journal *Phytomedicine* in 2003 identified compounds in Vitex agnus castus (AC) that were responsible for PMS relief.

Black Cohosh

Often chaste tree is taken together with black cohosh (Cimicifuga racemos), which was used medicinally by Native Americans and, later, American colonists for menstrual cramps and menopause. Black cohosh also contain phytoestrogens, which we've seen exert estrogenlike effects on the body. This can help ease symptoms.

Black cohosh has other amazing properties, too. Did you know that it's a natural analgesic? That's because it contains a natural salicylate, like you find in willow bark and in aspirin. It also helps regulate blood flow and relieve cramps. It's so effective that Germany's FDA counterpart,

Commission E, has given its stamp of approval for the use of black cohosh as a treatment for both PMS and menstrual cramps.

Licorice

Yes, you may think of licorice when you go to the movies. But did you know that licorice (Glycyrrhiza glabra), another phytoestrogen, has estrogenlike properties that can help soothe breast tenderness and other PMS symptoms like bloating? This herbal remedy has been tapped because of its "estrogenic" effects for thousands of years.

Dong Quai

Dong quai, a very popular herb in China, from the parsley family, also possesses estrogenic properties. For this reason, it is often called upon to ease PMS and other symptoms of hormonal fluctuations, such as hot flashes during menopause.

risky remedy!

It's important to note that it's not okay to use licorice if you have high blood pressure, diabetes, or kidney, heart, or liver disease, or if you are pregnant. If you have any questions, see your doctor.

Have a Cup of Herbal Tea

Finally, using herbal tea to relax can ease PMS. Valerian tea is great for destressing and can also be good for insomnia. Dandelion leaf tea can act as a mild diuretic, making you feel less bloated. For this reason, don't mix it with any prescription diuretic medicines you may already be taking, such as Lasix (furosemide).

natural news

If you have painful cramps, Agatha M. Thrash, M.D., the co-founder of the Uchee Pines Lifestyle Center in Seale, Alabama, recommends hydrotherapy, either a hot sitz bath or a nice hot foot bath. Use water at 105°F to 112°F (very hot) for 15 minutes if flow is slight and for 4 minutes if flow is heavy (in which case, the hot bath should be immediately followed by a hot vaginal douche at 104°F). Teas such as red raspberry, chamomile, catnip, and partridge berry are often helpful, too, says Dr. Thrash.

Ah, Aromatherapy!

Breathe deep of lavender, rosemary, and lemon balm, and you'll soothe the stress of PMS. You can also put any of these oils in a diffuser to help you relax. Lemon balm essential oil is not only a stress-buster, but it's also good for herpes, which some women get around their period. It's an antiviral, so you can apply it topically or use it in a bath. Rosemary in a bath or dabbed on your wrist can help boost concentration and ease fatigue.

Flower Power

Bach Flower Remedies (see Chapter 5) are made from a "sun tea" of specific wildflowers or trees known for their healing properties, then diluted (similar to homeopathic remedies, in that regard). They work to balance negative emotions, freeing the body's energy to heal itself. You can take the remedy under the tongue, or add a few drops to a glass of water and sip it. Nancy Buono, a Bach Foundation Registered Practitioner (BFRP) and Director of Bach Flower Education, recommends these Bach remedies to help with PMS. For more information, visit www.bachflowereducation.com.

Condition	Bach Flower Remedy
Mood swings	**Scleranthus,** to restore a sense of balance and poise
Irritability, easily annoyed	**Impatiens,** to deal with circumstances patiently and calmly
PMS, general	**Walnut,** to assist in adapting to the monthly hormonal changes

Exercise to Ease PMS

We know that one of the best ways to reduce PMS is through aerobic exercise, whether it's walking, jogging, swimming, or cycling. Aerobic training is more effective with PMS than weight training because it works on the cardiovascular system and reduces stress. "Regular exercise has also been shown to improve concentration and relieve cramps, pain, and water retention," says Dr. Wiancek. "It lowers estrogen levels because it gets estrogen moving out of the liver and improves glucose tolerance. It also increases endorphins, which help with mood."

To increase the chances you'll stick with the exercise you pick, choose something you actually enjoy. What a concept! If you love the outdoors, take trail walks. If you're hooked on TV, get an elliptical trainer or treadmill and set it up in front of the tube. Whatever you do, aim for an hour of aerobic exercise five times a week.

natural news

It's important to remember that we have the ability to feel more during PMS. "We don't want to act on our feelings, but we want to own them and understand them as ours," says Dr. Lucille. "Being able to do relaxation exercises or meditation, or have psychotherapy on board is important to help you to understand and identify your deeper feelings."

Natural R$_x$

Black cohosh: 80 mg twice daily—capsules and tablets; use at least two to three months to see results; avoid during pregnancy or while nursing.

Calcium: 500–1,500 mg daily.

Chaste tree: As directed; for menstrual problems, take during the last 14 days of the cycle after ovulation for three to four months; different brand formulations are available.

Cramp bark (Viburnum opulus): As directed. Relieves menstrual cramps.

Dandelion leaf: Tea, 1 TB. per cup of water, 3 cups daily; acts as diuretic and reduces water tension and breast tenderness associated with PMS; contains potassium; take on an empty stomach.

Dong quai (Angelica sinensis, also called tang-kuei): 100–200 mg daily—capsules and tablets; for PMS, start on day 14 and continue until menstruation starts.

Evening primrose: 500 mg three times daily—capsules.

Lavender: Add essential oil to a bath, apply to temples, and/or use in an aromatic diffuser. Visit www.leydenhouse.com for more information about oils and diffusers.

Lemon balm (Melissa officinalis): Cream, apply topically to treat herpes.

Licorice (Glycyrrhiza glabra): Tincture, ½ tsp., 40 drops, or 2.5 mL three times daily; cream: apply topically to treat herpes; has potent soothing, anti-inflammatory, and antiviral effects.

Magnesium: 300–700 mg daily.

Multivitamin: As directed.

Oat grass (Avena sativa): Tincture, ½ tsp., 40 drops, or 2.5 mL three times daily; can help fight osteoporosis through its rich calcium content.

Omega Woman: Nordic Naturals, as directed.

Rosemary: Add essential oil to bath or dab on wrists.

Tea tree oil: Use as an essential oil or salve.

Valerian: Tea, 1 TB. per cup of water, 3 cups daily.

Vitamin B complex: As directed.

Vitamin C: 200–500 mg daily.

Vitamin D: 1,000-2,000 IU daily.

Zinc: 15–50 mg daily.

Sinusitis

If you've ever had sinusitis, you know how painful it can be. When the sinuses, the hollow places behind your cheeks, nose, and eyes, are working the way they should, the mucous membranes inside them help to moisten and warm the air and filter out germs. But when your sinuses can't drain, it can be like the La Brea Tar Pits: nothing much is moving. It's also a prime spot for infection to set in, which is what sinusitis is.

You get sinusitis when a virus or bacteria decides to set up shop in your nasal passages. In acute cases, this is the result of a cold and the blocked sinuses that result. Still, if you don't fully recover, sinusitis can become chronic, as 37 million Americans know. Either way, symptoms can include pain and pressure in your sinus cavities, fever, cough, fatigue, and general malaise.

 dial your doc

> If you don't feel better within a few days, or if you have a low-grade fever of 99°F to 100°F, facial pressure or pain, a headache, congestion, thick yellow-green nasal discharge, bad breath, and/or pain in the upper teeth, call your doctor. You'll most likely be prescribed an antibiotic to eliminate the bacteria causing the infection.

Addressing the Diet

Did you know that the mucous membrane of the sinuses and the nose is the same membrane that extends all the way down the throat and into the gut? This means that, ultimately, sinusitis is all about the diet, says Greg Nigh, N.D. LA.c., who practices at the Nature Cures Clinic in Portland, Oregon (www.naturecuresclinic.com). "You always need to look at what contributes to the healthy ecology of the nose. You want healthy bacteria to grow in the digestive tract so they populate the whole mucous membrane."

If you want to get to the cause, you have to figure out what is creating inflammation in the sinuses. One of the best ways to do this is by practicing an elimination diet. Get major allergens out of your diet for about three weeks, says Dr. Nigh, and reintroduce them one by one to get a really good picture of which foods or food groups are giving you symptoms. Wheat and dairy are the most common culprits.

It's common for people with chronic sinus issues to have a reaction to a food that is predisposing them to a bacterial or fungal overgrowth. In fact, research at the Mayo Clinic in 1999 showed that the immune response to fungus causes most chronic sinusitis.

Natural Nasal Sprays

One of the best antifungal nutrients is garlic. Dr. Nigh uses a nasal spray with a garlic extract from a compounding pharmacy. "A pharmaceutical spray kills good and bad bugs. Garlic will kill fungus, but it won't kill the good bugs. The spray is carried deep into the cells." To get this garlic nasal spray from a compounding pharmacy, you'll need a prescription from your natural health practitioner.

You don't need a prescription for grape seed extract nasal spray. The phyto or plant compounds in grape seeds are good for sinusitis because of their antioxidant and anti-inflammatory effects and the ability to tone and protect capillaries in the nose. One brand is Nutribiotic Nasal Spray. You can buy it at www.herbalremedies.com. You can also use Xlear (www.xlear.com) to flush bacteria out of the nasal passages. It contains Xylitol (a natural sweetener), purified water, saline, and grapefruit seed as a preservative.

Natural Nutrients

Besides picking up a nasal spray and using it regularly, you can boost your immunity by focusing on antibacterial herbs to battle the bacteria that is generated with a sinus infection. These include oregano oil (also an antifungal herb), goldenseal, garlic, Oregon grape, and sage. You can also try an antiviral herb like echinacea and licorice. Barbara S. Silbert, D.C., N.D., a naturopathic doctor who practices in Bethel, Vermont, recommends general immune-stimulating and demulcent (soothing) herbs such as red clover and fenugreek.

NAC

To clear the pipes and get things moving again, you may want to try N-Acetylcysteine (NAC), an amino acid and antioxidant. This nutrient helps sinuses drain by thinning mucus. A review of research in the *European Respiratory Journal* in 2000 showed NAC's effectiveness in improving the symptoms of chronic bronchitis (another condition where mucus is generated) without side effects.

Bromelain

Recent research has been promising when it comes to the effects of bromelain, an enzyme derived from pineapple, on sinusitis, according to a study in *Otolaryngology*, the official journal of the American Academy of Otolaryngology. Bromelain helps to break down mucus, which gets it flowing out of the sinuses and relieves pressure.

Quercetin

Think of the bioflavonoid quercetin as a natural antihistamine. (Bioflavonoids give fruits and vegetables their unique color, as with green tea.) This natural remedy (especially when taken with bromelain) can help stop the release of histamine from tissues that can cause inflammation and congestion in the sinus passages. Quercetin stabilizes the immune system and enhances the effects of vitamin C, an anti-inflammatory and antioxidant, which also helps boost immunity. So does vitamin A, so include it, too.

natural news

Dr. Silbert recommends kosher salt packs as a remedy for sinusitis. Buy an empty pack that fits over your forehead and cheeks, which you can safely warm in an oven. Fill it with kosher salt, put it on a cookie sheet, and bake it in a warm oven until it is at a comfortable temperature to put over your sinuses. (You can also warm it in a microwave.) Take it out and put it over your sinuses. Sit with a box of tissues, because it's common for mucus to liquefy and drain.

Homeopathy

If you want to nip your sinus infection in the bud, try Sinusalia (www. boiron.com). Adults and kids 6 and over take two tablets every two hours up to six times a day, to find relief for sinus pain and other symptoms. That's because this gentle remedy contains pain-fighter belladonna to ease congestion, sanguinaria canadensis to stop pain and that runny nose, and spigelia anthelmia to put an end to post-nasal drip.

Hydrotherapy

One of Dr. Silbert's favorite immune-stimulating remedies is the cold, wet sock treatment. Just take a thin pair of cotton socks and run the foot part under cold water; wring them out very well, put them on your feet, and then put two pairs of thick wool socks over that and go to bed. "Most people dry the socks by morning and feel a lot better." This works best at the beginning of any cold, flu, or sinusitis by making the body mount an immune response: a fever or, at the very least, some good heat/sweating. If you wake up in the night and your feet are cold and wet, take off the socks, dry your feet, and go back to bed without them on. Some people dry the socks in a few hours, and some people need to do it two nights in a row to dry them out.

The Power of Acupuncture

Dr. Nigh is a big believer in acupuncture treatments for sinusitis. "It's a way of addressing the cause of the problem rather than just treating the symptoms." Usually people come into Dr. Nigh's office with congested sinuses, and after treatment their nose clears up almost immediately. "People can breathe much easier." The key is to practice this alternative therapy early and regularly. "Acupuncture always is better if you do several treatments initially," says Dr. Nigh. "But you need to be consistent with acupuncture to reap the benefits. In the long run, the price you pay for acupuncture in order to take care of sinusitis without using medication is pretty small."

Ah, Aromatherapy!

Holistic aromatherapist Jade Shutes, B.A., Diploma AT, recommends this remedy for sinusitis:

Steam inhalation

> 20 drops eucalyptus oil
>
> 16 drops rosemary oil
>
> 8 drops lemon oil
>
> 5 drops thyme oil

Combine the drops in a 5 mL amber bottle. Replace the cap and shake vigorously for two to four minutes. Label the bottle "Sinusitis synergy."

Bring 4 cups of water to a boil. Remove from stove and place two to three drops of the synergy into water. Immediately place a towel over your head and stand over the bowl of steaming water. Breathe in through the nose and out through the mouth. Be sure to close your eyes while doing this, to avoid eye irritation. Perform steam inhalation two to three times daily.

You can also get a prepared blend called Sinusitis Fighter from Leyden House (www.leydenhouse.com). This potent mixture contains lavender, eucalyptus, and peppermint essential oils. Put it in a diffuser and let it infuse the room to relieve sinus congestion. Your sinuses will thank you.

The Ayurvedic Perspective

Hilary Garavaltis, an ayurvedic practitioner and the dean of curriculum for the Kripalu School of Ayurveda at the Kripalu Center for Yoga & Health in Stockbridge, Massachusetts, recommends these ayurvedic practices for keeping the nasal passages clear and gently lubricated, allowing them to maintain their own strength and integrity against pathogens and pollutants:

◆ Use a neti lota pot, from the practice of yoga, to rinse your sinuses with warm saltwater. As a form of hydrotherapy, this clears out the sinuses and the salt also draws fluid out of swollen mucous membranes, allowing them to drain. This is especially helpful, Garavaltis says, during challenging allergy seasons or when you've been exposed to smoke, dust, or allergens.

◆ After nasal rinsing, always follow up with an oil lubricant. This can be just simple sesame oil or a blended "nasya" oil prepared with herbs that you can get from an ayurvedic practitioner.

◆ Regular breathing exercises can help keep the channels clear and open, and strengthen the lungs.

Dr. Silbert recommends a nasal lavage with a few drops of osha root tincture in the water. "It's similar to a neti pot, but with less fluid. Use an eyedropper instead of the neti pot." You can find ready-made saline mixes and neti pots at www.sinucleanse.com.

natural news

You can also open an acidophilus capsule and add the "friendly bacteria" into water in your neti pot, and let that circulate through the nose. "The more the good stuff is there, the less likely the fungus or other bacteria will be to populate the membrane," says Dr. Nigh.

Bust a Yoga Move

Here's how to practice the Dirga Pranayama, or the Yogic three-part breath, according to Stephen Hartman, the director of Professional Training and Association at the Kripalu Center for Yoga & Health in Stockbridge, Massachusetts:

1. Sit erect and relax your abdomen.

2. Place your palms on your belly and breathe into your lower lungs, feeling your diaphragm drop and your belly expend into your palms. Repeat several times.

3. Shift your palms to the sides of your ribcage and breathe into your chest, feeling your ribcage expand to the sides. Repeat several times.

4. Place your fingertips on the front of your chest just below the collarbones. Breathe into the upper part of your chest and feel your hands lifting. Repeat several times.

5. Combine all three in-breaths to make a Dirga Pranayama inhalation.

6. Exhale completely, gently contracting the abdomen to squeeze out residual air.

7. Repeat this cycle several times, moving your hands to the different parts of your body. Focus on filling and emptying your lungs completely.

8. Rest your hands in your lap and continue this breathing pattern for several minutes.

Natural R$_x$

Acidophilus bifidus: As directed.

Bromelain: 500 mg twice daily.

Echinacea: Tincture, ½ tsp, 40 drops, or 2.5 mL three times daily; capsules and tablets, 200 mg twice daily. Fights inflammation and viruses.

Fenugreek: ½ tsp, 40 drops, or 2.5 mL, three times a day; tea, 1 TB. per cup of water, three cups a day.

Flaxseed oil: 1 TB. daily. To reduce inflammation.

Garlic: Cloves, two or three daily; standardized extract, 400 mg two to three capsules daily.

Goldenseal: ½ tsp., 40 drops, or 2.5 mL, three times daily for a maximum of two weeks; capsules and tablets: 100 mg three times daily for a maximum of two weeks.

Grapefruit seed extract nasal spray: As directed. Antimicrobial.

Licorice: ½ tsp., 40 drops, or 2.5 mL, three times a day; tea, decoction, 1 TB. per cup of water, three cups a day.

Lycopodium homeopathic remedy: As directed.

Mercurius homeopathic remedy: As directed.

N-Acetylcysteine (NAC): 600–1,200 mg daily.

Oregon grape: ½ tsp, 40 drops, or 2.5 mL three times daily; tea, 1 TB. per cup of water, 2–3 cups daily.

Quercetin: 1,000 mg daily.

Red clover: ½ tsp., 40 drops, or 2.5 mL, three times a day; tea, 1 TB. per cup of water, three cups a day.

Sabadilla homeopathic remedy: As directed.

Sage: ½ tsp., 40 drops, or 2.5 mL, three times a day; tea, 1 TB. per cup of water, three cups a day.

Sinusalia: Take 2 tablets every two hours, up to six times daily. For children under 6, see your doctor about the correct dosage. www. boiron.com.

Vitamin A: 25,000 IU. Immune booster. If you are pregnant, check with your doctor first.

Vitamin C: 3,000 mg daily in divided doses. A natural anti-inflammatory nutrient.

Sprains and Strains

Sure, being active is a great way to stay in shape. But if you are overenthusiastic or just take a step in the wrong direction, a strain or sprain can result. A sprain means you've stretched or torn the ligament, a kind of giant elastic band attached to your bones that holds your joints where they should be. Ankle and knee sprains are the two most common ways we injure ourselves. Once you've sprained your ankle or knee, expect pain, swelling, and difficulty getting from point A to point B for up to 10 weeks. Severe sprains may require a cast.

dial your doc

If pain from an injury is severe or you suspect you have a fracture, call your doctor.

When you "pull a muscle," this is known as a strain. This can also be painful because you are stretching or tearing a muscle or tendon. You'll usually get these injuries in your back or a hamstring. Whether you've got a sprain or a strain, these natural remedies can help ease your discomfort and speed healing.

Relief Remedies

Want to cut your healing time in half? Try homeopathic arnica (Arnica montana), a member of the Asteraceae (daisy) family, immediately after an injury. Known as homeopathic aspirin, arnica jump-starts the healing of sprains and strains by relieving pain and swelling.

Use arnica massage oil before and after a workout to help loosen tight muscles and ease strains. (Avoid arnica on broken skin, as it may cause irritation.) Your sore muscles may also find relief from rosemary, birch, and fir essential oils. St. John's wort oil, salve, and liniment can be helpful if the pain you feel is throbbing or radiates out from the injured area.

To cool the fire of inflammation that occurs with sprains and strains, you can use licorice root, turmeric, and wild yam. You'll find them in teas, tinctures, and capsules. Natural compounds in hawthorn known as anthocyanidins and proanthocyanidins also help ease inflammation and reduce joint damage. The high vitamin C content in hawthorn can help improve blood circulation and relieve swelling.

natural news

Holly Lucille, N.D., a naturopathic doctor who practices in Los Angeles, recommends FlexAgility MAX, which includes clinically studied ingredients like bromelain, ginger, rhizome extract, Boswellia serrata gum extract, N-acetylcysteine (NAC), and antioxidants like vitamin C and green tea leaf extract; all relieve occasional pain and stiffness due to overuse. You can find FlexAgility MAX at your local health food retailer, or visit www.enzy.com.

Taking a Soak

To soothe sore muscles, Brigitte Mars, A.H.G., author of *The Desktop Guide to Herbal Medicine,* recommends taking an herbal bath and adding Epsom salts. That's because when the magnesium sulfate in Epsom salts is absorbed in the skin, it reduces swelling and relaxes muscles. Here's how to do it:

1. Add 2 to 4 cups of Epsom salts to a running bath.

2. Next, grab a colorful washcloth and put a handful of herbs, like calendula, juniper berries, and rosemary, inside. Tie it up tight with a hair tie. Throw it into the tub.

3. For sprains, you can also add 10 drops of tea tree oil to the water.

4. Fill the tub to the desired level, then allow the water to cool so you can climb in. This will also give the herbs more time to "steep."

5. Soak for at least 20 minutes.

One of the biggest mistakes you can make with a sprain is not following P.R.I.C.E.: protect, rest, ice, compression, and elevation. Once you know you've injured your ankle or knee, protect it by getting off your feet. Use crutches, a cane, or a splint to get around. Rest it by avoiding using your ankle or knee. Ice it and compress it with a bandage to limit swelling. Finally, elevate it to reduce swelling. If you don't see improvement after two or three days, see your doctor.

Nutrients You Need

The sea is full of wonderful nutrients. One of the most helpful for joint pain and inflammation is glucosamine sulfate, an easily absorbed source of glucosamine derived from shellfish. It can also stimulate the repair of damaged connective tissue and cartilage. For this reason, it can be helpful after a sprain or strain. A major component of joint cartilage, glucosamine also helps in the formation of skin, tendons, ligaments, and synovial (joint) fluids. It is often used to treat osteoarthritis.

When it comes to bruises, which occur when blood vessels are damaged or broken, choose vitamin C with bioflavonoids. That's because these nutrients build collagen and strengthen blood vessels. Both bromelain (an enzyme that comes from pineapple) and papain (an enzyme from papaya) can help with the swelling and inflammation that accompanies bruising. That's because these natural nutrients help break down protein and ease congestion in blood vessel walls.

Natural Rx

Arnica homeopathic remedy: As directed.

Arnica massage oil: As directed.

Birch essential oil: Topically as directed.

Calendula: As directed.

Epsom salts: 1 cup in the bath.

Fir essential oil: Topically as directed.

FlexAgility MAX: As directed. www.enzy.com

Glucosamine sulphate: As directed.

Juniper berries: As directed.

Licorice root: Tincture, ½ tsp, 40 drops, or 2.5 mL, three times daily; tea, decoction: 1 TB. per cup of water, 3 cups daily; capsules, as directed.

Rosemary: As directed.

Rosemary essential oil: Topically as directed.

St. John's wort: Apply as oil, salve, or liniment.

Turmeric: Tincture, ½ tsp, 40 drops, or 2.5 mL, three times daily; standardized extract, one 400–600 mg capsule [100 percent curcumin] three times daily.

Vitamin C with bioflavonoids: 200–500 mg daily.

Wild yam: Tincture, ½ tsp, 40 drops, or 2.5 mL, three times daily; capsules and tablets, 100 mg three times daily.

Sunburn

When it comes to the sun, a little bit goes a long way. Although sunshine helps the body manufacture vitamin D, an important nutrient, overexposure to ultraviolet rays can be harmful and can cause *sunburn* and even *skin cancer* if you become overexposed. Melanin, the pigment in our skin, protects us from sunburn, but it can only do so much. If you are fair (think Cinderella), you'll burn in less than half an hour. If you are dark-skinned (think Sleeping Beauty), you can stay in the sun for a while longer.

You know you have sunburn when you turn that classic shade of pink. You may also get blisters if you've really baked yourself, along with fever, aches, and/or chills. But you may not see the full effect the sun has had on your skin for 24 hours or longer.

def•i•ni•tion

Sunburn is an inflammation of the skin caused by too much exposure to the sun or a tanning lamp. Symptoms include pink skin, pain, and blisters.

When you get too much sun exposure, you can damage your DNA and increase your risk for **skin cancer.** According to the Centers for Disease Control, if you have a history of sunburn with blisters, it doubles your risk of malignant melanoma, the fastest-increasing type of skin cancer.

Lower Your Risk

One of the best ways to lessen your risk of sunburn and skin cancer is to avoid the sun when the rays are the most intense, which is from 11 A.M. to 4 P.M. When you do go out, wear a hat that covers your face, use an umbrella, and sit or walk in the shade whenever possible. Wear sunglasses, especially at high altitudes, because the sun can burn your retina. (You can actually get a melanoma of the eye.) Use a natural lip balm (no petroleum products, please!) with sun protection so you don't develop cold sores from too much sun exposure. Of course, nix tanning parlors.

Use Sunscreen the Right Way

Besides reducing your exposure, change the way you think about sunscreens. Using one doesn't mean you are protected from skin cancer or that you have carte blanche to stay in the sun all day. This kind of thinking is a big part of the reason why the skin cancer rate is increasing every year.

dial your doc

Contact your doctor right away if you have signs of shock, heat exhaustion, dehydration, or other serious reactions, including faintness or dizziness; rapid pulse or rapid breathing; extreme thirst, no urine output, or sunken eyes; pale, clammy, or cool skin; nausea, chills, or rash; eyes that hurt and are sensitive to light; or severe, painful blisters.

You will want to choose a sunscreen with a high SPF to boost your protection. Choose a waterproof sunscreen with a minimum of 30 SPF (preferably, 50 SPF), with both UVA and UVB block, and apply it generously 30 minutes before sun exposure. Pay special attention to your face, nose, ears, and shoulders. Reapply every hour or after you go in the water. Use a sunscreen on a regular basis, including on cloudy days, since 80 percent of the sun's UV rays pass through the clouds.

Also, it's extremely important to choose a sunscreen that is paraben, or PABA, free because parabens are known carcinogens, substances that can cause cancer. Good brands of PABA-free sunscreen include Jason and Aubrey.

Some sunscreens now contain green tea. Farmers in Asia don't have the skin cancer rate we have in the United States, and the thinking is it's because they drink a lot of green tea. Studies show that the nutrients in green tea actually protect against skin cancer, so it's a good idea to add some to your diet, too.

Sunscreen Pills?

You heard right. Polypodium leucotomos extract (it comes from ferns that grow in the Honduran jungles) can keep you from looking like a lobster by protecting DNA and immune cells. A study in the medical journal *Photodermatology, Photoimmunology & Photomedicine* (1997) showed that Heliocare (Polypodium leucotomos) extract prevents acute sunburn. It's important to use a sunscreen when taking this supplement. You can find Heliocare in major pharmacies across the United States or at www.heliocare.com. It also contains green tea extract, which helps protect DNA, and the antioxidant beta carotene.

natural news

If you shun the sun completely, you lack a very necessary nutrient that helps the body absorb calcium, keeps bones strong, and nourishes tissues and cells—vitamin D. "A significant number of people don't meet the adequate intake," says Karen Collins, M.S., R.D., a registered dietitian and nutrition consultant to the American Institute for Cancer Research. When we don't get enough vitamin D, we put our bones at risk for osteoporosis. Research now also suggests that vitamin D may help lower the risk for pancreatic, breast, colon, lung, and prostate cancer. Collins explains, "Vitamin D plays a role in keeping cells in a normal or noncancerous form and controls their growth and reproduction."

To maximize the benefits and get vitamin D safely from the sun, aim for 15 minutes three times a week with hands, face, and arms exposed each day. For northern climates in the winter, supplement with foods rich in vitamin D, like Norwegian cod liver oil, salmon, mackerel, egg yolks, milk and fortified juices, breakfast cereals, and soy milk. You can also supplement with vitamin D to meet your needs.

The other sunscreen pill, a superoxide dismutase (SOD) supplement called GliSODin, alleviated the severity of redness associated with sunburn by almost 10 percent, according to a recent report in the *European Journal of Dermatology*. Discovered in 1968, SOD is considered to be more potent than other antioxidant vitamins because it forces the body to produce its own antioxidants. GliSODin is a combination of SOD extracted from cantaloupe and wheat gliadin.

Aloe and Other Herbal Remedies

Okay, you've done your best, but you still ended up with a sunburn. What do you do? One of the best natural remedies is aloe vera because this anti-inflammatory plant contains compounds similar to aspirin.

This means it helps ease the pain and redness of sunburn. Aloe also stimulates blood flow, improving healing time. Ideally, you have an aloe vera plant handy. If you do (if not, why not get one now?), slice open one of the spiky leaves from the plant lengthwise and slather the gel on the burn. Do this several times a day until you feel better. If you are going to buy a ready-made aloe vera gel, look for one that is pure aloe, for best results. A good brand to try is Burt's Bees Aloe & Linden Flower After Sun Soother, at www.burtsbees.com.

Lavender essential oil is great for burns (see "First Aid"), including sunburn. "Doing cool compresses of lavender essential oil can really help take the sting out of sunburn," says Courtney Gilardi, N.D., a naturopathic physician at the Kripalu Center for Yoga & Health in Stockbridge, Massachusetts. Three of her other favorites are calendula, chickweed, and St. John's wort in salve and tea form. "You just make a nice herbal tea and put it on a compress and let it sit on the skin; it's amazing how healing this can be."

You can also use black tea externally to take the sting out of sunburn. If you're in a pinch when you're traveling and you've spent too much time in the sun, use black tea bags from room service to soothe a sunburn. A cool bath in black tea is very soothing. You'll find many remedies for the skin, including Burn Relief RX, at www.healingcove.com.

risky remedy!

St. John's wort can make you more vulnerable to sunburn.

Homeopathic Help

Beverly Yates, N.D., a naturopathic doctor and founder of the Naturopathic Family Health Clinic in Mill Valley, California, recommends the homeopathic remedy Cantharis (Spanish fly) for sunburn. "It's amazing. It's something you really want in your home kit, for sure." If you have blisters, itching or burning, or severe pain with a sunburn, it can help.

The Future with Black Raspberries

Soon you may be able to use black raspberry cream after sun exposure to help prevent skin cancer. When researchers at Ohio State University made a compound of black raspberries and applied it to the skin of mice, it helped to slow the growth of squamous cell carcinoma, the second-leading cause of skin cancer. We think this is because black raspberries contain antioxidants called anthacyanins, which help stop the inflammation (from DNA damage) and oxidative stress (from free radicals) that happen when you get a sunburn. Ultimately, the researchers' aim is to make the extract into a gel or lotion to quell inflammation and reduce skin cancers.

natural news

If there is damage externally, there is damage internally, reminds Dr. Gilardi, who says it's also really important to eat high-antioxidant foods like blueberries to help the body heal. Drink plenty of water, too, to rehydrate yourself.

Natural Rx

Aloe vera: Apply topically.

Burn Relief RX: Apply topically.

Calendula salve: Apply topically.

Calendula/chickweed/St. John's wort: Use as a compress.

Chickweed salve: Apply topically.

GliSODin: As directed. www.glisodin.com and www.swansonvitamins.com.

Heliocare (Polypodium leucotomos extract): As directed. www.heliocare.com.

Homeopathic Cantharis: 3 or 4 30C pellets every two to three hours until symptoms improve.

Lavender essential oil: Apply topically.

Thyroid Disorders

If you're feeling blue, have zero energy, or can't fit into your skinny jeans, you may have *hypothyroidism*, which means your thyroid isn't producing enough thyroid hormone. Other symptoms of hypothyroidism include brain fog or difficulty concentrating, dry skin and hair, depression, constipation, increased sensitivity to cold, and heavier-than-normal menstrual periods. Untreated mild hypothyroidism also increases the risk for a heart attack because having low thyroid levels can increase cholesterol and blood pressure. It can also cause infertility and chronic pain.

The most common cause of hypothyroidism is Hashimoto's thyroiditis, a type of autoimmune disease in which antibodies mistake the thyroid gland as "other than the body" and begin to attack it. Ack! Women are more likely to experience hypothyroidism than men.

def•i•ni•tion

Hypothyroidism occurs when the body doesn't produce enough thyroid hormone. Hyperthyroidism occurs when the body produces too much.

Hyperthyroidism, on the other hand, occurs when the body produces too much thyroid hormone. It is much less common, affecting fewer than 1 in 10 people with thyroid problems, and results in symptoms like a speedy heart rate, high blood pressure, anxiety, diarrhea, and difficulty sleeping. It's like having 10 cups of coffee all the time! Hyperthyroidism can happen at any time, either slowly or suddenly, but it's usually triggered by Graves disease, which is, like Hashimoto's thyroiditis, an autoimmune disease.

Experts aren't sure what causes hyperthyroidism, but they think it's some combination of factors, including genetics and toxic environmental exposures. According to Mary Shomon, author of *Living Well with Graves' Disease and Hyperthyroidism*, there is more evidence that major physical or emotional stress, such as a divorce or a death in the family, is a factor when it comes to triggering Graves' disease.

You can also develop hyperthyroidism because you are taking too much thyroid medicine or because you have nodules in your thyroid that start producing thyroid hormone on their own. A few drugs can spur hyperthyroidism as well. One is a heart drug, amiodorone (brand name Pacerone). A small percentage of pregnant women can develop temporary hyperthyroidism that causes them to have terrible morning sickness.

Metabolism Regulator

When the thyroid, a small butterfly-shaped gland located at the base of the neck, is working the way it should, it regulates every aspect of our metabolism, from the rate at which the heart beats to how quickly we burn calories. This is truly an amazing feat, and one we don't think about unless it's not working the way it should. The thyroid gland sends out hormones that control virtually *every* organ. It's the thermostat for your body and regulates all the bodily systems.

The thyroid affects our energy, appetite, body weight, and body temperature. Almost every tissue in the body is dependent on thyroid hormones. The thyroid responds to the master gland just below the brain, the pituitary, which signals it via thyroid-stimulating hormone (TSH). It makes thyroid cells produce more thyroid hormone.

A crucial constituent of thyroid hormone is being able to read the DNA in your cell nucleus, says Richard L. Shames, M.D., author of *Feeling Fat, Fuzzy, or Frazzled?* "It allows your cells' machinery to read your genetic information—in other words, to read the book of life." Thyroid hormone is also key to mitochondria function, the place in the cell where main energy production occurs.

1-2-3 Testing

Hypothyroidism tends to run in families. If one of your parents has it, you have a very significant chance of having it, too. The American Thyroid Association recommends that everyone be tested for low thyroid function at age 35. After the age of 50, ask for a blood test every 5 to 10 years to screen for thyroid disease. Several tests can help evaluate whether you have hypothyroidism. A TSH test measures the level of thyroid-stimulating hormone in the blood. If you have a high TSH, it means you have low thyroid function.

Since thyroxine (T4) is the major hormone the thyroid gland produces, a test called a free thyroxine (FT4) measures the amount of this hormone in the blood. Cells convert T4 to its active form, called T3, which affects our cells directly. A free thyroxine (FT3) test measures the level of this hormone in the blood. Thyroperoxidase antibody tests help to diagnose Hashimoto's thyroiditis. To get a more complete understanding of your current thyroid function, ask your doctor for a TSH, free thyroxine (FT4), free thyroxine (FT3), and thyroperoxidase antibody tests. (Overactive thyroid is also diagnosed by measuring blood levels of thyroid hormones.)

You might even want to consider some advanced testing that you can get without a doctor's order. A simple home test can help you find answers. Dr. Shames says, "The newer, more sophisticated tests can be more accurate than the older blood tests." Often doctors order only a TSH test, but if you would like get a clearer picture of your thyroid results (TSH, FT3, FT4, and peroxidase antibodies), visit Dr. Shames's website, www.feelingfff.com, to order a home test kit. You collect and mail samples to the lab; using a password and a code number, you can then obtain your results online. To test only your TSH, visit www.thyroid-info.com/diet/tshtest.htm.

Beyond Testing

Be aware that blood tests are not always the final word. The American Academy of Clinical Endocrinologists has established that anyone with a TSH over 3 has a low thyroid, but many doctors still use 5 or higher as a diagnostic indicator. "Find a doctor who will treat you, not the blood test," says Jacob Teitlebaum, medical director of the Fibromyalgia and Fatigue Centers nationally and author of *From Fatigued to Fantastic!* "Just because it's in the normal range doesn't mean you don't need to be treated. Over 13 million Americans with thyroid disease remain undiagnosed, and the majority of those receiving treatment are not being dosed appropriately."

To assess the possibility of hypothyroidism, ask yourself if it's a new symptom for you, if it has persisted for more than two weeks, and if it occurs in conjunction with other symptoms of hypothyroidism, such as weight gain and sensitivity to cold. Talk to your doctor and visit www. thryoid-info.com, www.drbrownstein.com, www.feelingfff.com, and www.vitality101.com for more information.

If you have hypothyroidism, your doctor will probably prescribe the synthetic thyroid hormone levothyroxine (Levoxyl, Levothroid, or Synthroid) to restore adequate hormone levels in the body. You'll need to take it daily on an empty stomach half an hour before you eat. (Don't take it with calcium and iron because they block absorption.) But some do better with Armour Thyroid, a more natural version, made from desiccated (freeze-dried) porcine thyroid. Armour Thyroid contains a mixture of thyroid hormones T4 (thyroxine) and T3 (triiodothyronine).

"The decision has to be made with your doctor," says Shomon. "Usually the first thing that's offered is the synthetic version, like Synthroid, but some doctors feel strongly about providing a natural option. It's not a one-size-fits-all solution. It's more trial-and-error process, depending which you feel best on. The key thing is awareness that there is an alternative, that there are natural drugs available."

 risky remedy! _____

Shomon warns about self-medicating with nonprescription over-the-counter thyroid glandular formulas. "You can get them at any health food store on the Internet. The problem is, we don't know how much thyroid is in any one of them, so you're not getting a consistent dosage of thyroid in it, and there are a lot of concerns about the purity of those products because they involve animal processing. The biggest fear, but the least likely, is mad cow disease. Many of these products come from abroad, and they may not necessarily be porcine; they may be bovine." Her advice is not to take them unless it's under the direction of a holistic doctor who specifies a particular brand.

Supplements for Thyroid Health

Autoimmune diseases like Hashimoto's thyroiditis and Graves' disease create a lot of oxidative stress in the body. For this reason, says Dr. Shames, it's important to have antioxidants in your arsenal. Good nutritional support enables thyroid hormone to work better as well.

You can build a good foundation with a multivitamin, extra vitamin C, extra antioxidants, and omega-3 essential fatty acids.

In addition, Dr. Shames says one specifically designed thyroid product for hypothyroidism is MedCaps T-3 (available at www.xymogen.com/2007/formulas.asp, sold only to health practitioners). It includes thyroid-empowering ingredients like rosemary extract, zinc, and vitamin D, all co-factors in thyroid functions. It also contains selenium, which studies show can convert T4 into active T3.

natural news _____

Dr. Shames says it's important to keep in mind that many of the multiple vitamins and antioxidant preparations that are available at health food stores and discount health food stores do not have the purity or the potency to be maximally helpful for a thyroid candidate. That's why it's important to buy supplements directly from a top-rated nutraceutical company that uses only hypoallergenic, easily assimilated, absorbable items. Often these top companies will sell only to doctors or clinics.

If you have hypothyroidism, it can be smart to take tyrosine, an amino acid that is a building block for thyroid hormone. Iodine is also an issue, says Shomon. One quarter of Americans are iodine deficient. This can impact the thyroid because you don't have enough of the basic building blocks to produce thyroid hormone; this can lead to inactivity and the development of a goiter. For less risk, use iodized salt.

Omega-3 essential fatty acids can be important, especially if you have Hashimoto's thyroiditis or Graves' disease, in the case of hyperthyroidism, since both are autoimmune diseases. Fatty acids can help particularly when it comes to the hair and skin.

Another herbal supplement that's very popular with holistic doctors for thyroid patients is an ayurvedic remedy known as Guggul (guggulsterone). According to Shomon, it works to help prevent sluggish metabolism, increase oxygen uptake, and improve the conversion of thyroid hormone in the muscles and in the tissues. Also, Dr. Shames recommends regularly including rosemary in your diet or taking 75 to 100 mg of rosemary leaf extract daily to help.

Correct Use of Natural Remedies

"If you have mild hyperthyroidism, there are different nutrients that can help you lower your thyroid function, that are safer than medicine and act in a less permanent way than radioactive iodine or surgery," says Dr. Shames. Using natural remedies can also help minimize the amount of antithyroid drug you have to be on. The lower the dosage of prescribed medication, the lower the chance of any side effects from those drugs. If you have severe hyperthyroidism, natural remedies can be used as an adjunct to prescription medicines. But even though these remedies are natural, you'll need to be under the care of a doctor who is familiar with Graves' disease first. He or she will most likely want to put you on some sort of antithyroid drug until your overactive gland begins to calm down.

Once that begins to happen, you can add more items. First, start with a good multivitamin that contains high amounts of B vitamins and calcium. Then you may want to add nutrients like high-dose L-carnitine. It has a thyroid-lowering effect, especially with high doses of quercetin (3,000 to 4,000 mg daily of each).

Those with hypothyroidism should avoid soy products, but they can be helpful with hyperthyroidism because they can slow thyroid production. Taking 75 mg of soy isoflavones (at your health food store) can lower thyroid function.

Fluoride also can lower thyroid function. Yes, you're used to finding it in your toothpaste, but you can also take fluoride tablets. People who use fluoride tablets as part of an oral hygiene program generally take 1 mg daily. For therapeutic action against hyperthyroidism, take 2 to 3 mg daily.

Hyperthyroidism is often quite stressful in adrenal function. Herbs that can help support the adrenal (stress) glands are lemon balm and licorice. (Acupuncture has also been shown to be very effective in helping to balance both under- and overactive thyroid.)

Foods to Avoid

If you have hypothyroidism, don't put goitrogens (foods that suppress thyroid function) on your grocery list. Goitrogens include foods like soy, cauliflower, broccoli, and kale. If you eat them raw in large quantities (some are sensitive to even small quantities), they have an antithyroid effect. A chemical component in them slows the thyroid and causes goiters, enlarging the thyroid. Avoid soy, especially in edamame and in its unfermented form.

If you have hyperthyroidism, you should eliminate smoking, caffeinated beverages, sugar, and alcohol.

Natural R\x

Hypothyroidism

Ashwaganda root: 100 mg daily. Helps convert T4 to an active form of T3 that the body can use.

B-complex vitamin: 50 mg.

Multivitamin with minerals: As directed, daily.

Omega-3 essential fatty acids: 1,000 mg.

Omega-6 essential fatty acids: 500 mg.

Rosemary leaf extract: 75–100 mg.

Selenium: 200 mcg.

Vitamin C: 1,000 mg.

Zinc: 15–50 mg daily.

For added convenience and high quality, all of these "Natural R$_x$" nutrients for hypothyroidism are combined in two Xymogen products available at www.xymogen.com:

Active Essentials: 1 packet daily.

MedCaps T3: Four capsules daily.

Hyperthyroidism

Alpha lipoic acid: 600 mg daily.

Fluoride: 1 mg, 2–3 tablets daily.

L-carnitine: 4,000 mg daily.

Lemon balm: Tincture: ½ tsp, 40 drops, or 2.5 mL daily; tea, 1 TB. per cup of water, 2–3 cups daily.

Licorice: Tincture: ½ tsp, 40 drops, or 2.5 mL daily.

Quercetin: 4,000 mg daily.

Soy isoflavones: 75 mg.

Tinnitus

Is that the phone ringing or is it your ears? That hissing or buzzing sound you hear is tinnitus, a truly annoying condition that can happen when we overuse nonsteroidal anti-inflammatory drugs like aspirin (notice a connection between those headaches and that ringing?), are exposed to loud noises (at a rock concert recently?), have wax in the ears, or suffer allergies. It's hard to say which is worse, having tinnitus all the time or on and off. Either way, you may be miserable. What can help is to increase circulation to the ear and decrease inflammation. Check out these natural rescue remedies.

What Hurts and What Helps

Allergic to dairy? If so, you'll need to eliminate it from your diet to decrease fluid in the ear that can cause tinnitus. You also may want to try avoiding caffeine, salt, sugar, and alcohol, as they can all make symptoms worse. And we don't want that!

One of the best herbs for tinnitus is ginkgo because it improves circulation to the inner ear. Will someone please answer that phone? High doses of ginger (300 mg twice daily) may be helpful. The herb feverfew has anti-inflammatory properties, which is important when it comes to tinnitus. Often used to help prevent and alleviate migraines, you may find that it helps alleviate your tinnitus, too. Omega-3 essential fatty acids can also make a difference, taken as both fish oil and flaxseed oil, because they decrease inflammation as well.

You may also want to try a few homeopathic remedies. Do you have a low humming in your ear? Try Natrum salicylicum. Ringing or roaring noise in your ears? Try Kali carbonicum. Sensitive to noise? Try Cimicifuga. Feel like Jimmy Stewart in *Vertigo*? Try Calcarea carbonica. You'll find these and others at your health food store.

natural news

As we said before, excess earwax can contribute to tinnitus. Too much earwax can be caused by high levels of fat in the diet. But you can use olive oil to clear it out. Heat olive oil to body temperature (put it on your hand first, to ensure it's not burning). Drop a few drops of lukewarm oil in your ear two or three times a day for a few days, and it will melt the wax. Don't use a Q-tip to get it out; it will just push the wax farther into your ear and could damage your eardrum. If you experience problems, see your doctor.

Alternative Therapies

You may want to venture further afield. With craniosacral therapy, developed in the 1970s by osteopathic physician and surgeon John E. Upledger, a practitioner uses light pressure to release restrictions in the craniosacral system (the membranes that surround the brain and spinal cord) by monitoring the rhythm of the cerebrospinal fluid as it flows through the system. This technique is designed to work with the body's own inclination to heal itself.

dial your doc

It's important to see your health care provider to get an accurate diagnosis before using any alternative treatments for tinnitus.

Or you can go the do-it-yourself route with a new biofeedback program you can install on your home computer, called Healing Rhythms, created by Deepak Chopra, M.D.; Dean Ornish, M.D.; and Andrew Weil, M.D. Many folks have found it very helpful for stress reduction. You can find it at www.wilddivine.com.

Natural R_x

B complex: 100 mg daily. A deficiency may cause symptoms.

Calcarea carbonica homeopathic remedy: As directed.

Cimicifuga homeopathic remedy: As directed.

Feverfew: As directed.

Flaxseed oil: 1 TB. daily.

Ginger: 300 mg twice daily.

Ginkgo: 40 mg three times daily.

Kali carbonicum homeopathic remedy: As directed.

Magnesium: 500 mg.

Multivitamin/mineral supplement with zinc: As directed.

Natrum salicylicum homeopathic remedy: As directed.

Omega-3 fatty acids (fish oil): 3,000–4,000 mg.

Vitamin C: 1,000 mg twice daily.

Varicose Veins

If you have varicose veins, you know they can make your legs look like a road map with twisting, turning streets complete with bulges and bumps, usually of a purplish or blue hue. You also know how painful they can be. Varicose veins occur because the valves in your veins that allow blood to flow to the heart become weak and don't work the way they should. When this happens, the blood flows backward and pools in the veins in the back of the calves or the inside of the legs, resulting in the winding road we just talked about.

Spider veins are tiny versions of varicose veins that can occur in capillaries and can stretch like a web across your leg or face. Whether over a large or small area, you'll find spider veins closer to the surface of the skin than varicose veins.

Women usually get varicose veins more than men—in fact 1 out of 2 folks over 50 are affected. Family history, age, hormonal changes, pregnancy, and obesity can cause varicose veins. Sun exposure can cause spider veins.

dial your doc

If you have varicose veins, consult your physician. Your health-care practitioner will do a physical exam and may also run tests to see how well your veins function. You may need an ultrasound test to look for blood clots.

The Power of Bioflavonoids

When it comes to relieving the symptoms of varicose veins, like swelling in the legs and aching pain, one of the best places to start is with bioflavonoids. That's because the powerful antioxidant (scavenging free radicals that do cell damage) and anti-inflammatory properties of bioflavonoids help to strengthen blood vessel walls, which started this whole problem in the first place. You can start with bioflavonoids in foods like citrus fruits, berries, red grapes, and plums. It's also smart to take a bioflavonoid supplement with rutin. That's because bioflavonoids like rutin strengthen the walls of veins, improving function.

Soothing Herbs and Remedies

You'll definitely want to include herbs in your varicose veins remedy kit. Horse chestnut is number one (more about this in a minute), but yarrow, bilberry, gotu kola, and ginkgo can all be beneficial. Research in the medical journal *Drugs Under Experimental and Clinical Research* showed that taking butcher's broom alone or in combination with vitamin C and hesperidin helped to safely relieve the symptoms of varicose veins, including pain, leg cramps, itching, and swelling. Studies show that taking a plant extract from the bark of the French maritime tree, a powerful antioxidant (brand name Pycnogenol), has also been proven effective in easing varicose vein symptoms. For more information, visit www.pycnogenol.com.

Homeopathic Help

The homeopathic remedy Hamamelis can help if your veins are sore and bruised. Other homeopathic remedies such as Arnica montana, Lachesis homeopathic remedy, and Pulsatilla can also provide relief. You can find more information about homeopathic remedies for varicose veins at www.1-800Homeopathy.com.

natural news

Eating a high-fiber diet, plenty of fruits and vegetables, and whole grains (see the chapter on constipation for more ideas); drinking plenty of water; exercising regularly (biking is great!) standing for shorter periods; and maintaining a healthy weight can all help reduce the symptoms of varicose veins.

Topical Treatments

Horse chestnut cream is a number-one pick because it strengthens capillaries, improves circulation, and has been proven through research to relieve the symptoms of varicose veins. Massage it in gently, though, so you don't loosen a blood clot if you have one. In 1999, German researchers observed more than 5,000 patients who used horse chestnut cream and found that pain, fatigue, itching, and swelling in the leg were all relieved.

In 2002, a study in the medical journal *International Angiology* concluded that horse chestnut seed extract taken orally was a safe and effective treatment for varicose veins. Other research shows it can be as helpful as wearing compression stockings in boosting blood flow to the heart. You can find horse chestnut cream and horse chestnut seed extract at health food stores. Witch hazel and yarrow tea applied topically can also be very soothing.

> **risky remedy!**
> Don't take bilberry if you are on a prescription diuretic, and don't take gotu kola if you have liver disease.

Natural Rx

Arnica montana homeopathic remedy: As directed.

Bilberry, standardized extract: One 80–160 mg capsule of 25 percent anthocyanosides, three times daily.

Bioflavonoid complex: As directed.

Burdock: Tincture, ½ tsp, 40 drops, or 2.5 mL three times daily; tea, 1 TB. per cup of water, 3 cups daily.

Butcher's broom: 150 mg three times daily.

Calcarea carbonica homeopathic remedy: As directed.

Flaxseed oil: 1 TB. or 1,000 mg daily.

Ginkgo: Tincture, ¼ tsp, 20 drops, or 1.3 mL three times daily, or one 40–80 mg capsule containing 24 percent glycosides and 6 percent lactones three times daily.

Gotu kola: Tincture, ½ tsp, 40 drops, or 2.5 mL three times daily, or 200 mg capsules two to four times per day, standardized to contain 10 percent asiaticosides.

Hamamelis homeopathic remedy: Three or four 30C pellets twice daily.

Hesperidin: As directed.

Horse chestnut: Topical salve containing 20 percent aescin.

Horse chestnut seed extract: 250 mg two times daily.

Lachesis homeopathic remedy: As directed.

Pulsatilla homeopathic remedy: As directed.

Pycnogenol: 50-100 mg three times daily. www.pycnogenol.com.

Rutin, a bioflavonoid: 500 mg two times daily.

Witch hazel: Topical cold compress.

Yarrow: Tea, 1 TB. per cup of water; or apply topically as a cold compress.

Vitamin C: 200–2000 mg daily in divided doses.

Vitamin E: 800 IU daily.

Weight Loss

Dread stepping onto the scale? You're not alone. Approximately 34 million Americans are at least 20 percent over their ideal weight, and this can contribute to a wide variety of problems, including heart disease and diabetes. How exactly do you lose weight? One of the best ways is by looking at what didn't work before and making positive changes.

Starting Over

"The number-one step is to figure out your relationship with food," says Holly Lucille, N.D., a naturopathic doctor whose practice is in Los Angeles, California. "Do you use it to comfort you, for example? Or to get rid of stress? Then do a diet autopsy to figure out what didn't work before so you don't repeat your mistakes."

To do so, take out a pen and get writing. Putting down your past experiences in a journal can be a valuable way to figure out what worked and what didn't when you last tried to shed a few pounds. Perhaps you hated the way you felt when you deprived yourself. Maybe you need to add more exercise and do it in a more moderate fashion this time. Maybe deep-seated emotional issues drive you to overeat. In this case, it can be very helpful to work with a trained therapist. (Find one who has experience with food issues.) Regardless, the key to lifelong weight loss is a sensible plan you can live with—one day at a time.

natural news

To motivate yourself to try again, make a list of all the reasons why you want to lose weight. What is really important to you? Being healthier? Keeping up with your kids? Once you have your reasons, write them down in black and white on index cards, suggests Judith Beck, Ph.D., author of *The Beck Diet Solution*. Doing so will help you stay on track by helping you remember why you want to lose weight when faced with temptation or when you have sabotaging thoughts, like, "I've had a hard day and I deserve this cookie." Find out more about *The Beck Diet Solution* at www.beckdietsolution.com.

Begin with Breakfast

Start by eating breakfast. Yes, you heard right. According to the May 2008 issue of the *Harvard Heart Letter*, eating breakfast, especially if it includes a whole-grain, high-fiber cereal like steel-cut oatmeal; or a whole-grain English muffin with, say, peanut butter; or a smoothie with added oat bran, ground flax seeds, or wheat germ can help keep you from overeating and gaining weight. In fact, a 2008 study in the medical journal *Pediatrics* showed that the more often kids eat breakfast, the less likely they are to be overweight.

Research in *The British Journal of Nutrition* recently showed that when we eat fat, protein, and carbs in the morning, it keeps us satisfied longer. Breakfast also keeps our blood sugar and insulin more stable. It even reduces the risk for diabetes, heart attack and stroke, and heart failure.

Keep Your Tank Full

Nothing sabotages weight-loss efforts faster than getting too hungry (okay, starving!) and then eating your way through the fridge or the cupboard. You get the idea. To avoid this dire situation, never let yourself get into this state, where blood sugar plummets and chaos reigns. To keep your sanity, have a snack every few hours, whether it is a piece of low-fat string cheese, dried fruit, or a handful of unsalted nuts, or even a meal, especially if it's been four to five hours since you've last eaten.

When you do eat a meal, include protein. A study at Purdue University showed that when women followed a reduced-calorie diet with higher protein content, about 30 percent of total calories, they felt fuller and in a better state of mind. They also lost 18 pounds over a period of 12 weeks! Good sources of lean protein include chicken, fish, black beans, chickpeas, nonfat dairy products, and edamame.

natural news

Eating foods with a high fluid content, like fruits and veggies, and foods with air, like whipped shakes and puffed cereals, can make you feel full longer and help you stick to your weight-loss goals!

Consider the Glycemic Index

When it comes to losing weight, it's important to find a plan that will allow you to lose weight slowly and steadily. Aim for 1 to 2 pounds a week. You can either choose an established diet plan like Weight Watchers or the South Beach Diet, or DIY (do-it-yourself) by cutting back on portion size, cutting out overindulgence on sweet treats, and getting more active. After all, dieting isn't rocket science; it's just expending more energy than you take in!

Regardless, when you make choices about meals, it's important to pick foods that are low on the *glycemic index* (GI). "Choosing low-GI carbs, ones that produce only small fluctuations in your blood glucose and insulin levels, can help reduce your risk of heart disease and diabetes," says Beverly Yates, N.D., a naturopathic doctor whose practice is the Naturopathic Family Health Clinic in Mill Valley, California. "This is key for sustainable weight loss."

def•i•ni•tion _____

The **glycemic index** (GI) is a ranking system for carbohydrates based on their effect on blood glucose levels. Carbohydrates that break down rapidly during digestion have a high glycemic index. Carbohydrates that break down slowly, releasing glucose gradually into the bloodstream, have a low glycemic index.

Generally, soft foods, like cotton candy, are higher on the GI, while hard foods, like whole-wheat pasta, are lower. Foods higher in fiber, like whole-wheat pasta, also keep you feeling fuller longer! A 2005 study in the *Journal of the American Dietetic Association* showed that when girls aged 9 to 19 ate high-fiber breakfast cereal, they had a lower BMI, or body mass index, a number calculated from height and weight that indicates body fat. You can find a whole list of the GI of foods at www. glycemicindex.com.

Deal with Cravings

When you're trying to lose weight, one of the biggest traps is cravings, whether it's for an ice cream sandwich or a chocolate bar. Fortunately, a natural remedy is at hand. Called 5-Hydroxytryptophan, or 5-HTP, it's an amino acid that helps boost serotonin levels and curb carb cravings. "If your serotonin is normal, you're less likely to reach for food," says Dr. Lucille. "5-HTP promotes a satiated feeling and decreases carbohydrate cravings." You can buy 5-HTP at your local health food store.

Chromium is also a key craving nutrient. If you take it with meals throughout the day (it's best absorbed with food), it can help with sugar cravings and with insulin resistance, which means the body is able to handle whatever sugar you eat in a more efficient way.

When you do want sugar, reach instead for stevia (Stevia rebaudiana), a South American herb that the Guarani Indians of Paraguay have used as a sweetener for centuries. Stevia satisfies your sweet tooth and doesn't interact with your blood sugar, so you get a lot of bang for your buck, says Dr. Yates. In fact, it's about 30 times sweeter to the sweet taste buds than regular sugar. (Avoid chemical sweeteners because they can actually cause you to crave more sweets by upsetting blood sugar levels.)

natural news

Eating slowly is one of the best ways to lose weight and keep it off, says Marc David, author of *The Slow Down Diet*. And what could be more natural? When we eat too fast, it's like doing anything else in overdrive: it stresses us, so we produce the stress hormones cortisol and insulin, which slash our calorie-burning power and make us more likely to gain weight, especially in the midsection. Eating fast also means we're more likely to overeat because our brain doesn't register the food we've taken in, so we just want more. Instead, double the time you eat. Turn off the TV. Take the time to experience the taste and smell. *Enjoy your food!*

Nature's Weight-Loss Secrets

Want to get fat burning? Eat Malabar Tamarind (Garcinia cambogia), a small, highly acidic fruit that resembles a miniature pumpkin, used in India, Pakistan, and Sri Lanka as both a food and a medicine. Research has provided mixed results about Garcinia cambogia's weight-loss effects, but you may want to try it for yourself. You can find it at your health food store or at www.nutriherb.net.

Green Tea

Caffeine is another great fat burner. "Anything with caffeine will help in making the body more efficient at fat burning or thermogenesis," says Dr. Yates. "The beauty of green tea is that, unlike coffee, it has a lot of healthy benefits, including antioxidants and only a modest amount of caffeine. Of all the caffeinated products, this is the best by far for weight management and weight loss." You may also want to try Yerba Mate tea from South America (www.yerbamatetea.com). It boosts energy and helps suppress the appetite.

natural news

Research published in the *American Journal of Clinical Nutrition* in 2005 showed that drinking tea, which is rich in catechins, is a good habit to cultivate. In a 12-week, double-blind study, the men who drank 1 bottle of oolong tea containing 690 mg of catechins daily saw a decrease in body weight, BMI, waist circumference, body fat mass, and subcutaneous fat area!

Chitolean

Amy Greeson, R.Ph., a licensed pharmacist in Thomasville, North Carolina (www.healingseekers.com), says that Chitolean may be helpful in your weight-loss efforts. Chitolean is a combination of rice bran and Chitosan, a natural source of fiber (from the exoskeletons of shrimp) that is believed to bind and remove fats from food after ingestion. "I like to also use it in patients who need to lower their cholesterol," she says. You can find out more about Chitolean from Da Vinci Laboratories (www.davinci.com).

A Note About Hoodia

You've probably heard of hoodia, the African cactuslike plant that may be an appetite suppressant. The Bushmen in the desert have used it for centuries to stave off hunger during long hunting trips. Basically, it fools the brain into thinking you've eaten when you haven't. Pretty clever, huh? Animal studies have also shown its effectiveness. Unfortunately, it's very difficult to find a supplement that contains

100 percent hoodia gordononii, the variation needed for best effects. The active ingredient is called P57. With better regulation, supplements in the future may come in more effective products.

dial your doc

If you think you have an endocrine disorder like hypothyroidism, this condition can lead to a sluggish metabolism that makes it very difficult to lose weight. Contact your doctor and see the section on thyroid disorders for more information.

Cleanse Your Body

A whole-body cleanse can be a good way to kick-start your diet, says Dr. Lucille, because the enzymes that break down storage fat are located in your liver. A cleanse initiates the breakdown of these fats. "It stimulates weight loss and makes you more conscious of what you've been putting in your body," says Dr. Lucille.

An easy do-it-yourself cleanse that Dr. Lucille recommends is called Enzymatic Therapy Whole Body Cleanse (www.enzy.com). This is one of the only companies in the nutraceutical business that is registered as an FDA-standard pharmaceutical-grade manufacturing facility, and it is also organically certified. The cleanse is a simple two-week program that uses a soothing herbal blend to support detoxification for the whole body, including the intestines, liver, gallbladder, and circulatory and lymphatic systems. Milk thistle is part of the mix to help eliminate toxins and support liver function. Visit www.wbcleanse.com for more information.

natural news

A recent study in *The International Journal of Obesity* shows the value of including seafood in a diet plan. Researchers in London found that including lean or fatty fish or fish oil in a diet for young overweight men helped them lose more weight than a diet without seafood. This led researchers to conclude that including seafood can boost weight loss. It may help you, too!

Flower Power

Bach Flower Remedies (see Chapter 5) are made from a "sun tea" of specific wildflowers or trees known for their healing properties, then diluted (similar to homeopathic remedies, in that regard). They work to balance negative emotions, freeing the body's energy to heal itself. You can take the remedy under the tongue, or add a few drops to a glass of water and sip it. Nancy Buono, a Bach Foundation Registered Practitioner (BFRP) and director of Bach Flower Education, recommends these Bach remedies to help with the process of weight loss and self-acceptance. For more information, visit www.bachflowereducation. com.

Condition	Bach Flower Remedy
Poor self-image; feelings, of being toxic fat; self-disgust	**Crab Apple,** to cleanse and purify the body and outlook, and bring greater self-acceptance and self-love
Have tried many times to lose weight, but it keeps coming back	**Chestnut Bud,** to gain awareness and experience from past mistakes, to really learn how to go about the process properly
Eat to avoid uncomfortable feelings, to keep busy	**Agrimony,** to feel more comfortable and able to communicate about what troubles you

Move Away from Food

Of course, exercise is important when it comes to any weight-loss program. Don't fight it—you'll feel better once you begin! To get active, find something you like that you can do on a consistent basis every day. Many people find that walking works best (doesn't your dog want to go for a walk, after all?). "You've just got to expend more calories than you take in when you eat," says Dr. Yates. "It's just simple mathematics." And don't worry about being Olympic caliber. "You may not be able to run a marathon, but you can walk around a well-lit mall or your neighborhood and do that as your exercise," says Dr. Yates.

Start with a 40-minute walk six days a week. If you want to add weight training or aerobics, you may want to join a gym or work with a fitness trainer to get more guidance for your unique situation. If you have any health concerns, check with your doctor first.

natural news

Identifying sensitivities to foods like wheat, dairy, corn, or soy can help you lose weight—and keep it off. Dr. Yates suggests keeping a diet diary for a week and looking at what you are eating and how it affects you. You can also do an elimination diet for two weeks and avoid offending foods, and see how you feel. Naturopathic doctors and other alternative health practitioners can also order lab tests for delayed food sensitivities.

Natural Rx

5-HTP: As directed.

Burdock: Tincture, ½ tsp, 40 drops, or 2.5 mL three times daily; tea, 1 TB. per cup of water, 3 cups daily.

Cardamom: Seeds, chew five seeds three times daily after meals to aid in digestion; tincture, ½ teaspoon, 40 drops, or 2.5 mL three times daily.

Cayenne: As directed.

Chickweed: As directed.

Chitolean: As directed. www.davinci.com.

Chromium picolinate: 200–400 mcg daily with meals.

Cinnamon: Tea, 1 TB. per cup of water, 4 cups daily.

Cod liver oil: www.nordicnaturals.com. As directed.

Coenzyme Q10: 100–300 mg per day. Some studies show that a deficiency in this nutrient can lead to weight gain. Supplementation may help weight loss.

Conjugated linoleic acid (CLA): 1,000-2,000 mg three times daily with meals. Some research shows that it helps change fat to lean muscle.

Dandelion root: Tincture, ½ tsp, 40 drops, or 2.5 mL three times daily; tea, 1 TB. per cup of water, 3 cups daily.

Diet Rx: As directed. www.physicianformulas.com.

Enzymatic Therapy's Whole Body Cleanse: As directed. www.wbcleanse.com

Flaxseed oil: As directed.

Garcinia cambogia: As directed.

Ginger: Tincture, ½ tsp, 40 drops, or 2.5 mL three times daily; tea, 1 TB. per cup of water, 3 cups daily; capsules, 300 mg twice daily.

Green tea: 1 TB. per cup of tea, 3 cups daily; capsules, as directed.

Gurmar: As directed.

Hemp seed oil: 1 TB. daily.

Multivitamin and mineral with B complex: As directed.

Stevia: To taste.

Stinging nettles: Tea, 1 TB. per cup of water, 2–3 cups daily; capsules and tablets, 200 mg three times daily.

Yerba Mate: As directed.

Glossary

acidic   Having a pH less than 7.

alkaline   Having a pH greater than 7.

allergic contact dermatitis   Develops when the body's immune system reacts against a substance that comes into repeated contact with the skin.

antibodies   Type of protein produced by the immune system to identify and neutralize foreign substances or antigens such as bacteria and viruses.

arrhythmia   Irregular beat or any variation from the normal rhythm of the heartbeat.

atopic eczema   Common symptoms include itchiness, dryness of the skin, redness, and inflammation. In infected eczema, the skin may crack and weep, which is known as wet eczema.

aura   A visual disturbance that is characterized by bright flashes of light, jagged lines, and distortion of images, but not a complete loss of vision.

blood glucose or blood sugar   The main sugar found in the blood and the body's main source of energy.

blood pressure   Measure of the force of blood rushing through and pushing against arteries. Measured in millimeters of mercury (mmHg), systolic blood pressure, the top number in 120/80, indicates arterial pressure as the heart beats; the diastolic, the lower number, is the pressure between beats while the heart rests. Increased pressure on arteries damages those vessels and increases risk of heart attack and stroke.

bronchi   Large air tubes leading from the trachea that carry air to and from the lungs. *Bronchi* is plural for the Greek word *bronchos*, a conduit to the lungs.

carotenoid   A substance that makes certain vegetables yellow, orange, or red. The body makes some carotenoids, like beta carotene, into vitamin A. All carotenoids are antioxidants.

cluster headaches   Intense, severe headaches afflicting more men than women. The headache is brief, lasting 15 minutes to two hours on one side of the head. It occurs every day or multiple times a day for about two weeks to two months, and then spontaneously goes away. Whereas migraine sufferers are light sensitive, cluster headache sufferers get red, watery eyes. Capsaicin cream (the active component of cayenne pepper) can help cluster headaches by stimulating and blocking pain fibers by depleting them of the neurotransmitter substance P.

congestive heart failure   A special cardiac circumstance that refers to the inability of the heart to effectively pump enough blood.

cytokines   A group of proteins and peptides similar to hormones and neurotransmitters that enables cells to communicate with one another. Many types of cells release cytokines. Due to their central role in the immune system, cytokines are involved in a variety of immunological, inflammatory, and infectious diseases.

D-ribose   A naturally occurring carbohydrate.

diabetes type 1   Condition in which the body does not produce insulin, which is necessary for the body to be able to use sugar, the basic fuel for cells. Insulin takes the sugar from the blood into the cells.

diabetes type 2   Condition in which either the body does not produce enough insulin or the cells ignore the insulin. Insulin is necessary for the body to be able to use sugar.

duodenum   The first part of the small intestine, right after the stomach.

endometriosis   Growths that respond to a woman's monthly cycle. Every month, hormones cause the lining of a woman's uterus to build up with tissue and blood vessels. If a woman doesn't get pregnant, the uterus sheds this tissue and blood as her menstrual period. Unfortunately, each month, endometriosis growths add extra tissue and blood, too, and this results in inflammation, pain, and scar tissue that can block the ovaries and fallopian tubes and lead to infertility.

flavonoid (or bioflavonoid)   Compound found in fruits, vegetables, and certain beverages that has beneficial biochemical and antioxidant effects. Flavonoids have been reported to have antiviral, antiallergic, antiplatelet, anti-inflammatory, antitumor, and antioxidant activities.

glycemic index (GI)   A ranking system for carbohydrates based on their effect on blood glucose levels. Carbohydrates that break down rapidly during digestion have a high glycemic index. Carbohydrates that break down slowly, releasing glucose gradually into the bloodstream, have a low glycemic index.

helicobacter pylori   A bacterium that can damage stomach and duodenal tissue, causing ulcers. It is known as H. pylori for short.

insulin resistant   The insulin produced by the pancreas cannot connect with fat and muscle cells to let glucose inside and produce energy. The more obese a person becomes, the more fat stores impede the way insulin works in the body. So any weight loss—even 10 or 20 pounds—can reduce the risk of diabetes.

irritant contact dermatitis   Condition caused by frequent contact with everyday substances, such as detergents and chemicals, that are irritating to the skin.

jet lag   When the body's clock gets out of sync traveling across one or more time zones on a jet plane. That's because the daylight and darkness hours are different than what you're used to.

leukotrienes   A group of hormones that cause the symptoms of asthma. Inhibiting their formation can help ease asthma symptoms.

mitral valve   Valve that separates the left atrium from the left ventricle of the heart.

pH   A measure of the acidity or alkalinity of a solution. pH stands for "potential of hydrogen."

placebo effect   Occurs when a patient's symptoms are alleviated or exacerbated by an otherwise innocuous treatment, simply because the individual expects or believes that it will work.

prostaglandins   Substance discovered in human semen in 1935 by the Swedish physiologist Ulf von Euler, who named them mistakenly thinking that they were secreted by the prostate gland. Actually, they're a group of hormonelike substances found in virtually all tissues and organs that stimulate target cells into action. Prostaglandins act differently in different tissues. For example, omega-6 fatty acids, found in meats and most vegetable oils, stimulate the production of inflammatory prostaglandins, while the consumption of omega-3 fatty acids found in coldwater fish inhibits the production of these inflammatory prostaglandins.

sinus headache   Typically involves pain and pressure in the sinus area and discolored nasal discharge. When sinus infection is the cause of the headache, an accompanying fever is often present, and x-rays or a sinus CT scan indicate some sinus blockage. Often migraine suffers have sinus aggravation or irritation that seems like a sinus headache, but the migraine is the underlying cause of the pain. Once the migraine is treated, they feel better.

skin cancer   Develops mainly on areas of skin exposed to a lot of sun, including the scalp, face, lips, ears, neck, chest, arms and hands, and legs. Some types of skin cancer appear as a small growth or as a sore that bleeds, crusts over, heals, and then reopens. With melanoma, an existing mole may change or a new, suspicious-looking mole may develop.

substance P   In the central nervous system, substance P has been associated with the regulation of respiratory rhythm and the transmission of pain impulses.

sunburn   When ultraviolet light causes the skin to burn, bringing pain, redness, and swelling. Depending on the severity of the burn, the dead, damaged skin may peel away to make room for new skin cells. Sunburn can also damage the DNA of skin cells, which sometimes leads to skin cancer.

synovial fluid   A thick fluid found in the cavities of synovial joints that lubricates and cushions cartilage and other tissue in joints during movement.

tension-type headache   A bilateral band–type of headache without migrainelike symptoms (nausea and sensitivity to light, noise, or smells). Instead, the pain is dull or squeezing, like a tight vice on both sides of the head. Tension headaches are due to tight, contracted muscles in the shoulders, neck, scalp, and jaw, and are usually triggered by stress, anxiety, fatigue, or anger, or by clenching or grinding teeth. Supplements that can bring relief include valerian root. This is the second most common type of headache.

Appendix B

Resources

Online

Here you'll find a variety of websites of natural healing resources.

General

HealthRef.com
"Ask the Doctor," "Remedy of the Month," popular health topics, information on supplements, *The Complete Natural Medicine Reference* available on CD

Acupuncture

Acupuncture.com
www.acupuncture.com
Information about Chinese medicine, health, and wellness; online store.

Aromatherapy/Essential Oils

The Aroma Tree
139 South Eastbourne Avenue
Tucson, AZ 85716
1-866-276-6287
520-327-5456
info@thearomatree.com

Blessed Herbs
109 Barre Plains Road
Oakham, MA 01068
1-800-489-4372
www.blessedherbs.com

East-West School for Herbal and Aromatic Studies
Jade Shutes, Director of Education, Founder
919-892-7230
www.TheIDA.com

Essential Aura Aromatherapy
1935 Doran Road
Cobble Hill, BC V0R 1L0
250-758-9464
www.essentialaura.com
www.organicfair.com

Essential Wholesale
503-722-7557
www.essentialwholesale.com

Leyden House Limited
200 Brattleboro Road
Leyden, MA 01337
413-772-0858
1-800-754-0668
www.leydenhouse.com

Mountain Rose Herbs
85472 Dilley Lane
Eugene, OR 97405
1-800-879-3337
www.mountainroseherbs.com

Original Swiss Aromatics
P.O. Box 6842
San Rafael, CA 94903
415-459-3998
www.originalswissaromatics.com

Simplers Botanical Company
P.O. Box 2534
Sebastopol, CA 95473
1-800-652-7646
www.simplers.com

SKS Bottle
2600 7th Avenue, Building 60
West Watervliet, NY 12189
518-880-6980
www.sks-bottle.com

Specialty Bottle
5215 5th Avenue South
Seattle, WA 98108
206-340-0459
www.specialtybottle.com

Ayurvedic Medicine

The National Institute of Ayurvedic Medicine
www.niam.com
Books, products, and information

Flower Essences

Bach Flower Education
www.bachflowereducation.com
Bach Flower Remedy books, remedies, courses, and consultation information

Bach Original Flower Remedies
www.bachremedies.com
Website for the Nelsons, who manufacture and distribute the remedies internationally

Dr. Edward Bach Centre
www.bachcentre.com
Home page of Dr. Edward Bach; lists Bach Foundation Registered
Practitioners

Living Enrichment
www.bachremedystore.com
Remedies for sale

Meditation

Meditation Society of America
www.meditationsociety.com
The home of Meditation Station; information on meditation techniques
for beginners, intermediates, and experts; free newsletter

How to Meditate
www.how-to-meditate.org
Explains how and why to meditate

Self-Realization Fellowship
www.yogananda-srf.org/index.html
Yoga methods of meditation, home-study lesson series, meditation
centers

The Transcendental Meditation Program
www.tm.org
Information about this simple technique of meditation created by
Maharishi Mahesh Yogi; introductory videos; free e-zine

Wildmind Buddhist Meditation
www.wildmind.org
Meditation MP3s, CDs, and DVDs; online courses for learning meditation at home; free meditation newsletter

The World Wide Online Meditation Center
www.meditationcenter.com
A user-friendly site offering meditation instruction

Yoga

ABC-of-Yoga
www.abc-of-yoga.com
Yoga gear, DVDs, books, and audio

Gaiam
www.gaiam.com
A lifestyle company with products for wellness, green living, spirituality, fitness, yoga, and a healthy home

Kripalu Center for Yoga & Health
www.kripalu.org
Information, forums, videos, CDs, mats, and more

Yoga.com
www.yoga.com
Beginner's guide, news, articles, and forum

Yoga with Judith Hanson Lasater
www.judithlasater.com
Workshops and classes; books

Herbal Medicine

Brigitte Mars
www.brigittemars.com
Educational materials, books, tapes, and CDs from renowned herbalist Brigitte Mars

Michael Tierra's East West Herb Course & Planetary Herbs & Formulas
www.planetherbs.com/index.php
Website of Dr. Michael Tierra L.AC., O.M.D., founder of the American Herbalists Guild; seminars; herb store

Tree Farm Communications
www.treefarmtapes.com/catalog/speaker.asp?speakerid=156
Tapes on a variety of subjects featuring Amanda McQuade Crawford, Dip. Phyto., MNIMH, RH (AHG), founding member and first secretary of the American Herbalists Guild

Homeopathy

Boiron USA

www.boironusa.com

A world leader in homeopathy; wide range of homeopathic medicines; information about homeopathy

The National Center for Homeopathy

www.nationalcenterforhomeopathy.org

Homeopathy Today magazine and e-newsletter

Homeopathy Resource

www.homeopathyresource.com

Health articles and newsletter; e-mail consultation with a qualified homeopath

Hyland's Homeopathy

www.hylands.com

Wide range of homeopathic medicines; free e-newsletter

The Homeopathic Store

www.thehomeopathicstore.com

Just a store; health articles and newsletter; e-mail consultation with a qualified homeopath

Massage Therapy

Associated Bodywork and Massage Professionals

www.massagetherapy.com

Information about the benefits of massage, a massage and bodywork glossary, what to expect when you get a massage; help in finding a qualified massage therapist

Qigong

Spring Forest Qigong

www.springforestqigong.com

Information about Qigong and guided healing meditations

Books

The Blood Pressure Cure: 8 Weeks to Lower Blood Pressure Without Prescription Drugs, by Robert E. Kowalski (Wiley, 2007).

Born a Healer, by Chunyi Lin with Gary Rebstock (Spring Forest Publishing, 2003).

The Brain Diet, by Alan C. Logan, N.D., FRSH (Cumberland House, 2007).

Changing the Course of Autism: A Scientific Approach for Parents and Physicians, by Bryan Jepson, M.D., Katie Wright, and Jane Johnson (Sentient Publications, 2007).

Cholesterol Down: 10 Simple Steps to Lower Your Cholesterol in 4 Weeks— Without Prescription Drugs, by Janet Bond Brill, Ph.D., R.D. (Three Rivers Press, 2006).

The Clear Skin Diet: A Nutritional Plan for Getting Rid of and Avoiding Acne, by Alan C. Logan, N.D., FRSH, and Valori Treloar, M.D. (Cumberland House Publishing, 2007).

The Complete Natural Medicine Reference: A Software Health Guide, created by naturopathic physicians, www.HealthRef.com.

Creating and Maintaining Balance: A Woman's Guide to Safe, Natural, Hormone Health, by Holly Lucille, N.D., R.N. (Impakt Health, 2004).

The Desktop Guide to Herbal Medicine: The Ultimate Multidisciplinary Reference to the Amazing Realm of Healing Plants, in a Quick-Study, One-Stop Guide, by Brigitte Mars (Basic Health Publications, 2007).

Dr. Janson's New Vitamin Revolution, by Michael Janson, M.D. (Avery, 2000).

Feeling Fat, Fuzzy or Frazzled?: A 3-Step Program to Beat Hormone Havoc, Restore Thyroid, Adrenal, and Reproductive Balance, and Feel Better Fast!, by Richard Shames, M.D., and Karilee Halo Shames, R.N., Ph.D. (Plume, 2005).

Free Your Breath, Free Your Life: How Conscious Breathing Can Relieve Stress, Increase Vitality, and Help You Live More Fully, by Dennis Lewis (Shambhala, 2004).

The Fiber35 Diet: Nature's Weight Loss Secret, by Brenda Watson, C.N.C., and Leonard Smith, M.D. (Free Press, 2007).

From Fatigued to Fantastic!, by Jacob Teitelbaum (Avery/Penguin Group USA, 1996).

Heart Health for Black Women: A Natural Approach to Healing and Preventing Heart Disease, by Beverly Yates, N.D. (Marlowe & Co., 2000).

Hope and Help for Chronic Fatigue Syndrome and Fibromyalgia, by Alison C. Bested, M.D., FRCP(c), and Alan C. Logan, N.D., FRSH, with Russell Howe, LLB (Cumberland House, 2006).

Living Well with Chronic Fatigue Syndrome and Fibromyalgia, by Mary Shomon (Collins, 2004).

Living Well with Graves Disease and Hyperthyroidism, by Mary Shomon (HarperResource, 2005).

Living Well with Hypothyroidism, by Mary Shomon (HarperResource, 2005).

Natural Eye Care: Your Guide to Healthy Vision, by Marc Grossman, O.D., L.Ac., and Michael Edson, MS, L.Ac., www.naturaleyecare.com.

The Natural Healing Companion: Using Alternative Medicines: What to Buy, How to Take, and When to Combine for Best Results, by Deborah A. Wiancek, N.D. (Rodale, 2000).

The New 8-Week Cholesterol Cure, by Robert E. Kowalski (Collins, 2006).

The Okinawa Program: How the World's Longest-Lived People Achieve Everlasting Health—And How You Can, Too, by Bradley J. Willcox, M.D.; D. Craig Willcox, Ph.D.; and Makoto Suzuki, M.D. (Random House, 2002).

Pain 1-2-3: A Proven Program for Eliminating Chronic Pain Now, by Jacob Teitelbaum, M.D. (McGraw Hill, 2005).

Snooze…or Lose!, by Helene Emsellem, M.D. (Joseph Henry Press)

Take Two Apples and Call Me in the Morning: A Practical Guide to Using the Power of Food to Change Your Life!, by Judy Stone, CN, M.S.W. (Hara Publishing Group, 2002).

The Tao of Natural Breathing: For Health, Well-Being, and Inner Growth, by Dennis Lewis (Rodmell Press, 2006).

The Thyroid Diet: Manage Your Metabolism for Lasting Weight Loss, by Mary Shomon (Harper Thorsons, 2005).

The Thyroid Hormone Breakthrough: Overcoming Sexual and Hormonal Problems at Every Age, by Mary Shomon (Collins, 2006).

Thyroid Power: Ten Steps to Total Health, by Richard Shames, M.D., and Karilee Halo Shames, R.N., Ph.D. (Collins, 2002).

What Your Doctor May Not Tell You About Migraines, by Alexander Mauskop, M.D., and Barry Fox, Ph.D. (Grand Central Publishing, 2001).

Will Yoga & Meditation Really Change My Life?, edited by Stephen Cope (Storey Publishing, 2003).

A Woman's Guide to Sleep: Guaranteed Solutions for a Good Night's Rest, by Joyce Walsleben, M.D. (Crown, 2001).

Practitioners

General Natural Medicine

Alternative Medicine Directory
www.altmedicine.net

The American Association of Naturopathic Physicians
www.naturopathic.org

American Holistic Medical Association
www.holisticmedicine.org

Health World Online, Professional Referral Network
www.healthreferral.com

Healthy Alternatives
www.health-alt.com

Acupuncture

Acupuncture.com
www.acupuncture.com

American Academy of Medical Acupuncture
www.medicalacupuncture.org

Aromatherapy

East West School for Herbal and Aromatic Studies
Jade Shutes, Director of Education, Founder
919-892-7230
www.TheIDA.com

National Association for Holistic Aromatherapy
www.naha.org

Ayurvedic Medicine

The College of Maharishi Vedic Medicine
www.maharishi-medical.com

Kripalu Center for Yoga & Health
www.kripalu.org

The National Institute of Ayurvedic Medicine
www.niam.com

Flower Essences

Bach Foundation Registered Practitioners
www.bachcentre.com

Flower Essence Society
www.flowersociety.org

Chiropractic

American Chiropractic Association
www.amerchiro.org

Craniosacral Therapy

The Upledger Institute
www.upledger.com

Chronic Fatigue/Fibromyalgia

The Annapolis Center for Effective CFS/Fibromyalgia Therapies
Jacob Teitelbaum, M.D., medical director
410-573-5389
New patient appointments: 410-266-6958

Referrals to practitioners nationwide
www.fibroandfatigue.com
www.endfatigue.com

Herbal Medicine

American Herbalists Guild
www.americanherbalistsguild.com

Homeopathy

The Homeopathic Academy of Naturopathic Physicians
www.healthy.net/pan/pa/homeopathic/hanp

The National Center for Homeopathy
www.nationalcenterforhomeopathy.org

The North American Society of Homeopaths
www.homepathy.org

Massage Therapy

American Massage Therapy Association
www.amtamassage.org

Associated Bodywork & Massage Professionals
www.massagetherapy.com

Meditation

Kripalu Center for Yoga & Health
www.kripalu.org

The Transcendental Meditation Program
www.tm.org
1-888-532-7686

Reflexology

Reflexology Association of America
www.reflexology-usa.org

Qigong

National Qigong Association USA
www.nqa.org

Qigong Institute
www.qigonginstitute.org

Yoga

International Association of Yoga Therapists
www.yrec.org

Kripalu Center for Yoga & Health
www.kripalu.org

Expert Panel

Judith S. Beck., Ph.D, is the director of the Beck Institute for Cognitive Therapy and Research in suburban Philadelphia, clinical associate professor of psychology in psychiatry at the University of Pennsylvania, and author of *The Beck Diet Solution*.

Herbert Benson, M.D., is director emeritus at the Benson-Henry Institute for Mind-Body Medicine in Boston, Massachusetts.

Timothy Birdsall, N.D., is the vice president of integrative medicine for the Cancer Treatment Centers of America. Visit www.cancercenter.com.

Mary Ann Block, M.D., is the founder and director of The Block Center in the Dallas area of Texas. Visit www.theblockcenter.com.

Joshua Bomser, Ph.D., is an associate professor of nutrition in the Department of Nutrition at Ohio State University.

Janet Bond Brill, Ph.D., R.D., is the author of *Cholesterol Down: 10 Simple Steps to Lower Your Cholesterol in 4 Weeks Without Prescription Drugs.* Visit www.cholesteroldown.com.

Nancy Buono is a Bach Foundation Registered Practitioner (BFRP) and the director of Bach Flower Education. Visit www.bachflowereducation. com.

Barbara Close is the founder of Naturopathica Spa in East Hampton. Visit www.naturopathica.com.

Suzy Cohen, R.Ph., has a syndicated column, "Dear Pharmacist" which reaches nearly 24 million readers. She is also the author of *The 24-Hour Pharmacist: Advice, Options, and Amazing Cures from America's Most Trusted Pharmacist* (Collins Living).

Karen Collins, M.S., R.D., is a registered dietitian and nutrition consultant to the American Institute for Cancer Research in Washington, D.C.

Lisa Cowley, D.C., is a chiropractor at her practice, Alternative Healthcare, in Southold, New York.

Amanda McQuade Crawford, Dip. Phyto., MNIMH, RH (AHG), MNZAMH, is a founding member and the first secretary of the American Herbalists Guild, and a consultant medical herbalist in Los Angeles, California.

Marc David is a nutritional psychologist and founder of The Institute for the Psychology of Eating and author of *The Slow Down Diet: Eating for Pleasure, Energy & Weight Loss* (Healing Arts Press).

Roy Desjarlais is vice president of clinical services at the Upledger Institute.

Robert A. Duarte, M.D., is the director of the Long Island Jewish (LIJ) Pain and Headache Treatment Center in Manhasset, New York.

Nancy Eagles, is a chartered herbalist who lives in North Vancouver, British Columbia. Visit www.inannaherbs.com.

Helene Emsellem, M.D., is the director of the Center for Sleep & Wake Disorders in Chevy Chase, Maryland, and the author of *Snooze...or Lose!* Visit www.snoozeorlose.com.

Fred Freitag, D.O., is the associate director of the Diamond Headache Clinic in Chicago, Illinois. Visit www.diamondheadache.com.

Vincent Giampapa, M.D., F.A.C.S., is the author of *The Anti-Aging Solution* and *The Gene Makeover.*

Courtney Gilardi, N.D., is a naturopathic doctor practicing at the Kripalu Center for Yoga & Health in Stockbridge, Massachusetts. Visit www.kripalu.org.

Hilary Garavaltis is an Ayurvedic practitioner and the dean of curriculum at the Kripalu School of Ayurveda in Stockbridge, Massachusetts. Visit www.kripalu.org.

Amy Greeson, R.Ph., is a pharmacist in High Point, North Carolina, and president of Healing Seekers. Visit www.healingseekers.com.

Marc Grossman, O.D., L.Ac., is a doctor of optometry who practices in New Paltz, New York. Visit www.naturaleyecare.com.

Pamela Hannaman, N.D., M.S., C.P.C., earned her doctorate in naturopathic medicine from Bastyr University in Seattle. She currently does consulting as a health, wellness, nutritional, and life counselor in Ashland, Virginia. Visit www.hannaman-pittman.com.

Stephen Hartman is the director of professional training and association at the Kripalu Center for Yoga & Health Stockbridge, Massachusetts. Visit www.kripalu.org.

Michael Janson, M.D., is the author of *Dr. Janson's Vitamin Revolution.* Visit www.drjanson.com.

Bryan Jepson, M.D., is a physician at Thoughtful House in Austin, Texas, and author of *Changing the Course of Autism.* Visit www.thoughtfulhouse.org.

Dr. Joseph Keenan is a professor of family medicine at the University of Minnesota, and also holds a joint professorship in the University of Minnesota School of Food Science and Nutrition.

Christine Lay, M.D., is a neurologist at the Headache Institute at St. Luke's–Roosevelt Hospital Center in New York, New York. Visit www. wehealny.org/headache/index.html.

Dennis Lewis is the author of *The Breath of Presence: Awakening to Who You Really Are*. Visit www.authentic-breathing.com.

Phyllis Light, R.H., is a professional member of the American Herbalist Guild and the director of herbal studies at Clayton College of Natural Health in Birmingham, Alabama.

Chunyi Lin is the director of the Spring Forest Center for Health, Wellness & Empowerment and author of *Born a Healer.* (Spring Forest Qigong Company, Inc.)

Alan C. Logan is the author of *The Brain Diet* and *The Clear Skin Diet: A Nutritional Plan for Getting Rid of and Avoiding Acne with Valori Treloar.* Visit www.drlogan.com.

Margot Longenecker, N.D., is a naturopathic physician who practices in Branford and Wallingford, Connecticut. Visit www.drlongenecker. com.

Dr. Holly Lucille, N.D., R.N., is a naturopathic physician and the author of *Creating and Maintaining Balance: A Woman's Guide to Safe, Natural, Hormone Health.* Visit www.allheallucille.com or call 323-658-9151.

Brigitte Mars, A.H.G., is a renowned herbalist and the author of *The Desktop Guide to Herbal Medicine: The Ultimate Multidisciplinary Reference to the Amazing Realm of Healing Plants, in a Quick-Study, One-Stop Guide.* Visit www.brigittemars.com.

Keri Marshall, is a naturopathic doctor who practices in Dover, New Hampshire, at the Makai Naturopathic Center.

Alexander Mauskop, M.D., is a fellow of the American Academy of Neurology and is board certified in neurology and headache medicine. He is the director of the New York Headache Center and the author of *What Your Doctor May Not Tell You About Migraines.* Visit www. nyheadache.com.

Greg Nigh, N.D., L. Ac., practices at the Nature Cures Clinic in Portland, Oregon. Visit naturecuresclinic.com.

Gary Rebstock is the co-author with Master Chunyi Lin of *Born a Healer*. Visit www.springforestqigong.com.

Joel Saper, M.D., is the founder and director of the Michigan Headache & Neurological Institute. Visit www.mhni.com.

Richard Shames, M.D., is the author of *Feeling Fat, Fuzzy, or Frazzled?: A 3-Step Program to: Beat Hormone Havoc, Restore Thyroid, Adrenal, and Reproductive Balance, and Feel Better Fast!*. Visit www.feelingfff.com.

Mary Shomon is the author of *Living Well with Hypothyroidism* and *Living Well with Graves Disease and Hyperthyroidism*. Visit www.thryoid-info.com.

Jade Shutes is the director of education and the founder of the East West School for Herbal and Aromatic Studies. Visit www.TheIDA.com.

Barbara S. Silbert, D.C., N.D., is a naturopathic doctor who practices in Bethel, Vermont.

Judy Stone, CN, M.S.W., is a certified nutritionist and the author of *Take Two Apples and Call Me in the Morning: A Practical Guide to Using the Power of Food to Change Your Life!*. Visit www.nutritionmagician.net.

Jacob Teitelbaum, M.D., is a board-certified internist and the medical director of the national Fibromyalgia and Fatigue Centers, Inc., in Annapolis Maryland. He is the author of *From Fatigued to Fantastic!* and *Pain Free 1-2-3*. Visit www.endfatigue.com.

Agatha Thrash, M.D., is the medical director of The Uchee Pines Lifestyle Center in Seale, Alabama. Visit www.ucheepines.org.

Valori Treloar, M.D., CNS, is the co-author of *The Clear Skin Diet* with Alan C. Logan. Her practice, Integrative Dermatology, is in Newton, Massachusetts. Visit www.integrativedermatology.com.

Joyce Walsleben, Ph.D., is the Associate Professor of Medicine at the Sleep Disorders Center at the New York University School of Medicine and the author of *A Woman's Guide to Sleep: Guaranteed Solutions for a Good Night's Rest*.

Brenda Watson, N.D., C.N.C., is the author of *The Fiber35 Diet: Nature's Weight Loss Secret.* Visit www.fiber-35-diet.com.

Deborah Wiancek, N.D., is the director of the Riverwalk Natural Health Clinic in Vail, Colorado, and the author of *The Natural Healing Companion: Using Alternative Medicines: What to Buy, How to Take, and When to Combine for Best Results.* Visit www.healthref.com or call 970-926-7606.

Bradley J. Willcox, M.D., is a clinical scientist and geriatrician at the Pacific Health Research Institute at the University of Hawaii in Honolulu, and the co-author of *The Okinawa Program: How the World's Longest-Lived People Achieve Everlasting Health—and How You Can, Too.* Visit www.okinawaprogram.com.

Beverly Yates, N.D., is the director of the Naturopathic Family Health Clinic in Mill Valley, California, and the author *of Heart Health for Black Women: A Natural Approach to Healing and Preventing Heart Disease.* Visit www.naturalhealthcare.com, or call 415-381-4600 or 1-800-279-2430.

Index

B

C

E

F

P